Microspheres and Regional Cancer Therapy

Edited by

Neville Willmott, Ph.D.
Oncology Research
Celltech, Ltd.
Slough, United Kingdom

and

John Daly, M.D.
Department of Surgery
Hospital of the University of Pennsylvania
Philadelphia, Pennsylvania

CRC Press
Boca Raton Ann Arbor London Tokyo

Library of Congress Cataloging-in-Publication Data

Microspheres and regional cancer therapy/edited by Neville Willmott
and John M. Daly.
    p. cm.
    Includes bibliographical references and index.
    ISBN 0-8493-6952-5
    1. Cancer—Chemotherapy. 2. Microspheres (Pharmacy) 3. Isolation
perfusion (Physiology) I. Willmott, Neville. II. Daly, John M.
    [DNLM: 1. Microspheres. 2. Neoplasms—drug therapy.
3. Perfusion, Reginal—methods. QZ 267 M626 1993]
RC271.C5M52 1993
616.99'4061—dc20
DNLM/DLC
for Library of Congress   93-20500
                                                  CIP

No claim to original U.S. Government works
International Standard Book Number 0-8493-6952-5
Library of Congress Card Number 93-20500
Printed in the United States of America 1 2 3 4 5 6 7 8 9 0
Printed on acid-free paper

FOREWORD

From the very beginning of the modern history of chemotherapy, a "magic bullet," to use a favorite expression of Paul Ehrlich, has been sought to derive greater benefit from chemotherapeutic agents. In particular, this has been, and still is, a matter of urgent necessity in cancer chemotherapy. Apart from the rare success of the cis-platinum-based regimes in testicular and ovarian cancer, most solid tumors either are or become resistant to the currently available anticancer drugs.

A continuing effort is focused on developing new chemical entities which would either be toxic to tumor cells or inhibit their malignant phenotype, but absence, or possibly ignorance, of qualitative biochemical events characteristic of tumor cells makes the prospects of such an approach unclear. An alternative to overcoming the low therapeutic index of anticancer drugs is to localize these nonspecific drugs at the tumor site by associating them with carriers that possess some "affinity", defined in the broadest sense, for the tumor.

Carriers reaching solid tumor tissue via the blood supply may promote tumor localization of active agents by enhanced vascular permeability, reduction of rate of elimination, phagocytosis by stromal elements, or endocytosis by tumor cells themselves. In the 1970s, a variety of natural or synthetic substances such as deoxyribonucleic acid, immunoglobulin, erythrocytes, micron-sized microspheres, and liposomes were investigated as targetable anticancer drug carriers designed for systemic administration. Some promising results were obtained in *in vitro* and *in vivo* studies, such as a moderate decrease in systemic drug toxicity, most likely attributable to the slow release of active agents from the carrier. However, clinical application was precluded by the lack of substantial carrier-mediated tumor localization.

The use of antibodies against putative tumor antigens appears an attractive drug delivery modality; however, as pointed out by the editors in the final chapter, there are many complex problems to be addressed, for example, the heterogeneity or polyclonality of tumor cell populations, the generation of an immune response in the patient to the (generally) mouse antibody, the marked accumulation at sites other than the tumor, and the manufacturing costs involved with the production of biomolecules. Again, we cannot avoid the question of whether or not there are antigens that sufficiently distinguish tumor cells from normal cells: without them the concept of antibodies as carriers of cytotoxic drugs or therapeutic radionuclides appears flawed.

The theory underlying certain uses of microparticulates as targeting vehicles also has logical flaws. Thus, micron or sub-micron sized particles (microspheres, liposomes) administered intravenously should pass through capillaries (generally accepted to be of the order of 7 μm diameter) and remain in the systemic circulation until they encounter their target. In practice, the vast majority of particles of this size localize in the liver due to the resident phagocytic cells. When particles larger than the capillary diameter are administered intravenously they embolize in the first capillary bed encountered, the lung. Both of these situations can be readily visualized by radioisotopic imaging techniques that show solid tumors of liver and lung as "cold spots", indicating that the radioactive particles accumulate preferentially in normal liver and lung.

Targeting to solid tumors should be a sequential process of area followed by cell targeting: the active agent must first be restrictively distributed to the tumor area before adequate accumulation in tumor cells can be achieved. These considerations led us in 1978 to propose and apply the technique of transcatheter infusion of a microencapsulated anticancer drug into the feeding arteries of solid tumors. The infused microcapsules, being larger than capillary diameter, were entrapped in the tumor vasculature in accordance with their size and then released incorporated drug into the surrounding tumor tissue. In this way, treatment is confined to the tumor-bearing organ and systemic drug exposure is minimized. Because the therapeutic effect is due to both microembolization of drug carrier and sustained release of drug incorporated within the carrier, we termed this mode of treatment "chemo-embolization".

Our experience in over a thousand patients has convinced us that, where selective catheterization is possible, transcatheter arterial embolization with microparticles can be a reliable treatment for inoperable liver tumors, pain control of bone lesions, and as a preoperative adjuvant for locally invasive tumors.

The efficacy of therapeutic strategies based on embolization obviously depends on the properties of the drug-carrier combination, the technique of drug infusion, and the vascular architecture of individual tumors. We must assess drug-carrier systems with respect to biocompatibility and biodegradability, particle size, type of drug to be used, efficiency of drug loading, and mechanism and rate of drug release. *In vivo,* the degree of targeting achieved and methods of augmentation (vasoactive agents, magnetic control) are major concerns. Finally, although not addressed here, pharmaceutical considerations relevant to production of particulate material for clinical use, optimization of methods of storage (e.g. freeze-drying), and regulatory issues impinging on controlled release/targetable formulations may soon require discussion.

This volume edited by Drs. Willmott and Daly is both timely and relevant. The interested reader will benefit from the discussions on pharmaceutical, pharmacological, biological, and medical aspects of microparticulate systems used in regional cancer therapy. It is, of course, the case that because of the dissemination of many malignant tumors, micrometastases are beyond the scope of regional therapy. Clearly, when occult metastases are expected with a high degree of certainty, regional therapy should be complemented by systemic therapy. Lastly, it is important that the knowledge and technology generated from research on area-targeted drug delivery systems, such as that contained in this volume, be widely disseminated so that it can be applied to the development of systems designed to achieve the ultimate goal of tumor cell-targeting.

Tetsuro Kato, M.D.
Department of Urology
Akita University of Medicine
Akita, Japan

PREFACE

Although many excellent texts exist that treat the subject of drug delivery with a broad brush, this volume grew out of the editors' feeling that it was timely to produce a monograph that focused on a particular drug delivery system designed to treat a particular human disease state. The subject of the volume is an exciting one, bridging as it does basic and clinical science, and grew out of the editors' complementary interests and experience in these areas pertaining to the use of microspheres. Indeed, as we hope will be apparent, it is the collaborative efforts of basic scientists and clinicians that has advanced microspheres incorporating active anti-cancer agents from the status of attractive concept, via biodistribution studies in patients, to preliminary clinical evaluation.

Although the work falls into laboratory-based and clinical studies, it was decided not to divide the volume into sections along those lines in order to reflect the multidisciplinary nature of the subject. Indeed, some chapters include work that runs the gamut from fundamental science to application in patients. Thus, the subject matter of this volume covers the description and characterization of microspherical systems suitable for regional therapy, the disposition and fate of incorporated agents *in vivo,* and the targeting potential of these systems for solid tumors. Where possible, key points are illustrated by reference to data in patients. Animal studies, however, are frequently the only source of quotable data but should be of particular relevance in the targeting area because the basis is physicochemical rather than biochemical.

Multiauthor volumes tend to suffer two disadvantages. First, a lack of uniformity of style and, second, the lengthy editorial and publication processes mean they appear after publication of material in scientific journals. To avoid the first problem, we adopted a rigid editorial process that meant all original manuscripts were changed to a degree and some have been radically altered. As regards the second, we can only hope to emulate the English essayist and critic William Hazlitt (1778–1830) who "hated to fill a book with things that all the world knows."

THE EDITORS

Neville Willmott, Ph.D., is a Team Leader in Oncology at Celltech Ltd., one of the foremost biotechnology companies in the U.K. Dr. Willmott received his B.Sc. (Chemistry) from the University of Newcastle in 1971. He obtained his M.Sc. and Ph.D. degrees in 1972 and 1976 from the Universities of Newcastle and Edinburgh, respectively. Following extensive postdoctoral work at the Universities of Nottingham, Glasgow, and Strathclyde, he joined industry in 1991.

Dr. Willmott is a member of the Controlled Release Society, British Association for Cancer Research, European Association for Cancer Research, British Society for Cell Biology, and British Society for Immunology. He has been the recipient of Royal Society Study Grants to collaborate with researchers in Greece, Italy, and Australia and his research has attracted funding of almost £1/2 million from the Medical Research Council, Association for International Cancer Research, Imperial Cancer Research Fund, Cancer Research Campaign, Scottish Home and Health Department, and private industry.

Dr. Willmott is the author of 54 papers and 11 book chapters and reviews. His current research interests include pathogenesis of solid tumor development and spread, design and delivery of peptide mimetic drugs, and novel targets for therapeutic intervention in cancer.

John M. Daly, M.D., is Chief of the Division of Surgical Oncology at the Hospital of the University of Pennsylvania and the Jonathan E. Rhoads Professor of Surgery at the University of Pennsylvania School of Medicine, Philadelphia, PA.

Dr. Daly graduated in 1969 from LaSalle University, Philadelphia, PA, with an B.A. degree in Biology (cum Laude) and obtained his M.D. degree in 1973 from Temple University School of Medicine.

Dr. Daly is a Fellow of the American College of Surgeons and a member of the American Society for Parenteral and Enteral Nutrition, American Surgical Association, Association for Academic Surgery, Collegium Internationale Chirurgiae Digestivae, Society for Surgery of the Alimentary Tract, Society of Surgical Oncology, Society of University Surgeons, Surgical Infection Society, and the Halstead Surgical Society. He is the President of the American Cancer Society, Philadelphia Division and a Director of the American Board of Surgery. He has been the recipient of many awards and honors including the Florence Baron Lecture, Brigham and Womens Hospital, Harvard Medical School, 1992, the Tovee Lecturer, University of Toronto, 1992, and the Jonathan M. Wainwright Award, 1992, Moses Taylor Hospital. He is the Program Director of an NIH-sponsored Surgical Oncology Training Grant and the Principal Investigator in a number of other grants.

Dr. Daly is the author of more than 160 papers and has been the author or co-author of more than 60 book chapters. He has also been the editor or co-editor of two books. His current research interests include tumor immunology, nutrition of solid tumors, and novel treatment strategies for cancer.

CONTRIBUTORS

J. H. Anderson, M.D., F.R.C.S(S).
University Department of Surgery
Royal Infirmary
Glasgow, United Kingdom

Mark A. Burton, Ph.D.
Department of Surgery
University of Western Australia
Royal Perth Hospital
Perth, Australia

Yan Chen, Ph.D.
Department of Surgery
University of Western Australia
Royal Perth Hospital
Perth, Australia

T. G. Cooke, M.D., F.R.C.S.
University Department of Surgery
Royal Infirmary
Glasgow, United Kingdom

Jeffrey Cummings, Ph.D.
Imperial Cancer Research Fund
Medical Oncology Unit
Western General Hospital
Edinburgh, United Kingdom

J. M. Daly, M.D., F.A.C.S.
Department of Surgery
Hospital of the University of
  Pennsylvania
Philadelphia, Pennsylvania

H. J. Gallagher, F.R.C.S.I.
Department of Surgery
Hospital of the University of
  Pennsylvania
Philadelphia, Pennsylvania

John F. Smyth, M.D., F.R.C.P.
Imperial Cancer Research Fund
Medical Oncology Unit
Western General Hospital
Edinburgh, United Kingdom

**Jacqueline A. Goldberg, M.D.,
  F.R.C.S.**
University Department of Surgery
Royal Infirmary
Glasgow, United Kingdom

**Bruce N. Gray, Ph.D.,
  F.R.A.C.S., F.A.C.S.**
Department of Surgery
University of Western Australia
Royal Perth Hospital
Perth, Australia

P. K. Gupta, Ph.D.
Abbott Laboratories
North Chicago, Illinois

David G. Hirst, Ph.D.
CRC Gray Laboratories
Mount Vernon Hospital
Northwood, United Kingdom

C. T. Hung, Ph.D.
Zenith Technology Corporation Ltd.
Dunedin, New Zealand

Colin S. McArdle, M.D., F.R.C.S.
University Department of Surgery
Royal Infirmary
Glasgow, United Kingdom

**James H. McKillop, M.D.,
  F.R.C.P.**
University Department of
  Medicine
Royal Infirmary
Glasgow, United Kingdom

David Watson, Ph.D.
Department of Pharmaceutical
  Sciences
University of Strathclyde
Glasgow, United Kingdom

Neville Willmott, Ph.D.
Oncology Research
Celltech Limited
Slough, United Kingdom

ACKNOWLEDGMENTS

Part of the research described in this volume was conducted in Glasgow during the period of 1982 to 1991. The subject progressed to a stage worthy of publication in book form due to stable financial support, particularly from the Medical Research Council, Association for International Cancer Research, Imperial Cancer Research Fund, and Cancer Research Campaign. This support enabled the establishment of vital collaborations between scientists and clinicians that was the hallmark of the program. The contributions of Jeff Cummings, Colin McArdle, Jim McKillop, Rodney Bessent, Jacqueline Goldberg, John Anderson, Sandy Florence, and David Kerr are acknowledged. I had some fun: I hope they did.

I must pay tribute to those who lightened the editorial load. P. K. Gupta and Mark Burton willingly gave of their time to review submitted chapters: their comments were perceptive and valuable. Although the final version bears their stamp, they are not responsible for any deficiencies. The editorial process was long and hard, but considerably less than it might have been due to Tina Jones' indexing skills, Apple Macintosh, Microsoft Corporation's Microsoft Word, and Claris' MacWrite II. I am sincerely grateful to all of the contributors for their industry, patience, and forbearance, without which the editorial process would have been meaningless.

Finally, I know that without the formative influence of my parents, Emma and Harry, and the support and encouragement of my dear wife, Janis, and two adorable children, Ewan and Neil, the project could not have been realized: they contributed more than they knew.

TABLE OF CONTENTS

Chapter 1

PHARMACEUTICAL AND METHODOLOGICAL ASPECTS OF MICROPARTICLES

Yan Chen, Mark A. Burton, and Bruce N. Gray

TABLE OF CONTENTS

0-8493-6952-5/94/$0.00 + $.50
© 1994 by CRC Press, Inc.

1

I. INTRODUCTION

The past decade has seen a major effort to redefine the ability of cytotoxic drugs to cause tumor regression in terms of the total exposure of the tumor to the particular drug (defined as the area under the concentration-time curve) rather than the administered dose, which may be modified because of toxic side effects. This has helped to clarify some of the variation in response between individual patients when treated with cytotoxic chemotherapy. It is now apparent that in many of the earlier studies, patients, and hence their tumors, were not exposed to sufficiently high drug concentrations to cause meaningful tumor regression. Thus, the main requirements for effective cell killing are for the target cells to be exposed to a sufficiently high drug concentration for an adequate period of time to ensure irreversible changes that lead to cell death. The main dose-limiting factor for cytotoxic drugs is the tolerance of normal tissues. Systemically administered drugs will always cause damage to normal healthy tissues, although this varies between different agents. Therefore, it is not possible to simply use higher drug doses to achieve clinically useful destruction of the cells comprising a solid tumor.

Direct administration of cytotoxic agents into the environment of the tumor has the potential to increase target cell exposure while at the same time decreasing exposure of normal tissues. This principle has been widely applied by administering cytotoxic drugs either directly into tumors or into body cavities, such as the peritoneal or pleural space. Similarly, administration of cytotoxic drugs into the arterial blood supply of solid tumor-bearing organs will result in the target organ receiving a higher peak concentration of drug than when given systemically. This technique has been widely used for treating primary and secondary malignant tumors in liver, isolated limbs, and head and neck cancer. Although regional organ perfusion does increase peak drug concentrations to the target tissues, this exposure advantage is restricted to the first pass of blood through the perfused organ. That fraction of drug not removed on the first pass recirculates as if given systemically.

The greatest advantage would be obtained by a drug delivery system that not only enhanced delivery of the drug to the target organ but also prevented loss of the drug in the efferent venous drainage from that organ. Microspheres and microcapsules, collectively referred to as microparticles, have been described for delivery of active agents to target organs.[1] Due to their size they are trapped in the microvasculature of tissues, when administered via the regional artery, where they release their drug payload. The procedure is termed chemoembolization. Microspheres are monolithic and may contain dispersed drug molecules either in solution or solid form, whereas microcapsules consist of drug concentrated in a central core inside a polymer-rich wall or shell. Figure 1 illustrates the basic structures of these two microparticles, although variations have been described.[2]

Administration of the drug microsphere system will effectively localize the drug to the target organ and the release profile of the drug from the system can be chosen to obtain a specified duration of exposure. The ability to design drug microsphere systems with a variety of release profiles has opened up a whole new area for cytotoxic drug delivery. There are certain basic requirements for this form of therapy

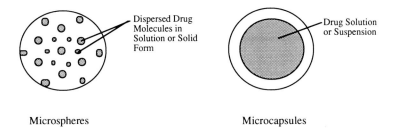

Microspheres   Microcapsules

FIGURE 1.   A schematic representation of microspheres and microcapsules.

to be effective. First, there is a need to localize sufficient quantities of the drug at the target site to have the desired cytotoxic effect. Second, there is a need to control the rate of delivery into the tumor milieu that will cause maximal cell destruction.

The use of targeted drug delivery by microspheres has particular attraction for treating tumors within isolated organs that have a single afferent arterial blood supply, such as the liver. Moreover, it is obviously of most value in those circumstances in which the tumor in the target organ is the sole site that requires treatment. It would thus have little application in treating patients with widespread cancer. However, there are many clinical situations in which tumor is localized to one area that cannot be effectively treated by conventional techniques. In addition, if general toxicity can be reduced by targeted drug delivery, it may be possible to combine systemic treatments for disseminated disease with regional treatments for known, isolated tumors.

The main objective of this chapter is to describe the materials used and the methods employed for the preparation of microparticulate carriers for regional cancer therapy. Contrasting methodologies will be examined with respect to both pharmaceutical characteristics and therapeutic strategies. The emphasis on particular systems reflects their frequency of appearance in the literature as vehicles for regional cancer therapy. A review of microspherical systems designed for other applications is not intended, and such systems are only considered by way of illustrating specific points.

II. SELECTION OF MATRIX/WALL MATERIALS FOR MICROPARTICLES

Microspheres and microcapsules can be prepared from numerous natural and synthetic materials. However, the choice of matrix material and methodology for use in regional cancer therapy, or indeed any other application, should be informed by the following considerations:

1.   Size and structure of particles required
2.   Physicochemical properties of the drug, such as water solubility
3.   Surface properties of particles, such as shape and charge
4.   Degradability of the matrix and its toxicity

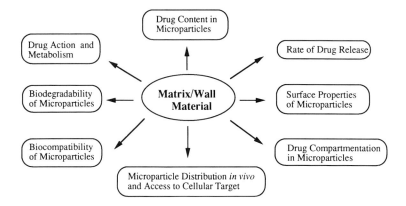

FIGURE 2.   Interrelationship between matrix material and microparticle performance.

5.   Desired level of drug incorporation and release rate of drug from the matrix
6.   Stability of the drug during formulation, storage, and use
7.   Stability of the microparticle matrix during storage and use
8.   Antigenicity

Once fabricated, the primary function of the matrix/wall constituents (i.e., polymer materials) of microparticles is to protect the drug and optimize its pharmacokinetic and pharmacodynamic profile. The interrelationship between polymer material and *in vivo* performance of microparticles is described in Figure 2.

A variety of materials have been employed, including both biodegradable and nonbiodegradable polymers. Table 1 lists those reported in the literature: although not all are used for preparation of microparticles for use in regional chemotherapy, they are included to illustrate the versatility of this approach to drug delivery.

A. PROTEINS

The use of proteins as matrix/wall materials has received a great deal of attention. This is not surprising because proteins are biodegradable natural polymers and they possess functional groups, such as −COOH and −NH$_2$, which are useful in forming different types of bond in the formulation of drug delivery systems. Among proteins, albumin is the most widely used material.[3-9] It has many favorable features, such as a high stability and biodegradability, and can be easily processed (heat denatured or chemical cross-linked) to produce a variety of drug release profiles.

The disadvantage of albumin as a microsphere matrix is its low drug-carrying capacity. Efforts have been made to blend albumin with polyamino acids of opposite charge to the drug to increase drug loading through ionic binding.[13,14] Similarly, Cremers et al.[15] described a technique using a mixture of albumin and heparin for the preparation of doxorubicin-loaded microspheres. Under physiological conditions heparin is negatively charged due to the carboxylic acid, sulfate, and sulfamate groups in its structure. Therefore, it forms ionic linkages with doxorubicin in the ionic form. Their results showed that the addition of heparin increased the drug-

TABLE 1
Polymer Materials Used in the Formulation of Microparticles

Matrix/wall material	Substance(s) entrapped	Delivery system	Ref.
Natural Polymers			
Proteins			
Albumin	Doxorubicin	Microspheres	3, 4, 5, 6
	5-Fluorouracil	Microspheres	3, 7
	Mitomycin C	Microspheres	8, 10
	Mercaptopurine	Microspheres	9
	Cisplatin	Microspheres	11
Albumin/chitin	Cisplatin	Microspheres	12
Albumin/PAA[a]	Doxorubicin	Microspheres	13
Albumin/PGA[b]	Doxorubicin	Microspheres	14
Albumin/Heparin	Doxorubicin	Microspheres	15
Casein	Doxorubicin	Microspheres	16
Casein/PAA	Doxorubicin	Microspheres	16
Fibrinogen	5-Fluorouracil	Microspheres	17
Gelatin	Bleomycin	Microspheres	18
	Mitomycin C	Microspheres	18
	5-Fluorouracil	Microspheres	18
Hemoglobin	Doxorubicin	Microspheres	19, 20
Transferrin	Doxorubicin	Microspheres	19
Zein	Mitomycin C	Microspheres	21
	Daunomycin HCl	Microspheres	21
	Peplomycin sulfate	Microspheres	21
Polysaccharides			
Agarose	Mitomycin C	Microbeads	10
	Cytosine arabinoside	Microbeads	Cited in 10
Alginate	Liposomes	Microcapsules	22
6-*O*-Carboxymethyl chitin	Doxorubicin	Microspheres	23
Chitosan	Model drug	Microspheres	24
Chitosan/alginate	Microparticles	Microcapsules	25
Chitosan/alginate	Cells	Capsules	26
Dextran	Doxorubicin	Microspheres	14
Polyacryl starch	Proteins	Microparticles	27
Synthetic Polymers			
Polyesters			
Polylactic acid	Leuprolide acetate	Microcapsules	28
Poly(D,L-lactide)	Cisplatin	Microspheres	29
	CCNU[c]	Microspheres	30
Poly(glycolic acid)	Prednisolone-21-acetate	Microspheres	31
	Methylene blue	Microspheres	32
Poly(lactic/glycolic) acid	Leuprolide acetate	Microcapsules	28
	Muramyl dipeptide	Microspheres	33
PLG[d]	Hormone	Microspheres	34
PLG-GLU[e]	Bromocriptine	Microspheres	35
Poly(β-hydroxybutyrate)	CCNU	Microspheres	30

TABLE 1 (Continued)
Polymer Materials Used in the Formulation of Microparticles

Matrix/wall material	Substance(s) entrapped	Delivery system	Ref.
Synthetic Polymers			
Polyamides			
Nylon	pH indicators	Microcapsules	39
Polyanhydrides			
PCPP-SA[f]	Bethanechol	Microspheres	40
Acrylate polymers			
Eudragit™	5-Aminosalicylic acid	Microspheres	41
HEMA-MMA[g]	Cells	Microcapsules	38
Poly(methyl methacrylate)	Pseudoephedrine	Microspheres	36
Others			
Ethylcellulose	Cisplatin	Microcapsules	11, 42
	Mitomycin C	Microcapsules	43
Cellulose acetate butyrate	Pseudoephedrine	Microspheres	36
	Paracetamol	Microcapsules	37
HPC[h]-ethylcellulose	Piretanide	Microcapsules	44
Polyglutaraldehyde	Doxorubicin	Microspheres	45
Polystyrene	Fe_3O_4	Microspheres	46
	Doxorubicin	Microspheres	47
Carnauba wax	5-Fluorouracil	Microspheres	48
Polydimethylsiloxane (silastic)	Model drug	Microparticles	49
Polyphosphazene	Melphalan	Microspheres	50
	Melphalan methyl ester	Microspheres	50

  [a]   Poly(L-aspartic acid).
  [b]   Poly(L-glutamic acid).
  [c]   1-(2-Chloroethyl)-3-cyclohexyl-nitrosourea.
  [d]   Poly(D,L-lactide-co-glycolide).
  [e]   Poly(D,L-lactide-co-glycolide-D-glucose).
  [f]   Poly(*bis*(p-carboxy-phenoxy) propane) anhydride/sebacic acid.
  [g]   Hydroxyethylmethacrylate-methyl methacrylate.
  [h]   Hydroxypropylcellulose.

loading capacity of albumin by up to fourfold, although as with polyamino acids,[13] release of doxorubicin incorporated via ionic binding was rapid.

    Albumin also has the ability to form covalent linkages with drugs, such as doxorubicin, through cross-linking agents, such as glutaraldehyde.[45,51] This covalent binding results in drug complexation within microspheres allowing sustained release and altered biological fate within tumor tissue (see Chapter 5).

    Other proteins, such as gelatin, hemoglobin, transferrin, and casein, have also been used in the formulation of microparticles. Gelatin is readily available, of low antigenicity, and is used as a plasma substitute. In comparison with albumin, gelatin is more versatile in that it can be processed into microparticles by both emulsion stabilization and aqueous phase separation techniques.[18,52] Microspheres prepared from transferrin and hemoglobin exhibit many similarities to those made from albumin.[13,19] However, casein microspheres are different from their albumin counterparts in that they incorporate a higher proportion of doxorubicin in the form of a covalent complex with matrix protein (Chapter 5) and degrade more slowly *in vivo*.[53,54]

B. POLYSACCHARIDES

Polysaccharides, such as starch and dextran, are another group of biodegradable polymers that have been extensively investigated. One application has been their use as emboli for vascular blockade of target organs. When administered simultaneously with anticancer drugs this has the effect of delaying transit of the drug through the capillary network of the target organ, resulting in increased exposure of the target organ to the drug[55,56] (see also Chapter 7).

More recently polysaccharides, such as chitin and chitosan, have been investigated as drug carriers.[12,23] They are hydrophobic and may chelate with metals, which is useful in formulation of sustained release carriers for metal-based drugs, such as cisplatin. Nishioka et al.[12] demonstrated that addition of chitin into albumin microspheres, or treatment of the microspheres with chitosan, sustained the release of cisplatin. In addition, incorporation of chitin into albumin microspheres almost doubled cisplatin loading. Although chitin is biodegradable and is readily formulated into microspheres, its insolubility in water and most common organic solvents (except strong acids) limits its clinical application. In an attempt to overcome this, water-soluble derivatives, such as carboxymethyl-chitin and dihydroxypropyl-chitin, have been developed.[57] In particular, carboxymethyl-chitin has shown potential as a useful sustained release microparticulate carrier for proteins and anticancer drugs.[23]

C. SYNTHETIC POLYMERS

Synthetic biodegradable polymers, such as polyesters, polyamino acids, polyanhydrides, and polyamides have also been explored for use in microsphere/microcapsule preparation. The advantage of synthetic polymers is that their degradation rate can be controlled through adjusting the molecular weight of a homopolymer or hydrophilicity and composition of a co-polymer.[58]

Polyamides, such as nylon,[39] may be used for microencapsulation of large molecules, such as proteins and enzymes; however, microencapsulation of small molecular weight compounds needs inclusion of hard matrices, such as formalinized gelatin or calcium alginate, inside the nylon coating.[59] Not all compounds are suitable for incorporation into nylon microcapsules: the quaternary compounds, for example, cannot be formulated in this way because of their interference in the reaction to form nylon.

Other polymers, such as polyesters, are hydrophobic and therefore act as a good barrier for controlling drug release. Because biodegradation of synthetic polymers generally involves bulk erosion, drug release usually is diffusion-controlled prior to the erosion of polymer. However, once polymer erosion begins, the drug release mechanism becomes complex. Fast bulk erosion of the polymer can result in a burst release of drug *in vivo*. There is little information regarding the compatibility of these polymers with drug candidates; however, one polyester, poly(D,L-lactide-co-glycolide), has been reported to be chemically incompatible with some peptides.[60]

D. GLASS AND CERAMICS

The majority of the work performed on the development of ceramic or glass microspheres has been directed toward clinical utility for internal radiation therapy of hepatic metastases. The development of microparticles for radionuclide imaging,[61] for use as diagnostic aids[62] or for therapeutic purposes,[63] provides an interesting contrast to the requirements for drug delivery and release. Radioactive microparticles cannot allow significant diffusion of radionuclide from the matrix into surrounding tissue and hence into the systemic circulation. The application of radioactive microparticles in regional cancer therapy (radioembolization) is discussed elsewhere in this volume (Chapter 5).

Since the 1960s there have been a number of attempts to develop radioactive particles for intra-arterial administration in the treatment of hepatic malignancies. This began with the use of colloidal suspensions of ^{32}P, ^{198}Au, and proteinate aggregates of ^{90}Y,[64] but was soon developed into the manufacture of inert ceramic microspheres carrying ^{90}Y by the 3M Corporation.[65] These 40 to 60 μm diameter microspheres were chemically and physiologically inert, with a density of 3 g/ml and a melting point in excess of 1500°C.[66] However, the need to spheridize these ceramic microspheres at high temperatures with volatile high activity radionuclides was hazardous and expensive.[67]

During the 1970s small (0.9 to 1.43 μm) ^{90}Y microparticles were produced from fused clay aerosols,[68] but a group in Atlanta, Georgia also began development of glass microspheres containing stable ^{31}P or ^{89}Y, which could be activated relatively easily by neutron bombardment to the energetic isotopes ^{32}P and ^{90}Y. Thus, microspheres can conveniently be manufactured and stored while nonradioactive. Manufacture of glass microspheres involves melting the constituents at 1500°C with the ^{89}Y incorporated and then crushing the cooled ingot before spheridization through a flame sprayer and sizing in sieves.[67]

Radioactive glass microspheres have been examined in preclinical and clinical settings with a lack of hematological and pulmonary toxicity (indicating efficient localization) and tumor responses at the high absorbed dose of 320 Gy.[69,70] A major drawback of this system is the high particle density of approximately 3 g/ml, which promotes rapid sedimentation. This can be overcome prior to administration by maintaining microspheres as a homogeneous suspension. The effect of high density on homogeneity of microsphere dispersion when introduced into the hepatic artery, and its influence on particle distribution *in vivo,* is not known. Clinical application of ^{90}Y microspheres is discussed in Chapter 3.

Other groups have examined the utility of polystyrene resin microspheres incorporating ^{90}Y, which have a density much closer to whole blood (1.3 g/ml) and distribute intravascularly directly with the blood flow.[71-73] The latter microspheres were initially considered at risk of leaching the isotope into the systemic circulation, but this has not been the case with the microspheres developed by our group using an insoluble yttrium salt.[74]

III. TECHNIQUES FOR MICROPARTICLE PREPARATION

A variety of techniques have been reported for the manufacture of microspheres and microcapsules. These can be classified into the following groups:

A. EMULSION STABILIZATION

In this process the dispersed phase is drug dissolved or suspended in an aqueous polymer (e.g., protein) solution and emulsified in a water-immiscible continuous phase, usually an oil. The water-in-oil emulsion is then stabilized by heat or the addition of a chemical cross-linking agent. Free-flowing microparticles are recovered after washing, filtration, and drying of the hardened particles. This technique is generally used to produce microspheres. However, if the drug to be incorporated exists as solid particles of size less than the emulsion droplets, microcapsules will be formed.

The emulsion stabilization technique is generally used for water-soluble drugs but is also suitable for insoluble drugs able to be dispersed in the polymer solution. The polymer must be water soluble and capable of forming emulsions. Whether stabilization should be accomplished thermally or by the addition of chemical cross-linking agent is dependent on the heat stability of the drug, desired release characteristics, and degradation properties of microparticles. Factors, including temperature, concentration of cross-linking agent, and duration of stabilization, have a great influence on both drug release and degradation properties of microparticles. These will be addressed in Section IV. This technique is well known as the method for manufacturing protein, particularly albumin microspheres. Yapel[7] reviewed heat and chemical stabilization for preparation of albumin microspheres. Arshady[2] reviewed the manufacture of microspheres/microcapsules using various modifications of emulsion stabilization.

B. SOLVENT EVAPORATION

In this process the drug is dissolved or dispersed in a volatile, water-immiscible organic solvent that contains the matrix polymer. This solution or dispersion is emulsified in an aqueous solution containing a surfactant to form microdroplets. The organic solvent is then removed by evaporation at the water/air interface at atmospheric or reduced pressure. The hardened microparticles carrying drug are obtained after complete removal of organic solvent followed by filtration and drying. The rate of solvent evaporation is critical in controlling the porosity of microparticles and thus the release rate of the system.[75]

This technique is simple, economic, and easy to perform. Depending on the solubility of the active agent in the polymer solution, the product can be either homogeneous microspheres or heterogeneous microcapsules. The polymer used in this method must be water insoluble. It is normally used for hydrophobic drugs[76,77] because of the aqueous continuous phase involved in the process. However, more recently the technique has proved useful in the formulation as microspheres of cisplatin[29] (low water solubility) and leuprolide acetate[28] (high water solubility). In the latter case a water-oil-water multiple emulsion instead of oil-water emulsion was produced during the process. Increasing the viscosity of the inner water phase by adding gelatin, lowering the temperature, and including oil as a barrier (minimizing migration of drug from inner to outer phase) allowed formulation of microcapsules with a high drug incorporation (up to 71%). This technique is currently used to produce a clinically approved product as a monthly depot injection of leuprolide.

C. COACERVATION OR PHASE SEPARATION

This technique can be further divided into organic phase separation and aqueous phase separation according to the nature of the medium employed.

1. Organic Phase Separation

This technique has been used to encapsulate water-soluble anticancer drugs. The simplest method involves dispersion of active agent in a solution of polymer in a nonpolar solvent. Alternatively, the active agent can be first dissolved in an aqueous solution and then dispersed in the polymer solution in a nonpolar solvent to form a water-in-oil emulsion. The wall-forming polymer is precipitated (phase separation) around the active ingredient or the droplets of its aqueous solution by decreasing the polymer solubility through (1) addition of a polymer nonsolvent, (2) addition of a second polymer that is incompatible with the wall-forming polymer, or (3) lowering the temperature. The resultant microcapsules are then hardened by successive washing in mixtures of solvent and nonsolvent for the polymer with decreasing amounts of the solvent for polymer.[77]

Unlike solvent evaporation the organic phase separation method has the major drawback of being susceptible to aggregation of particles. It is the most common method employed to prepare ethylcellulose microcapsules, the vehicle in the first clinical use by Kato et al. of chemoembolization.[78] Benita and Donbrow[79] found that addition of polyisobutylene formed a protective colloid on the surface of ethylcellulose droplets, which controlled article aggregation. Other methods, such as slowly reducing the phase separation temperature, employing vigorous agitation, and washing the product with cold solvent, can also minimize aggregation.[77]

It should be pointed out that the phase separation process employed to precipitate the polymer can influence microparticle characteristics. In a related system, Sato et al.[80] compared three techniques: evaporation, freeze-drying, and extraction of solvent for precipitation of poly(glycolic acid) from the dispersed phase of an oil-in-water emulsion to form microspheres. For incorporation of the water-soluble marker methylene blue, it was found that freeze-drying and solvent extraction techniques produced a good yield of microspheres. Microspheres formed by these two methods also showed high porosity with a resultant rapid release of the marker.

2. Aqueous Phase Separation

As an example of this process, drug is dispersed in an aqueous solution containing a gellable and ionizable polymer. The dispersion is then mixed with another aqueous solution of either polyelectrolyte or ions of opposite charge (opposite charges may be conferred on the polyelectrolytes by adjusting pH). Where oppositely charged components are present their instant interaction forms colloidal particles that engulf the drug.

Like the solvent evaporation method, this technique works best for water-insoluble drugs and usually forms microcapsules containing drug particles. Typical examples are the preparation of gelatin/acacia and alginate/CaCl$_2$ microcapsules.[22,81] Based on the similar principle of ionotropic gelation of a charged polysaccharide, Bodmeier et al.[25] used chitosan/tripolyphosphate to microencapsulate nanoparticles and microparticles.

D. INTERFACIAL POLYMERIZATION

With this technique the drug is dissolved or dispersed in an organic solution of a monomer, which can be polymerized to a solid. The organic solution that serves as disperse phase is emulsified into a continuous aqueous phase. Polymerization at the interface of the oil/water emulsion is induced by either a catalyst added into the system or bases present in water. For example, nylon (polyamide) microcapsules are prepared from an interface reaction of a diamine and a diacid halide.[59] This method has also been used to prepare nanoparticles.[82]

E. EMULSION/DISPERSION POLYMERIZATION

Emulsion polymerization is a method most frequently employed for the preparation of nanoparticles (10 to 1000 nm), for example, polymethyl methacrylate and polyalkylcyanoacrylate nanoparticles. The technique involves emulsification of a hydrophobic monomer in an aqueous phase with the monomer polymerized using either a free radical initiator or high energy irradiation.[82]

Dispersion polymerization is a relatively new technique.[83] It is based on precipitation polymerization in which polymerization begins with a monomer **dissolved** in dispersion medium (rather than an emulsion as in emulsion polymerization) and ends with an insoluble polymer in spherical form. A polymer stabilizer is used during the reaction to help the formation of well-defined polymer particles free of aggregates. The advantage of this method over emulsion polymerization, which requires water as continuous phase, is that both water and organic solvents can be used in this respect; this markedly increases the range of monomers that can be polymerized to form microparticles. Moreover, it can produce not only nanoparticles but also microparticles with size up to 15 μm.[84] For both methods, the drug to be incorporated desired to incorporate can be added directly to the monomer in solution before polymerization or postloaded by addition to the disperse phase after polymerization. Further details of these two methods were described by Candau and Ottewill.[85]

F. MECHANICAL PROCESSING

Mechanical processing involves the use of apparatus, such as fluidized beds, centrifugal encapsulating nozzles, or spray dryers, to microencapsulate active ingredients. Because they have not been used in cancer therapy, the interested reader is referred to Ranney.[86]

G. OTHER TECHNIQUES

New techniques are continually being reported for preparing microparticles. Wichert and Rohdewald[87] described a method to produce polylactic acid microparticles without using organic solvent. Briefly, the polymer was melted in the presence of drug to obtain a homogeneous mixture. After cooling, the mixture was emulsified in a hot, buffered Tween 80 solution. Free-flowing particles were recovered by centrifugation of microspheres in ice-water or spray drying with addition of polyvinylpyrrolidone. The group reported that particles with mean size of 2 to 22 μm were produced by this method. A smooth surface was revealed with microparticles recovered by spray drying. For heat-stable drugs this method can be considered an alternative preparation method for polyester microparticles, which avoids the use of organic solvents.

Modifications of some of the processes described in Section III may be required for any particular drug and delivery system. For example, in the preparation of cisplatin albumin microspheres, Nishioka et al.[12] found that chitosan treatment of albumin microspheres prepared by the emulsion stabilization method significantly suppressed drug release from microspheres. Bodmeier and McGinity[88] demonstrated that altering the pH of the aqueous phase is an effective way to increase drug loading within microspheres when using the solvent evaporation method to incorporate ionizable drugs.

Certain methods listed herein can be used not only for preparing microparticles but also for coating microparticles.[52,89] For example, by controlling dispersion time during the solvent evaporation process one can produce coated microparticles with different coat stability and release characteristics (Figures 3 and 4).

IV. CHARACTERIZATION OF MICROPARTICLES

Microparticle properties are of importance in determining their disposition in the body as well as therapeutic effects of the incorporated drug. Characterization of particles is an important step in optimization of design and development of drug carrier systems. This section considers factors that influence the *in vivo* performance of microspheres and microcapsules.

A. SIZE

Particle size is one of the most important parameters influencing the targeting of microparticles in regional cancer therapy; therefore, controlling the size of microparticles during preparation is a primary concern. Size distribution of particles is affected by the size of emulsion droplets formed during the preparation; thus,

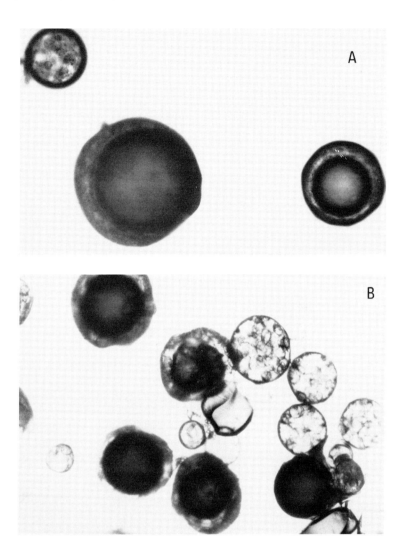

FIGURE 3. Effect of dispersion time during solvent evaporation on the stability of the coating. Particles were coated with a mixture of 1 part ethylcellulose and 3 parts of a copolymer of poly(hydroxybutyrate-hydroxyvalerate) containing 24 mol% hydroxyvalerate. (A) Dispersion time 1 h; the coatings are intact. (B) Mixing time 18 h; some of the coatings are interrupted. Average uncoated particle size is 120 μm (authors' unpublished results).

mixing speed during emulsification and the viscosity of the drug solution and organic phase can markedly influence particle size.[3] Particle size is smaller when the mixing speed or the viscosity of the organic phase (i.e., external phase) is high. On the contrary, a high viscosity drug solution leads to the formation of larger size microparticles. Additionally, the amount of drug incorporated into the microspheres

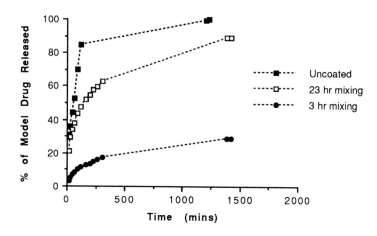

FIGURE 4.   Effect of dispersion time during solvent evaporation on the release of a model drug (potassium dichromate) from Dowex 50W-X4 ion-exchange resins coated with a copolymer of poly(hydroxybutyrate-hydroxyvalerate) (authors' unpublished results).

when the amount approaches the limit of drug solubility in the dispersed phase may also have an influence on the final size of the particles.[90] The higher the drug loading, the larger the size tends to be.[28,29]

Temperature during dispersion also has an influence on the size of microparticles depending on the phase to which heat is applied. In the case of emulsion stabilization of protein microspheres, increasing the temperature of the disperse phase to increase solvent power and reduce viscosity leads to the formation of smaller microspheres (unpublished observations). In the preparation of polyglycolic acid microspheres, raising the temperature of the continuous phase results in the production of larger microparticles.[80] If necessary, control of the size and size distribution of particles can be maintained by mechanical sieves.

B. DRUG INCORPORATION
1. Emulsion Stabilization

For systems in which drug and polymeric matrix material are mixed prior to microparticle formation (preloading), the extent of incorporation of drugs is controlled by the solubility of the drug, the chemical composition of the matrix material used, and the relative amount of both in the disperse phase.[91,92] Considering albumin microspheres prepared by emulsion stabilization, reduction in albumin concentration from 25% to 1% resulted in an increase in drug incorporation from 16% to 83% by weight.[90] However, this may alter particle size and stability, adversely affect drug release,[7] or change the structure and physicochemical properties of microspheres.[76] Changes in other process variables can increase drug loading. Gupta et al.[5] demonstrated increased incorporation of doxorubicin into albumin microspheres by lowering temperature and shortening heat stabilization times.

The importance of chemical composition of matrix material is illustrated by the contrast in doxorubicin incorporation into glutaraldehyde cross-linked microspheres prepared using either pure albumin or a mixture of albumin and polyaspartic acid as matrix material (Chapter 5). In the former case, doxorubicin was incorporated predominantly as a covalent complex with albumin, whereas in the latter case the drug was present in native form.

The use of postloading of microspherical systems is restricted to charged matrices and ionizable drugs with an opposite charge (being ionizable the problem of low water solubility does not arise). The most common drug incorporated into such systems is doxorubicin, which is positively charged at neutral pH. Goldberg et al.[14] used in ion-exchange principles to obtain microspherical systems with high drug loading and versatile release properties. The polymer with suitable ion-exchange properties was polyglutamic acid, which formed a stable polymer drug salt with the basic drug doxorubicin. Based on the same principle, others have used ion-exchange resins to incorporate doxorubicin with loadings of more than 35% (W/W) with polystyrene-based cation exchange resins.[47,93] It has further been demonstrated that drug incorporation into ionic resins can be affected by the resin's counter ion.[93]

A review of doxorubicin incorporation into microspherical systems shows that ion-exchange mechanisms with postloading of drug produce highest incorporation (Table 2).

2. Solvent Evaporation

Several factors have been identified that affect content of water-soluble drugs in microspheres during the solvent evaporation process using water as continuous phase.[50,88] For example, the glass transition temperature of the polymer and the residence time of the microspheres in water are two such factors. It is suggested that high glass transition temperature results in a markedly lower drug diffusion coefficient, thus limiting drug losses during the solvent evaporation process.[50] The use of reduced pressure speeds up evaporation of organic solvent, reducing the microsphere residence time in water.

Another approach to minimizing the partitioning of water-soluble, ionizable drugs into the aqueous continuous phase is to adjust the pH of the aqueous phase to reduce aqueous solubility of the incorporated agent.[88] Alternatively, the saturation of slightly water-soluble drugs in the aqueous phase and increasing the initial ratio of drug to polymer increases the incorporation of cisplatin into poly(D,L-lactide) microspheres tenfold.[29]

Particle size can also have effects on drug loading. Ogawa et al.[28] found that microparticles appeared to have variable drug loading in different particle size ranges of the same preparation. The smaller the size, the lower the drug loading. This may result from the increase in frequent contact between the outer water phase and inner water phase in smaller particles because of extended surface area of the water/oil emulsion. Alternatively, this phenomenon could be due to the fact that the larger

TABLE 2
Features of Doxorubicin-Loaded Microspheres

Microsphere matrix material	Stabilization technique	Drug loading (µg/mg MS)	Major binding mechanism	Ref.
PGLU[a]	Chemical cross-linking	19.6–27.2	Covalent	94
Cross-linked PVA[b]	Chemical cross-linking	8.9	Covalent	95
Albumin	Chemical cross-linking	6.3–9.1[e]	Covalent/physical	96
Albumin	Heat stabilization	10.8–45.7	Physical	97
Albumin	Chemical cross-linking	25.9–311.7[f]	Ionic	6
Albumin	Chemical + heat	130.0	Covalent/physical	4
Albumin	Chemical cross-linking	70.0	Covalent/physical	15
Albumin/heparin	Chemical cross-linking	250.0–300.0[f]	Ionic	15
Albumin/PGA[c]	Chemical cross-linking	180.0–460.0[f]	Ionic	14
Albumin/PAA[d]	Chemical cross-linking	29.8–42.4	Ionic	19
Casein	Chemical cross-linking	2.1–4.1[e]	Covalent/physical	16
Hemoglobin	Chemical cross-linking	7.1–10.1[e]	Covalent/physical	19
Transferrin	Chemical cross-linking	5.1–8.7[e]	Covalent/physical	19
Polystyrene resin	Polymerization	402.0–463.0[f]	Ionic	93

[a]   Polyglutaraldehyde.
[b]   Polyvinyl alcohol.
[c]   Polyglutamic acid.
[d]   Polyaspartic acid.
[e]   For these systems the drug loading quoted is for doxorubicin incorporated by noncovalent mechanisms (e.g., physical entrapment within matrix). Total incorporation of doxorubicin (i.e., covalently bound to matrix + physically entrapped within matrix) was approximately 30 µg/mg of microspheres (see Chapter 5).
[f]   The drug was loaded after microsphere preparation via ion-exchange interactions.

surface area associated with the smaller size particles takes more polymer; therefore, the drug loading is low.

C. DRUG RELEASE KINETICS

Release rate of drug from matrix is one of the most important characteristics of microspherical systems because it governs pharmacokinetic behavior and therefore efficacy. The release rate of a system is influenced by a number of factors: physicochemical/chemical properties of drug and polymer matrix material; interaction between polymer, drug, and cross-linking agent; method of preparation; drug payload; and size and density or porosity of microparticles.

Ruiz and Benoit,[98] working on a copolymer of poly(D,L-lactic acid) and glycolic acid as a biodegradable carrier for peptides, found that the overall polymer hydrophobicity affected the release rate of the incorporated peptide. A decrease of hydrophobicity of the polymer (by the presence of oligomers or gamma irradiation) led to rapid hydration of the polymer, resulting in a considerable increase in the porosity of the microsphere matrix with consequent increase in peptide release.

The effect of the chemical nature of the drug on the release characteristics of microspheres was demonstrated by Goedemoed et al.[50] They reported that polyphosphazene microspheres containing melphalan methyl ester showed sustained release, whereas the melphalan-loaded microspheres prepared from the same polymer exhibited high initial release that was not sustained. For a given matrix material, this illustrates the significant role the chemical properties of a drug play.

Yapel[7] reported that particles of small size (1 to 5 μm) exhibited faster drug release than the same weight of large microspheres (50 to 100 μm) due to the larger specific surface area and short diffusion path associated with smaller sized particles (see also Ponpaibul et al.[99]). However, the inverse relationship between particle diameter and incorporated drug release rate is not a universal finding: with doxorubicin-loaded microcapsules, Kawashima et al.[100] found that release rate was constant at least over a small size range (mean diameter 100 to 220 μm).

Drug loading has been identified as another factor influencing release from microparticles. Bodmeier and McGinity[88] reported that for the release of quinidine from microspheres the burst effect due to drug leaching and pore diffusion was more prominent at higher drug loading (43 to 52%) but eliminated at lower drug loading (6.3%).

The effect of stabilization of albumin microspheres on their drug release has been well studied. It is agreed that, in the case of heat stabilization, increased temperature and prolonged time of heat treatment result in more dense microspheres and slower release rate compared with those prepared at lower temperatures or for shorter times.[3,7,97,101] However, using chemical cross-linking agents to stabilize microspheres has produced inconsistent results. Some reports have demonstrated that with increased concentrations of the cross-linking agent, glutaraldehyde, in microsphere preparations a decrease in drug release rate *in vitro* ensues.[51,96] Others have found no evidence of such an inverse relationship.[101,102] Albumin and casein microspheres exhibit decreased drug release when glutaraldehyde concentration is increased from 1.0% (W/V) to 1.6% but no further change when concentration is increased to 2.2% (Figure 5).[53]

To interpret the mechanism of doxorubicin release from albumin microspheres stabilized by glutaraldehyde cross-linking a compartmentation model has been proposed. In this model, doxorubicin is considered to be incorporated into microspheres in discrete compartments or forms and is released at corresponding rates, each with its own rate constant (Figure 6).[13,53,97] First is native drug superficially located and loosely attached. Second is native drug strongly but noncovalently bound to the matrix material via forces, such as ionic bonding through the protonated amino group on the sugar ring of doxorubicin. Third is drug covalently bound to albumin matrix via glutaraldehyde (complexed and immobilized). Only doxorubicin in the first and second compartments can be released *in vitro*. It is believed that the release of doxorubicin from the first compartment results in the burst effect observed in release studies. Release from the second compartment is responsible for the sustained release of doxorubicin seen *in vitro*. Doxorubicin in the third compartment can only be released through biodegradation and contributes to the biological activity of microspheres *in vivo* (Chapter 5).

This model may explain why increasing the concentration of glutaraldehyde slows down the release rate of the drug in the initial phase and, once the cross-

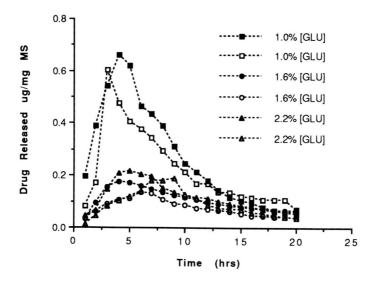

FIGURE 5. The influence of glutaraldehyde concentration on the release of doxorubicin from casein microspheres (differential release curve); 200 mg casein was used in the microsphere preparation. Glutaraldehyde (GLU) concentration (% w/v) in disperse phase. (From Chen, Y., Ph.D. thesis, 1989. With permission.)

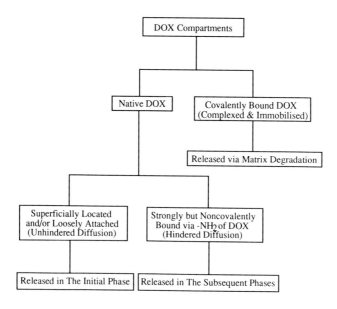

FIGURE 6. A proposed model of doxorubicin (DOX) compartmentation within microspheres. Compartments correspond to the forms in which doxorubicin is incorporated into microspheres.

linked network reaches its maximum density, further increasing the concentration of glutaraldehyde has little effect on the overall release of the drug (Figure 5) but increases the proportion of the drug in the third compartment (Chapter 5). Three compartments correspond to the three binding mechanisms described by Goldberg et al.:[14] (1) physically associated drug for fast release by desorption, (2) ionic bonding for moderate release by dissociation, and (3) covalent bonding for slow release after matrix degradation.

D. SURFACE PROPERTIES

Surface properties, including charge and hydrophilicity/hydrophobicity, are important factors determining microparticle dispersion and biological fate. Tomlinson and Burger[90] reported that the magnitude of the zeta potential of albumin microspheres was dependent on both the medium in which the particles were suspended and the presence of ionized drug. The latter has implications for detecting ionized drug on the microsphere surface. By measuring the mobility of microparticles at neutral pH using a microelectrophoresis technique, Chen[53] examined doxorubicin disposition on the surface of microspherical systems of defined release rate. It was found that doxorubicin-loaded protein microspheres with the least negative charge showed fastest initial release rate. This was interpreted as the result of positively charged doxorubicin on the surface of microspheres neutralizing the intrinsic negative charge of the protein matrix and suggests a method for estimating superficially located ionized drug in microspheres.

With regard to altering the hydrophobicity/hydrophilicity balance of the microsphere surface, Longo and Goldberg[103] developed a method for the preparation of hydrophilic albumin microspheres by steric stabilization of an aqueous albumin dispersion in an organic polymer solution. Davis and Illum[104] studied surface modification of particles using hydrophilic nonionic surfactants, such as poloxamer 338 and poloxamine 908. The effects of these polymers on biodistribution of surfactant-coated microspheres were significant. Uncoated particles localize mainly in the liver. Those microspheres coated with poloxamer 338 were diverted from liver to bone marrow, whereas those coated with poloxamine 908 remained almost exclusively in the circulation. This may be the result of surface-adsorbed hydrophilic polymers acting as a steric barrier to interaction between particles and opsonins (blood components involved in recognition and clearance of foreign particles).

Other studies have also shown that modifying the surface characteristics of particles can lead to a change in anatomical distribution of colloids.[105,106] Although such studies are of some interest as a precursor to the use of microspheres as a targeting vehicle, the problems of localizing active agents in pathological lesions, in adequate amount, still remain.

E. BIODEGRADABILITY

Biodegradability influences stability of the carrier system *in vivo* and therefore affects drug release rate and clearance of carrier from the body. For biodegradable microspheres made of protein, the rate of biodegradation is a function of the type of matrix and additives and the relative amount of protein and cross-linking agent used (or the temperature and length of heat treatment). When concentration of the cross-linking agent is too high, the particles can become resistant to enzymic digestion.[107] Davis et al.[108] described their *in vivo* studies on the biodegradation of glutaraldehyde cross-linked albumin microspheres after intramuscular injection. They demonstrated that biodegradability is directly related to the density of the microsphere matrix so that the higher the concentration of glutaraldehyde, the slower the degradation observed. They also reported that, in muscle tissue, the degradation process of microspheres prepared from 5% glutaraldehyde is first order with a half-life of 3.5 days.

A similar observation was reported by Willmott et al.[54,109] who showed that albumin microspheres began to erode in the lung 24 h after intravenous administration and by 2 days 50% of embolized microspheres had disappeared. After hepatic artery administration it took 3.6 days for half the amount of embolized microspheres to be removed from the liver. Under comparable conditions 50% of casein microspheres were lost after 3.5 days (lung) and 6.8 days (liver). Although examination of biodegradability of protein microparticles when exposed to enzymes can be conducted *in vitro,* it should be emphasized that this is a rapid process relative to that *in vivo*[53,107] and the rate of degradation is also enzyme specific.[3] This was confirmed by Willmott et al.[54] who demonstrated that, although casein microspheres were more sensitive to trypsin digestion than albumin microspheres *in vitro,* the casein system was more resistant to enzyme digestion after embolization in lung and liver.

For biodegradable microparticles prepared from polyesters, degradation can be affected by the hydrophobicity and the crystallinity of the polymer[98,110] and the presence of plasma proteins.[111] Thus, a high degree of hydrophobicity or crystallinity can slow the process of hydration and water penetration, resulting in slow degradation. Copolymerization destroys a polymer's crystallinity, which may produce more readily degradable matrices.[110] In a systematic study of the relationship between proportion of polylactate/polyglycolate and degradation rate, it was found that the copolymer of lactic acid and glycolic acid (1:1) showed the maximal biodegradation rate *in vivo.*[112] With regard to the presence of plasma proteins, their adsorption on the surface of poly(L-lactide) microcapsules causes an increase in H^+ concentration at the surface as well as increases the solubility of the polymer. In turn, these accelerate the degradation of poly(L-lactide) microcapsules.[111]

In a recent publication, Kissel et al.[35] described how the biodegradation rate of poly(D,L-lactide-co-glycolide)(PLG) was affected by the steric structure of the copolymers. They found that the *in vivo* release profile of agents incorporated into microspheres prepared from the linear PLG was biphasic: this was thought to be due to an initial burst effect then subsequent polymer degradation. Using a novel biodegradable terpolymer, which was prepared by grafting linear copolymers of PLG onto a core molecule containing a suitable functionality, degradation of the microspheres was accelerated and pharmacokinetic pattern of incorporated drug was changed.

The numerous examples cited herein demonstrate that the characteristics and performance of microparticles are determined by interactions between the drug load, the polymer matrix, and the preparation technique. The resultant drug-loaded microparticles are not just the sum of their parts but may be a new entity with properties that are difficult to predict from consideration of the original constituents.

V. NOVEL STRATEGIES

Although targeting of microspheres to tumor deposits can be efficient in the regional context (Chapters 3 and 8), drug release rates of the devices described herein are predetermined and not responsive to the external environment. The disadvantages of this type of system are as follows: (1) initiation of release of the drug cannot be controlled once the microparticles are administered, and (2) release rate of the drug either varies with time or is a constant function of time. There is no way to change or modulate the release rate once release has started.

These points present obstacles to the effective use of microparticles as chemotherapeutic drug carriers because they can lead to suboptimal delivery or release of drug. The use of external modulators of drug release can be considered as a means of improving the delivery of drug to the target tissue; thus, for example, a reliable external on/off stimulus could avoid repeat administration by providing pulses of drug at the desired time. In addition, if spatial control of drug release is needed (e.g., at the solid tumor site) and the on/off stimulus can be focused on defined anatomical areas, then drug release could be selectively initiated.

Approaches using magnetic control to enhance both targeting and regulation of drug release have been proposed.[91,113] Utilization of magnetic microparticles to improve targeting of drug carrier systems have been extensively studied[114-117] (see also Chapter 4). However, the idea of regulating drug release by exposing the magnetic particle-impregnated matrix to an externally applied oscillating magnetic field to promote the diffusion of drug through, and release from, the matrix has received relatively little attention.[118,119] If realized, this concept may be the means of regulating the release of anticancer drugs in tumor deposits so that the local concentration of the drug can be controlled to maximize therapeutic effects.

A supplementary role for microparticles has been suggested by several studies of hyperthermia and thermochemotherapy in cancer treatment at temperatures in excess of 42°C. The phenomenon of reduced blood flow consequent on microsphere embolization[55,56] (see also Chapter 5) can be used in concert with hyperthermia.[120] Locally applied hyperthermia of solid tumors is significantly improved if the cooling effect of the tumor blood supply is diminished. This allows accumulation of heat in the tumor and also combines therapeutically with embolic hypoxia and acidosis resulting from the presence of microparticles.

Other approaches have utilized increased temperature either as a direct therapeutic agent or as a mediator of drug delivery. A variety of polymer types have been developed that swell when exposed to increased temperature and subsequently release incorporated drug.[121] Temperature-sensitive liposomes carrying anticancer

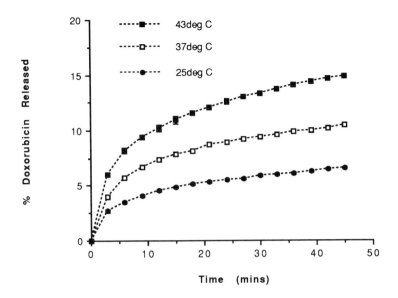

FIGURE 7. Effect of release medium temperature on the *in vitro* release profile of doxorubicin from ion-exchange microspheres. Each point represents the mean of three samples. (From Burton, M. A., Chen, Y., Atkinson, H., Codde, J. P., Jones, S. K., and Gray, B. N., *Int. J. Hyperthermia*, 8, 485, 1992. With permission.)

drugs have also been described that release drugs at faster rates *in situ* during the application of local hyperthermia.[122]

Ion-exchange microspheres have been shown to release drug more slowly when loaded under the influence of increased temperature.[52] More recently, Burton et al.[123] described the effects of elevated temperature on both the loading and release of doxorubicin. The rate of drug loading significantly increased as the temperature was elevated from 4 to 43°C, but the higher temperature also induced spontaneous aggregation of microspheres. The rate of release also increased with increasing temperature of the release medium in *in vitro* studies (Figure 7), and this resulted in a significant improvement in the therapeutic response of a solid rat tumor treated with microspheres and subsequently heated to 43°C for 30 min (Figure 8). Having different mechanisms of cytotoxicity the two modalities may be complementary: hyperthermia acting primarily on the semivascular internal areas of the tumor while the drug is released in the vicinity of the well vascularized growing edge of the tumor where the microspheres are embolized.

Ultrasound has also been used as an external modulator of drug release from a variety of polymers. Kost et al.[124] demonstrated a five-fold, reversible increase in degradation rates of polyanhydrides, polyglycolides, and polylactides resulting in a 20-fold increase in release rate of incorporated agents in an ultrasonic bath at 75 kHz. During ultrasonic radiation at 20 kHz for 1 h increased release rates were also recorded in *in vivo* experiments with biodegradable polymers implanted into

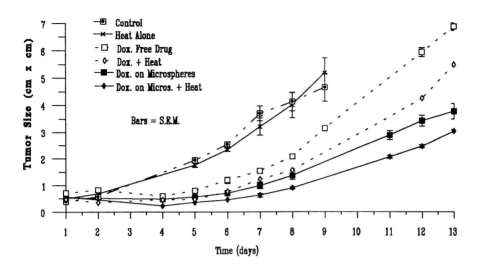

FIGURE 8. Therapeutic response of a hind limb salivary carcinoma implant in rats to treatment with hyperthermia, conventional doxorubicin treatment, and doxorubicin on ion-exchange microspheres. Group sizes were greater than five rats while chemotherapy was by intra-arterial (descending aorta) bolus injection of 6 mg/kg in each case. Hyperthermia was administered by hind limb immersion in hot water at 43°C for 30 min (authors' unpublished results).

rat hind limbs. This concept provides a significant opportunity for enhancing therapeutic responses where combined ultrasound, at intensities producing tissue hyperthermia,[125] and microsphere chemotherapy may be utilized in concert. The effects may be even further improved because it has been demonstrated that many anticancer agents can produce enhanced responses under the influence of ultrasound and temperature. Mechanisms for this effect may include increased cellular uptake, increased sensitivity, or altered distribution[126] and have been described for doxorubicin and hematoporphyrins.[127]

REFERENCES

1. **Willmott, N.,** Drug delivery strategies in malignant disease of the lung, *Adv. Drug Delivery Rev.,* 5, 133, 1990.
2. **Arshady, R.,** Albumin microspheres and microcapsules: methodology of manufacturing techniques, *J. Controlled Release,* 14, 111, 1990.
3. **Morimoto, Y. and Fujimoto, S.,** Albumin microspheres as drug carriers, *Crit. Rev. Therapeutic Drug Carrier Systems,* 2, 19, 1985.
4. **Jones, C., Burton, M. A., and Gray B. N.,** Albumin microspheres as vehicles for the sustained and controlled release of doxorubicin, *J. Pharm. Pharmacol.,* 41, 813, 1989.

5. **Gupta, P. K., Hung, C. T., and Lam, F. C.,** Factorial design based optimization of the formulation of albumin microspheres containing adriamycin, *J. Microencapsulation,* 6, 147, 1989.

6. **Sawaya, A., Benoit, J.-P., and Benita, S.,** Binding mechanism of doxorubicin in ion-exchange albumin microspheres, *J. Pharm. Sci.,* 76, 475, 1987.

7. **Yapel, A. F. Jr.,** Albumin microspheres: heat and chemical stabilization, in *Methods in Enzymology,* Vol. 112, Widder, K. J. and Green, R., Eds., Academic Press, Orlando, 1985, 3.

8. **Fujimoto, S., Miyazaki, M., Endoh, F., Takahashi, O., Shrestha, R. D., Okui, K., Morimoto, Y., and Terao, K.,** Effects of intra-arterially infused biodegradable microspheres containing mitomycin C, *Cancer,* 55, 522, 1985.

9. **Kramer, P. A.,** Albumin microspheres as vehicles for achieving specificity in drug delivery, *J. Pharm. Sci.,* 63, 1646, 1974.

10. **Hashida, M. and Sezaki, H.,** Specific delivery of mitomycin-C: combined use of prodrugs and spherical delivery systems, in *Microspheres and Drug Therapy, Pharmaceutical, Immunological and Medical Aspects,* Davis, S. S., Illum, L., McVie, J. G., and Tomlinson, E., Eds., Elsevier, Amsterdam, 1984, 281.

11. **Nishioka, Y., Kyotani, S., Okamura, M., Mori, Y., Miyazaki, M., Okazaki, K., Ohnishi, S., Yamamoto, Y., and Ito, K.,** Preparation and evaluation of albumin microspheres and microcapsules containing cisplatin, *Chem. Pharm. Bull.,* 37, 1399, 1989.

12. **Nishioka, Y., Kyotani, S., Masui, H., Okamura, M., Miyazaki, M., Okazaki, K., Ohnishi, S., Yamamoto, Y., and Ito, K.,** Preparation and release characteristics of cisplatin albumin microspheres containing chitin and treated with chitosan, *Chem. Pharm. Bull.,* 37, 3074, 1989.

13. **Willmott, N., Chen, Y., and Florence, A. T.,** Haemoglobin, transferrin and albumin/polyaspartic acid microspheres as carriers for the cytotoxic drug adriamycin, II: *in vitro* drug release rate, *J. Controlled Release,* 8, 103, 1988.

14. **Goldberg, E. P., Iwata, H., and Longo, W. E.,** Hydrophilic albumin and dextran ion-exchange microspheres for localized chemotherapy, in *Microspheres and Drug Therapy, Pharmaceutical, Immunological and Medical Aspects,* Davis, S. S., Illum, L., McVie, J. G., and Tomlinson, E., Eds., Elsevier, Amsterdam, 1984, 309.

15. **Cremers, H. F. M., Feijen, J., Kwon, G., Bae, Y. H., Kim, S. W., Noteborn, H. P. J. M., and McVie, J. G.,** Albumin-heparin microspheres as carriers for cytostatic agents, *J. Controlled Release,* 11, 167, 1990.

16. **Chen, Y., Willmott, N., and Florence, A. T.,** Comparison of albumin and casein microspheres as a carrier for doxorubicin, *J. Pharm. Pharmacol.,* 39, 978, 1987.

17. **Miyazaki, S., Hashiguchi, N., Sugiyama, M., Takada, M., and Morimoto, Y.,** Fibrinogen microspheres as novel drug delivery systems for antitumor drugs, *Chem. Pharm. Bull.,* 34, 1370, 1986.

18. **Jeyanthi, R. and Rao, K. P.,** Release characteristics of bleomycin, mitomycin C and 5-fluorouracil from gelatin microspheres, *Int. J. Pharm.,* 55, 31, 1989.

19. **Chen, Y., Willmott, N., Anderson, J., and Florence, A. T.,** Haemoglobin, transferrin and albumin/polyaspartic acid microspheres as carriers for the cytotoxic drug adriamycin, I: ultrastructural appearance and drug content, *J. Controlled Release,* 8, 93, 1988.

20. **Levy, M., Rambourg, P., Levy, J., and Potron, G.,** Microencapsulation, IV: cross-linked haemoglobin microspheres, *J. Pharm. Sci.,* 71, 759, 1982.

21. **Suzuki, T., Sato, E., Matsuda, Y., Tada, H., Unno, K., and Kato, T.,** Preparation of zein microspheres conjugated with antitumor drugs available for selective cancer therapy and development of a simple colorimetric determination of drug in microspheres, *Chem. Pharm. Bull.,* 37, 1051, 1989.

22. **Igari, Y., Kibat, P. G., and Langer, R.,** Optimization of a microencapsulated liposome system for enzymatically controlled release of macromolecules, *J. Controlled Release,* 14, 263, 1990.

23. **Watanabe, K., Saiki, I., Uraki, Y., Tokura, S., and Azuma, I.,** 6-O-carboxymethyl-chitin (CM-chitin) as a drug carrier, *Chem. Pharm. Bull.,* 38, 506, 1990.

24. **Gallo, J. M. and Hassan, E. E.,** Receptor-mediated magnetic carriers: basis for targeting, *Pharm. Res.,* 5, 300, 1988.

25. **Bodmeier, R., Chen, H., and Paeratakul, O.,** A novel approach to the oral delivery of micro- or nanoparticles, *Pharm. Res.,* 6, 413, 1989.

26. **Daly, M. M. and Knorr, D.,** Chitosan-alginate complex coacervate capsules: effects of calcium chloride, plasticizers, and polyelectrolytes on mechanical stability, *Biotechnol. Prog.,* 4, 76, 1988.

27. **Artursson, P., Edman, P., Laakso, T., and Sjoholm, I.,** Characterisation of polyacryl starch microparticles as carriers for proteins and drugs, *J. Pharm. Sci.,* 73, 1507, 1984.

28. **Ogawa, Y., Yamamoto, M., Okada, H., Yashiki, T., and Shimamoto, T.,** A new technique to efficiently entrap leuprolide acetate into microcapsules of polylactic acid or copoly(lactic/ glycolic) acid, *Chem. Pharm. Bull.,* 36, 1095, 1988.

29. **Spenlehauer, G., Veillard, M., and Benoit, J. P.,** Formation and characterization of cisplatin loaded poly(*d,l*-lactide) microspheres for chemoembolization, *J. Pharm. Sci.,* 75, 750, 1986.

30. **Bissery, M. C., Valeriote, F., and Thies, C.,** *In vitro* and *in vivo* evaluation of CCNU-loaded microspheres prepared from poly(±-lactide) and poly(β-hydroxybutyrate), in *Microspheres and Drug Therapy, Pharmaceutical, Immunological and Medical Aspects,* Davis, S. S., Illum, L., McVie, J. G., and Tomlinson, E., Eds., Elsevier, Amsterdam, 1984, 217.

31. **Redmon, M. P., Hickey, A. J., and Deluca, P. P.,** Prednisolone-21-acetate poly(glycolic acid) microspheres: influence of matrix characteristics on release, *J. Controlled Release,* 9, 99, 1989.

32. **Kanke, M., Morlier, E., Geissler, R., Powell, D., Kaplan, A., and Deluca, P. P.,** Interaction of microspheres with blood constituents, II: uptake of biodegradable particles by macrophages, *J. Parenter. Sci. Technol.,* 40, 114, 1986.

33. **Tabata, Y. and Ikada, Y.,** Protein precoating of polylactide microspheres containing a lipophilic immunpotentiator for enhancement of macrophage phagocytosis and activation, *Pharm. Res.,* 6, 296, 1989.

34. **Sanders, L. M., Kent, J. S., McRea, G. I., Vickery, B. H., Tice, T. R., and Lewis, D. H.,** Controlled release of a luteinizing hormone-releasing hormone analogue from poly(D,L-lactide-co-glycolide) microspheres, *J. Pharm. Sci.,* 73, 1294, 1984.

35. **Kissel, T., Brich, Z., Bantle, S., Lancranjan, I., Nimmerfall, F., and Vit, P.,** Parenteral depot-systems on the basis of biodegradable polyesters, *J. Controlled Release,* 16, 27, 1991.

36. **Bodmeier, R., Chen, H., Tyle, P., and Jarosz, P.,** Pseudoephedrine HCl microspheres formulated into an oral suspension dosage form, *J. Controlled Release,* 15, 65, 1991.

37. **Sprockel, O. L. and Prapaitrakul, W.,** A comparison of microencapsulation by various emulsion techniques, *Int. J. Pharm.,* 58, 123, 1990.

38. **Crooks, C. A., Douglas, J. A., Broughton, R. L., and Sefton, M. V.,** Microencapsulation of mammalian cells in a HEMA-MMA copolymer: effect on capsule morphology and permeability, *J. Biomed. Mater. Res.,* 24, 1241, 1990.

39. **Cuff, G. W., Combs, A. B., and McGinity J. W.,** Effect of formulation factors on the matrix pH of nylon microcapsules, *J. Microencapsulation,* 1, 27, 1984.

40. **Langer, R.,** Polymer implants for drug delivery in the brain, *J. Controlled Release,* 16, 53, 1991.

41. **Watts, P. J., Davies, M. C., and Melia, C. D.,** Encapsulation of 5-aminosalicylic acid into Eudragit RS microspheres and modulation of their release characteristics by use of surfactants, *J. Controlled Release,* 16, 311, 1991.

42. **Okamoto, Y., Konno, A., Tagawa, K., Kato, T., Tamakawa, Y., and Amano, Y.,** Arterial chemoembolization with cisplatin microspheres, *Br. J. Cancer,* 53, 369, 1986.

43. **Nemoto, R. and Kato, T.** Microencapsulation of anticancer drug for intra-arterial infusion and its clinical application, in *Microspheres and Drug Therapy, Pharmaceutical, Immunological and Medical Aspects,* Davis, S. S., Illum, L., McVie, J. G., and Tomlinson, E., Eds., Elsevier, Amsterdam, 1984, 229.

44. **Tsujiyama, T., Suzuki, N., Kuriki, T., Kawata, M., and Goto, S.,** Pharmacological evaluation of hydroxypropylcellulose-ethylcellulose microcapsules containing piretanide, *J. Pharm. Dyn.,* 13, 1, 1990.

45. **Tokes, Z. A., Ross, K. L., and Roger, K. E.,** Use of microspheres to direct the cytotoxic action of adriamycin to the cell surface, in *Microspheres and Drug Therapy, Pharmaceutical, Immunological and Medical Aspects,* Davis, S. S., Illum, L., McVie, J. G., and Tomlinson, E., Eds., Elsevier, Amsterdam, 1984, 139.

46. **Ugelstad, J., Rembaum, A., Kemshead, J. T., Nustad, K., Funderud, S., and Schmid, R.,** Preparation and biomedical applications of monodisperse polymer particles, in *Microspheres and Drug Therapy, Pharmaceutical, Immunological and Medical Aspects,* Davis, S. S., Illum, L., McVie, J. G., and Tomlinson, E., Eds., Elsevier, Amsterdam, 1984, 365.

47. **Jones, C., Burton, M. A., and Gray, B. N.,** *In vitro* release of cytotoxic agents from ion exchange resins, *J. Controlled Release,* 8, 251, 1989.

48. **Benita, S., Zouai, O., and Benoit J.-P.,** 5-Fluorouracil: carnauba wax microspheres for chemoembolization: an *in vitro* evaluation, *J. Pharm. Sci.,* 75, 847, 1986.

49. **Golomb, G., Fish, P., and Rahamin, E.,** The relationship between drug release rate, particle size and swelling of silicone matrices, *J. Controlled Release,* 12, 121, 1990.

50. **Goedemoed, J. H., Mense, E. H. G., deGroot, K., Claessen, A. M. E., and Scheper, R. J.,** Development of injectable antitumor microspheres based on polyphosphazene, *J. Controlled Release,* 170, 245, 1991.

51. **Sokoloski, T. D. and Royer, G. P.,** Drug entrapment within native albumin beads, in *Microspheres and Drug Therapy, Pharmaceutical, Immunological and Medical Aspects,* Davis, S. S., Illum, L., McVie, J. G., and Tomlinson, E., Eds., Elsevier, Amsterdam, 1984, 295.

52. **Irwin, W. J., Belaid, K. A., and Alpar, H. O.,** Drug delivery by ion-exchange, IV: coated resinate complexes of ester pro-drugs of propranolol, *Drug Dev. Ind. Pharm.,* 14, 1307, 1988.

53. **Chen, Y.** *In vitro* Characterisation and *In Vivo* Evaluation of Microspheres as Carriers for the Anticancer Drug Adriamycin, Ph.D. thesis, University of Strathclyde, Strathclyde, Scotland, 1989.

54. **Willmott, N., Chen, Y., Goldberg, J., and Florence, A. T.,** Biodegradation rate of protein microspheres in lung, liver and kidney of rats, *J. Pharm. Pharmacol.,* 41, 433, 1989.

55. **Gyves, J. W., Ensminger, W. D., Van Harken, D., Niederhuber, J., Stetson, P., and Walker, S.,** Improved regional selectivity of hepatic arterial mitomycin by starch microspheres, *Clin. Pharmacol. Ther.,* 34, 259, 1983.

56. **Burk, M., Schoppe, W. D., Miller, A. A., Jungblut, R. M., and Schneider, W.,** Dextran particle use in regional chemotherapy: problems of monitoring, in *Progress in Regional Cancer Therapy,* Jakesz, R. and Rainer, H., Eds., Springer-Verlag, Berlin, 1990, 105.

57. **Tokura, S., Nishi, N., Tsutsumi, A., and Somorin, O.,** Studies on chitin VIII some properties of water soluble chitin derivatives, *Polym. J.,* 15, 485, 1983.

58. **Linhardt, R. J.,** Biodegradable polymers for controlled release of drugs, in *Controlled Release of Drugs,* Rosoff, M., Ed., VCH, New York, 1989, 53.

59. **McGinity, J. W., Martin, A., Cuff, G. W., and Combs, A. B.,** Influence of matrices on nylon-encapsulated pharmaceuticals, *J. Pharm. Sci.,* 70, 372, 1981.

60. **Johnson, R. E., Lanaski, L. A., Gupta, V., Griffin, M. J., Gaud, H. T., Needham, T. E., and Zia, H.,** Stability of atriopeptin III in poly(D,L-lactide-co-glycolide) microspheres, *J. Controlled Release,* 17, 61, 1991.

61. **Willmott, N., Murray, T., Carlton, R., Chen, Y., Logan, H., McCurrach, G., Bessent, R. G., Goldberg, J. A., Anderson, J., McKillop, J. H., and McArdle, C. S.,** Development of radiolabeled albumin microspheres: a comparison of gamma-emitting radioisotopes of iodine (^{131}I) and indium (^{111}In/^{113m}I), *Int. J. Radiat. Appl. Instrum. B,* 18. 687, 1991.

62. **Al-Janabi, M. A. A., Heyam, Y. A., and Al-Salem, A. M.,** Preparation, analysis and application of [^{99m}Tc] human albumin microspheres ([^{99m}Tc]HAM) for lung scanning, *Int. J. Appl. Radiat. Isot.,* 35, 209, 1984.

63. **Burton, M. A., Gray, B. N., Klemp, P., Kelleher, D., and Hardy, N.,** Selective internal radiation therapy; distribution of radiation in the liver, *Eur. J. Cancer Clin. Oncol.,* 25, 1487, 1989.

64. **Ariel, I. M.,** The treatment of metastases to the liver with interstitial radioactive isotopes, *Surg. Gynecol. Obstet.,* 110, 739, 1960.

65. **Ariel, I. M.,** Radioactive isotopes for adjuvant therapy, *Arch. Surg.,* 89, 244, 1964.
66. **Ariel, I. M.,** Treatment of inoperable primary pancreatic and liver cancer by the intra-arterial administration of radioactive isotopes (Y90-radiating microspheres), *Ann. Surg.,* 162, 267, 1965.
67. **Ehrhardt, G. J. and Day, D. E.,** Therapeutic use of ^{90}Y microspheres, *Int. J. Radiat. Appl. Instrum. B,* 14, 233, 1987.
68. **Mauderly, J. L., Pickrell, J. A., Hobbs, C. H., Benjamin, S. A., Hahn, F. F., Jones, R. K., and Barnes, J. E.,** The effects of inhaled ^{90}Y fused clay aerosol on pulmonary function and related parameters of the beagle dog, *Radiat. Res.,* 56, 83, 1973.
69. **Herba, M. J., Illescas, F. F., Thirlwell, M. P., Boos, G. J., Rosenthall, L., Atri, M., and Bret, P. M.,** Hepatic malignancies: improved treatment with intra-arterial Y-90, *Radiology,* 169, 311, 1988.
70. **Houle, S., Yip, T.-C., Shepherd, F. A., Rotstein, L. E., Sniderman, K. W., Theis, E., Cawthorn, R. H., and Richmond-Cox, K.,** Hepatocellular carcinoma: pilot trial of treatment with Y-90 microspheres, *Radiology,* 172, 857, 1989.
71. **Grady, E.,** Internal radiation therapy of hepatic cancer, *Dis. Colon Rectum,* 22, 371, 1979.
72. **Mantravadi, R. V. P., Spigos, D. G., Tan, W. S., and Felix, E. L.,** Intra-arterial yttrium 90 in the treatment of hepatic malignancy, *Radiology,* 142, 783, 1982.
73. **Gray, B. N., Burton, M. A., Kelleher, D. K., Klemp, P., and Matz, L.,** Tolerance of the liver to the effects of yttrium-90 radiation, *Int. J. Radiat. Oncol. Biol. Phys.,* 18, 619, 1990.
74. **Burton, M. A., Gray, B. N., Kelleher, D. K., and Klemp, P. F.,** Selective internal radiation therapy: validation of intraoperative dosimetry, *Radiology,* 175, 253, 1990.
75. **Moldenhauer, M. G. and Nairn, J. G.,** The effect of rate of evaporation on the coat structure of ethylcellulose microcapsules, *J. Controlled Release,* 17, 49, 1991.
76. **Benoit, J. P., Benita, S., Puisieux, F., and Thies, C.,** Stability and release kinetics of drugs incorporated within microspheres, in *Microspheres and Drug Therapy, Pharmaceutical, Immunological and Medical Aspects,* Davis, S. S., Illum, L., McVie, J. G., and Tomlinson, E., Eds., Elsevier, Amsterdam, 1984, 91.
77. **Fong, J. W.,** Microencapsulation by solvent evaporation and organic phase separation processes, in *Controlled Release Systems: Fabrication Technology,* Vol. 1, Hsieh, D., Ed., CRC Press, Boca Raton, FL, 1988, 81.
78. **Kato, T.,** Encapsulated drugs in targeted cancer therapy, in *Controlled Drug Delivery, Clinical Applications, Vol. 2,* Bruck, S. D., Ed., CRC Press, Boca Raton, FL, 1983, 189.
79. **Benita, S. and Donbrow, M.,** Coacervation of ethylcellulose: the role of polyisobutylene and the effect of its concentration, *J. Colloid Interface Sci.,* 77, 102, 1980.
80. **Sato, T., Kanke, M., Schroeder, H. G., and Deluca, P. P.,** Porous biodegradable microspheres for controlled drug delivery, I: assessment of processing conditions and solvent removal techniques, *Pharm. Res.,* 5, 21, 1988.
81. **Motycka, S. and Nairn, J. G.,** Preparation and evaluation of microencapsulated ion-exchange resin beads, *J. Pharm. Sci.,* 68, 211, 1979.
82. **Kreuter, J.,** Nanoparticle-based drug delivery systems, *J. Controlled Release,* 16, 169, 1991.
83. **Barrett, K. E. J., Ed.,** *Dispersion Polymerisation in Organic Media,* Wiley, London, 1975.
84. **Williamson, B., Lukas, R., Winnik, M. A., and Croucher, M. D.,** The preparation of micronsize polymer particles in nonpolar media, *J. Colloid Interface Sci.,* 119, 559, 1987.
85. **Candau, F. and Ottewill, R. H., Eds.,** *Scientific Methods for the Study of Polymer Colloids and Their Applications,* NATO ASI series C: Mathematical and Physical Science, Vol. 303, Kluwer Academic, Dordecht, 1990, chap. 1 and 2.
86. **Ranney, M. W.,** *Microencapsulation Technology,* Noyes Development, Park Ridge, NJ, 1969, 120.
87. **Wichert, B. and Rohdewald, P.,** A new method for the preparation of drug containing polylactic acid microparticles without using organic solvents, *J. Controlled Release,* 14, 269, 1990.
88. **Bodmeier, R. and McGinity, J. W.,** The preparation and evaluation of drug-containing poly(d,l-lactide) microspheres formed by the solvent evaporation method, *Pharm. Res.,* 4, 465, 1987.

89. **Motycka, S., Newth, C. J. L., and Nairn, J. G.**, Preparation and evaluation of microencapsulated and coated ion-exchange resin beads containing theophyline, *J. Pharm. Sci.*, 74, 643, 1985.

90. **Tomlinson, E. and Burger, J. J.**, Incorporation of water-soluble drugs in albumin microspheres, in *Methods in Enzymology*, Vol. 112, Widder, K. J. and Green, R., Eds., Academic Press, Orlando, 1985, 27.

91. **Widder, K. J., Senyei, A. E., and Ranney, D. F.**, Magnetically responsive microspheres and other carriers for the biophysical targeting of antitumor agents, *Adv. Pharmacol. Chemother.*, 16, 213, 1979.

92. **Tomlinson, E., Burger, J. J., Schoonderwoerd, E. M. A., and McVie, J. G.**, Human serum albumin microspheres for intra-arterial drug targeting of cytostatic compounds: pharmaceutical aspects and release characteristics, in *Microspheres and Drug Therapy, Pharmaceutical, Immunological and Medical Aspects*, Davis, S. S., Illum, L., McVie, J. G., and Tomlinson, E., Eds., Elsevier, Amsterdam, 1984, 75.

93. **Chen, Y., Burton, M. A., Napoli, S., Martins, I., and Gray, B. N.**, Evaluation of ion-exchange microspheres as carriers for the anticancer drug doxorubicin: *in vitro* studies, *J. Pharm. Pharmacol.*, 44, 211, 1992.

94. **Tokes, Z. A., Rogers, K. E., and Rembaum, A.**, Synthesis of adriamycin-coupled polyglutaraldehyde microspheres and evaluation of their cytostatic activity, *Proc. Natl. Acad. Sci., USA*, 79, 2926, 1982.

95. **Wingard, L. B., Tritton, T. R., and Egler, A.**, Cell surface effects of adriamycin and carminomycin immobilised on crosslinked polyvinyl alcohol, *Cancer Res.*, 45, 3529, 1985.

96. **Willmott, N., Cummings, J., and Florence, A. T.**, *In vitro* release of adriamycin from drug-loaded albumin and haemoglobin microspheres, *J. Microencapsulation*, 2, 293, 1985.

97. **Gupta, P. K., Hung, C. T., and Perrier, D. G.**, Albumin microspheres. II. Effect of stabilisation temperature on the release of adriamycin, *Int. J. Pharm.*, 33, 147, 1986.

98. **Ruiz, J. M. and Benoit, J. P.**, *In vivo* peptide release from poly(d,l-lactic acid-co-glycolic acid) copolymer 50/50 microspheres, *J. Controlled Release*, 16, 177, 1991.

99. **Ponpaibul, Y., Price, J. C., and Whitworth, C. W.**, Preparation and evaluation of controlled release indomethacin, *Drug Dev. Ind. Pharm.*, 10, 1597, 1984.

100. **Kawashima, Y., Lin, S. Y., Kasai, A., Takenaka, K., Matsunami, K., Nochida, Y., and Hirose, H.**, Drug release properties of the microcapsules of adriamycin hydrochloride with ethyl cellulose prepared by a phase separation technique, *Drug Dev. Ind. Pharm.*, 10, 467, 1984.

101. **Burgess, D. J., Davis, S. S., and Tomlinson, E.**, Potential use of albumin microspheres as a drug delivery system, I: preparation and *in vitro* release of steroids, *Int. J. Pharm.*, 39, 129, 1987.

102. **Ratcliffe, J. H.**, Evaluation of Biodegradable Polymers for Intra-articular Drug Delivery, Ph.D. thesis, University of Nottingham, Nottingham, England, 1984.

103. **Longo, W. and Goldberg, E. P.**, Hydrophilic albumin microspheres, in *Methods in Enzymology*, Vol. 112, Widder, K. J. and Green, R., Eds., Academic Press, Orlando, 1985, 18.

104. **Davis, S. S. and Illum, L.**, Polymeric microspheres as drug carriers, *Biomaterials*, 9, 111, 1988.

105. **Leu, D., Manthey, B., Kreuter, J., Speiser, P., and Deluca, P. P.**, Distribution and elimination of coated poly(methyl 2-^{14}C-methacrylate) nanoparticles after intravenous injection in rats, *J. Pharm. Sci.*, 73, 1433, 1984.

106. **Douglas, S. J., Illum, L., and Davis, S. S.**, Particle size and size distribution of poly(butyl-2-cyanoacrylate) nanoparticles. II. Influence of stabilizers, *J. Colloid Interface Sci.*, 103, 154, 1985.

107. **Sheu, M. T., Moustafa, M. A., and Sokoloski, T. D.**, Entrapment of bioactive compounds within native albumin beads. II. Effects of rate and extent of crosslinking on microbead properties, *J. Parenter. Sci. Tech.*, 40, 253, 1986.

108. **Davis, S. S., Mills, S. N., and Tomlinson, E.**, Chemically crosslinked albumin microspheres for the controlled release of incorporated rose bengal after intramuscular injection into rabbits, *J. Controlled Release*, 4, 293, 1987.

109. **Willmott, N, Cummings, J., Stuart, J. F. B., and Florence, A. T.,** Adriamycin-loaded albumin microspheres: preparation, *in vivo* distribution and release in the rat, *Biopharm. Drug Disposition,* 6, 91, 1985.

110. **Thies, C.,** Dispersed systems for parenteral administration, in *Controlled Release of Drugs: Polymer and Aggregate Systems,* Rosoff, M., Ed., VCH, New York, 1989, 97.

111. **Makino, K., Ohshima, H., and Kondo, T.,** Effects of plasma proteins on degradation properties of poly(L-lactide) microcapsules, *Pharm. Res.,* 4, 62, 1987.

112. **Miller, R. A., Brady, J. M., and Cutright, D. E.,** Degradation rates of oral resorbable implants (polylactates and polyglycolates): rate modification with changes in PLA/PGA copolymer ratios, *J. Biomed. Mater. Res.,* 11, 711, 1977.

113. **Edelman, E. R., Kost, J., Bobeck, H., and Langer, R.,** Regulation of drug release from polymer matrices by oscillating magnetic fields, *J. Biomed. Mater. Res.,* 19, 67, 1985.

114. **Widder, K. J., Senyei, A. E., and Scarpelli, D. G.,** Magnetic microspheres: a model system for site-specific drug delivery *in vivo, Proc. Soc. Exp. Biol. Med.,* 158, 141, 1978.

115. **Morimoto, Y., Okumura, M., Sugibayashi, K., and Kato, Y.,** Biomedical applications of magnetic fluids, II: preparation and magnetic guidance of magnetic albumin microspheres for site-specific drug delivery *in vivo, J. Pharm. Dyn.,* 4, 624, 1981.

116. **Widder, K. J. and Senyei, A. E.,** Magnetic microspheres: a vehicle for selective targeting of drugs, *Pharmacol. Ther.,* 20, 377, 1983.

117. **Rettenmaier, M. A., Stratton, J. A., Berman, M. L., Senyei, A. E., Widder, K. J., White, D. B., and Disaia, P. J.,** Treatment of a syngeneic rat tumor with magnetically responsive albumin microspheres labeled with doxorubicin or protein A, *Gynecol. Oncol.,* 27, 34, 1987.

118. **Hsieh, D., Langer, R., and Folkman, J.,** Magnetic modulation of release of macromolecules from polymers, *Proc. Natl. Acad. Sci. USA,* 78, 1863, 1981.

119. **McCarthy, M., Soong, D., and Edelman, E.,** Controlled drug release from porous matrices impregnated with magnetic beads: a proposed mechanism and model for enhanced release, *J. Controlled Release,* 1, 143, 1984.

120. **Akuta, K., Abe, M., Kondo, M., Yoshikawa, T., Tanaka, Y., Yoshida, M., Miura, T., Nakao, N., Onoyama, Y., Yamada, T., Mukoujima, T., and Tsukada, K.,** Combined effects of hepatic arterial embolization using degradable starch microspheres (DSM) in hyperthermia for liver cancer, *Int. J. Hyperthermia,* 7, 231, 1991.

121. **Okanoa, T., Bae, Y. H., Jacobs, H., and Kim, S. W.,** Thermally on-off switching polymers for drug permeation and release, *J. Controlled Release,* 11, 255, 1990.

122. **Tomita, T., Watanabe, M., Takahashi, T., Kumai, K., Tadakuma, T., and Yasuda, T.,** Temperature-sensitive release of adriamycin, an amphiphilic antitumor agent, from dipalmitoylphosphatidylcholine-cholesterol liposomes, *Biochim. Biophys. Acta,* 978, 185, 1989.

123. **Burton, M. A., Chen, Y., Atkinson, H., Codde, J. P., Jones, S. K., and Gray, B. N.,** *In vitro* and *in vivo* thermal responses of doxorubicin on ion exchange microspheres, *Int. J. Hyperthermia,* 8, 485, 1992.

124. **Kost, J., Leong, K., and Langer, R.,** Ultrasound-enhanced polymer degradation and release of incorporated substances, *Proc. Natl. Acad. Sci. USA,* 86, 7663, 1989.

125. **Moros, E. G., Roemer, R. B., and Hynynen, K.,** Pre-focal plane high temperature regions induced by scanning focused ultrasound beams, *Int. J. Hyperthermia,* 6, 351, 1990.

126. **Saad, A. H. and Hahn, G. M.,** Ultrasound enhanced drug toxicity on chinese hamster ovary cells *in vitro, Cancer Res.,* 49, 5931, 1989.

127. **Yumita, N., Nishigaki, R., and Umemura, K.,** The increase of generation of superoxide radicals and the inhibitory effect in Yoshida sarcoma of anthracycline antitumor agents by ultrasound, *J. Jpn. Soc. Cancer Ther.,* 24, 63, 1989.

Chapter 2

BLOOD FLOW AND ITS MODULATION IN MALIGNANT TUMORS

David G. Hirst

TABLE OF CONTENTS

0-8493-6952-5/94/$0.00 + $.50

I. CHARACTERISTICS OF TUMOR VASCULATURE

A. MORPHOLOGY

The relationship between malignant tumors and their vascular supply is both complex and highly abnormal. Most blood vessels in tumors show characteristics that are seen only infrequently in normal tissue vasculature and the combination of these properties in tumors gives their vasculature a characteristic appearance. The pattern and density of blood vessels in tumors are dependent on the type, size, and site of growth in the host.[1-5] For most tumors larger than a few millimeters, capillary diameter and length are greater than in the host tissue of origin,[6,7] leading to greater intercapillary distances[8] and ultimately to necrosis. Vessels in normal tissues display a distinct hierarchy along the vascular network from arteries, arterioles, capillaries, venules, and veins. These categories can even be subdivided further.[9] Resistance to blood flow is greatest at the level of the arterioles; so it is through the vessels at that level (and precapillary sphincters) that the control of tissue blood flow by modulation of smooth muscle tone is most effective. This orderly arrangement is rarely found in tumors. In particular, arteriovenous anastomoses, sinusoidal venules, and blood channels lacking any apparent endothelial cell lining are commonly seen. There are also very few contractile vessels of the arteriolar type, leading some observers to conclude that tumor neovasculature is mostly of venous origin; smooth muscle is often almost entirely absent from tumor vessels, leading to the hypothesis that alterations in tumor blood flow are mostly passive, resulting from a steal phenomenon or diversion of blood to or from normal vessels. Incorporated, preexisting normal vasculature may be an exception to this rule in some tumors.

Flow characteristics through tumor vessels must be less than ideal for tissue perfusion. Perhaps most significantly the dearth of true capillaries and the relatively large diameter of tumor vessels reduce the possibility for facilitated passage of red blood cells (Fahraeus-Lindqvist effect), a process that markedly reduces flow resistance in normal vessels of small diameter.[10]

The vascular system is a highly complex network that has evolved to supply effectively the resting metabolic requirements of all the body's tissues and to provide a reserve capacity to cope with periodic increases in demand in organs, such as heart, muscle, and gut. The concept of reserve capacity can also be applied in another way, i.e., proliferative reserve. The cellular elements of blood vessels in most normal tissues show low rates of proliferation,[11,12] probably reflecting the replacement of cells lost through wear and tear. This rate can be increased dramatically, particularly in the endothelium to effect repair of damaged tissue (granulation tissue). In tumors, however, the endothelial proliferation rates are extremely rapid so that little or no reserve capacity exists.[12,13] We may think, then, of the blood flow through most tumors as being maximal and because of the unreactive nature of most tumor vessels we might assume that it would be difficult to manipulate tumor vasculature and blood flow. As we shall see, this is only partially true. We are now beginning to understand some of the mechanisms involved sufficiently to control tumor blood flow to therapeutic advantage.

B. SIGNIFICANCE FOR MICROSPHERE DELIVERY

As with all tissues, the delivery of substances to the target cells in malignant tumors is dependent on many physiological factors. These include absorption (if administration is by a route other than vascular), delivery by the vascular system, transport across the vessel walls, and through the interstitium.[14] Of these components, vascular transport is perhaps the most readily manipulated and is obviously the most relevant to a microsphere-based therapeutic approach. The aim of most of these approaches is to trap the maximal fraction of injected microspheres in tumors compared with normal tissues, thus permitting the biggest differential in radiation exposure (isotope loaded) or chemotherapy (drug delivery). In common with many other forms of cancer therapy, targeted microspheres are totally dependent on the blood supply for their delivery. We must consider, then, the factors that could affect the transport and distribution of microspheres throughout the vascular network of tumors. Their trapping within the vascular network is a purely passive process, but the numbers delivered to a tumor relative to sensitive normal organs will be proportional to the relative distribution of the cardiac output. This property has been exploited as a means of measuring organ blood flow[15-18] and in that application the aim of maximal trapping is the same as for the therapeutic approach. The effectiveness of trapping is highly dependent on the size of the spheres, and even where trapping is complete it occurs at different levels along the vascular network, e.g., in the hamster cheek pouch microvasculature 15 μm spheres usually impact at the entrance to small arterioles, whereas 8 to 10 μm spheres lodge in the precapillary arterioles themselves.[19] In general then, large spheres will lodge in large vessels, limiting further access, whereas small spheres will pass right through the capillary network. What then is the optimal size and does it vary from one tissue to another? Several authors have addressed this question mostly as it relates to the use of microspheres as blood flow markers in normal tissues. It is probably reasonable to generalize and conclude that spheres larger than 10 to 12 μm are trapped completely, whereas smaller ones are not in most organs,[20,21] including myocardium,[22,23] kidney,[24,25] intestine,[26,27] and dental pulp.[28] This distinction was not seen in bone.[29]

There are fewer studies in tumors, although they present particular problems because of the heterogeneity and disorganization of their vasculature. Jirtle et al.[30] confirmed the theoretical prediction that spheres of intermediate diameter (25 μm compared with 50 μm or 15 μm) gave the greatest trapping of radiolabel in a variety of tissues in the rat, including a mammary adenocarcinoma. However, other authors[25,31] concluded that smaller microspheres were superior, perhaps because of their higher surface area-to-volume ratio. Song et al.[32] selected 15 μm spheres for their studies involving tumors on the basis that anything smaller might pass through the dilated tumor vessels.[34,35] Few direct comparisons have been made of the retention ratio between tumors and their host organ. Meade et al.[35] found tumor/liver ratios of 3:1 for 15 and 32.5 μm microspheres, but a ratio of 1:1 for larger (50 μm) ones (Table 1), and it was later reported that there was no significant difference between 15 and 25 μm spheres.[36] It is also possible to extract similar information from another study of rat tumors.[30] These authors also emphasized the importance

TABLE 1
**Comparison of the Distribution Characteristics of
15, 32.5, and 50 μm Microspheres between Tumor
and Normal Liver Tissue**

Microsphere size (μm)	Number of tumors	Tumor/liver ratio[a]	Difference (p value)
15	27	3.18 ± 3.4	>0.05
32.5	13	3.21 ± 3.2	
15	27	3.18 ± 3.4	<0.05
50	18	0.88 ± 0.83	
32.5	13	3.21 ± 3.24	<0.005
50	18	0.88 ± 0.83	

[a]   Values are mean ± SD.

From Meade, V. M., Burton, M. A., Gray, B. N., and Self, G. W.,
Eur. J. Cancer Clin. Oncol., 23, 37, 1987. With permission.

of tumor size, concluding that there was a greater probability of shunting of spheres through tissue in larger tumors with more dilated capillaries.[33,34] Thus, although 25 μm spheres might all be trapped by a small tumor (<2 g in their study), many would pass through a larger one.

Optimal trapping of microspheres is only one consideration. A point often overlooked in discussions of microspheres as delivery vehicles concerns extraction of drug molecules by vasculature of solid tumor tissue. For physiological reasons[14,37] solid tumors appear less efficient than normal tissue at extracting low molecular weight species from plasma, which results in lower drug uptake by tumor than would be expected purely from tissue blood flow. However, disposition of drugs incorporated within microspheres of suitable size for embolization will not depend on extraction by tumor tissue, at least for initial localization.

II. TUMOR PERFUSION AND ITS MODULATION

A. INTRODUCTION

In the simplest terms it seems self-evident that one of the most important factors affecting the accumulation of microspheres in tumor tissue is the total amount of blood passing through the tumor in a given time (usually expressed as ml/100 g/ min); indeed, as we have seen, labeled microspheres are used to measure tissue blood flow. This is, of course, an oversimplification and relative distribution between different organs and throughout the tumor mass must also be considered. Blood perfusion is known to be heterogeneous in tumors.[7,38,39] What is already known about tumor blood flow and its manipulation? We are fortunate in being able to refer to several recent reviews relating to this subject,[9,40,41] and part of what follows has been derived from these sources.

It has long been known that the use of certain vasoactive substances can permit preferential alterations in the blood flow of tumors compared with normal tissues in small rodents[42] and even in humans.[43] The effectiveness of this approach was seen to depend on the steal phenomenon whereby blood flow in unreactive tumor vessels may change in response to alterations in local blood pressure resulting from either constriction or dilatation of normal tissue vessels that are reactive to vasoactive drugs. Although this principle is consistent with the lack of smooth muscle in the walls of most blood vessels within tumors, it soon became clear that this effect could not be consistently relied upon and that some tumor vessels do react to vasoactive stimuli, particularly to vasoconstrictors, such as norepinephrine.[44,45] Numerous early studies used direct methods to determine the reactivity of tumor blood vessels to vasoactive agents[46,47] and in most cases some effect was found, again mainly with vasoconstrictors. A possible explanation for the responsiveness of tumor blood vessels to vasoconstrictors can be found in a more recent study of liver tumors in the rabbit.[48] They showed that the decrease in blood flow in these tumors after norepinephrine infusion was proportional to the resting flow. We may interpret this as indicating that those tumor vessels that were dilated had more potential for constriction.

This leads to the rather unsatisfactory conclusion that vasoconstrictors may alter the relative distribution of blood to some tumors but not to others; so it is not surprising that vasoactive drugs have been used largely in diagnostic radiology as a means of improving contrast in tumor angiography and not to modify therapy. The use of vasoactive intervention in cancer therapy is a much more challenging problem, in which consequences of producing the wrong effect, as in distributing anticancer drugs or increasing tumor oxygenation prior to radiotherapy, could be disastrous. A much better understanding of the effects of vasoactive drugs on relative and absolute tumor blood flow is needed before these approaches can be combined with a novel delivery system (such as microspheres) for therapeutic agents.

B. THE CHOICE OF VASOACTIVE AGENT

A wide variety of different compounds, both naturally occurring and synthetic, have been shown to alter either the relative or absolute blood flow through malignant tumors (see recent reviews[40,41]), although most attention has recently been focused on the arterial vasodilators hydralazine and 5-hydroxytryptamine, the vasoconstrictor angiotensin II, and the calcium channel blockers, such as nifedipine, flunarizine, and nisoldipine. There is also interest in nicotinamide. Although all of these agents have been shown to alter blood flow in a variety of tumor systems, we are still a long way from being able to predict with any accuracy their effects in particular human cancers.

The majority of recent studies of the effects of vasoactive drugs in tumors have therefore been motivated by one or more of the following experimental observations:

1. Vasoconstrictors can under some circumstances increase blood flow to tumors and improve the therapeutic efficacy of some conventional chemotherapy drugs.
2. Several arterial vasodilators (e.g., hydralazine) have been shown to produce a collapse in the blood flow to many experimental tumors, creating the extreme hypoxia that favors the activation of bioreductive cytotoxins.

3. Several calcium channel blockers have been shown either to increase or decrease tumor blood flow at doses at which systemic effects are minimal.
4. Nicotinamide increases tumor blood flow but in a specific way; it reduces the fluctuations in regional perfusion known to occur in many experimental tumors.

The experimental evidence to support these statements will now be considered along with an assessment as to whether some of these agents could have a role in improving microsphere distribution in tumors. As the evidence is reviewed, we should remember that because of the way that microspheres in the 15 μm range are trapped in the microcirculation, it is the relative distribution of blood flow between the tumor and surrounding normal tissue vasculature supplied by the same major vessel that will determine the relative numbers of microspheres accumulating in each tissue.

1. Vasoconstrictors
a. Catecholamines

This class of compound, mostly naturally occurring neurotransmitters, has been tested extensively for the ability to alter blood flow to malignant tumors. As long ago as 1964, Abrams[43] described the use of adrenaline as an adjunct to the angiography of renal neoplasms, and more recently similar effects have been reported with noradrenaline.[48] Grady et al.[49,50] showed that adrenaline could be used to improve the localization of radioactive microspheres in liver cancer. Although there is now a considerable body of evidence indicating differential effects in tumors and normal tissues, the results reported with this class of agent are rather inconsistent. Perhaps the most detailed series of studies with noradrenaline (a vasoconstrictor in most, though not all, vascular beds) was carried out in Goteborg[51-54] using ^{133}Xe wash out, ^{86}Rb extraction, and radiolabeled microspheres. They consistently showed that tumor perfusion was reduced in tumors to a similar extent to that seen in normal tissues. Other studies, however, using similar microsphere techniques and drug doses have shown that noradrenaline increased[55] or decreased[56,57] the perfusion of liver tumors relative to normal liver tissue. A study of sarcomas implanted in the rat kidney found a relative increase in tumor/normal kidney perfusion ratio,[58] whereas this ratio was decreased when comparing mammary adenocarcinoma perfusion with normal mammary gland (Figure 1).[40]

We might predict that the relative effect of noradrenaline on tumor and normal tissue vascular beds would depend on the abundance of smooth muscle and adrenergic nerve terminals. This has been looked at in several studies and although in general both were found to be absent from tumor vessels,[55,61] some incorporated normal vessels retained their muscle layers.[62] The inconsistency of the responses to noradrenaline, many measured with a microsphere-based technique, leads inevitably to the conclusion that this agent does not seem to be a likely candidate for improving the distribution of microspheres in tumors as a therapeutic strategy. This may have contributed to the shift in attention to other vasoconstrictors, such as angiotensin II, in the hope of obtaining a more consistent response.

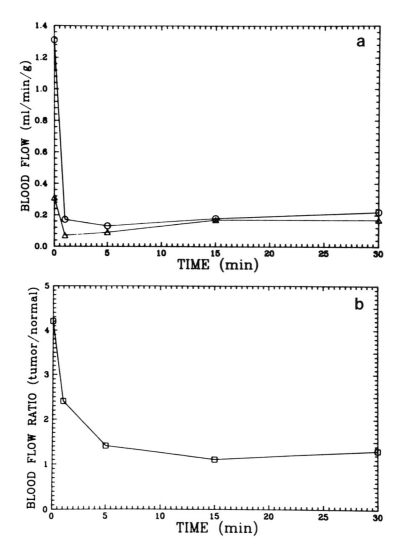

FIGURE 1. The effect of a continuous intra-arterial infusion of noradrenaline (1.4 μg/min) into W/ Fu rats bearing the MTW-9B mammary adenocarcinoma. (a) Blood flow measured by labeled micros-pheres in tumor (○) and normal mammary gland (△) as a function of duration of infusion. (b) The ratio of malignant to normal tissue blood flow (□). (From Jirtle, R. L., *Int. J. Hyperthermia*, 4, 355, 1988. With permission.)

b. *Angiotensin II*

This peptide is one of the most potent arteriolar vasoconstrictors known and is normally produced locally in the blood vessels by the action of renin and angiotensin-converting enzyme on angiotensin I. It is rapidly broken down to inactive constit-uents in the blood so that a bolus injection of the agent raises blood pressure for only a few minutes. More prolonged effects can be achieved by infusions, although tachyphylaxis may occur. An advantage, therefore, of its use is that it permits rather precise control of vasoconstriction and blood pressure.

Angiotensin II acts by binding to specific receptors on the smooth muscle cells of arterioles. It follows then that the vasculature supplying a given tissue must be sufficiently differentiated to have formed these structures before angiotensin II can exert its effects. The rationale for the use of angiotensin II to increase tumor blood flow is that it is generally supposed that the poorly differentiated structure of tumor vessels will be only weakly or not at all responsive to the agent. The reliability and clinical relevance of this assumption will be discussed later.

The first application of angiotensin II to oncology was as an aid to tumor imaging by angiography.[63-65] It was seen as a distinct improvement over the use of epinephrine as first reported by Abrams.[43] These authors[63-65] showed that vascular area was significantly increased by angiotensin II infusion in a variety of human tumors. Later reports emphasized the diagnostic value of angiotensin II in distinguishing between malignant and inflammatory lesions.

Results obtained in animal systems have been generally consistent. Jirtle[40] showed that the infusion of angiotensin II at a rate of 1.4 μg/min into tumor-bearing rats caused a fourfold increase in tumor blood flow relative to that seen in the surrounding mammary tissue, although the absolute blood flow to the tumor was actually reduced by about 30%. Suzuki et al.[66] showed in a subcutaneous rat hepatoma model not only that absolute blood flow through the tumor could be increased sixfold by the infusion of angiotensin II but that the antitumor effect of the cytotoxic drug mitomycin C was significantly enhanced. Similar results have also been reported by Hemingway et al.,[67] who observed liver tumor/normal liver ratios of 2:1 in rats. Recent studies in liver tumors in a variety of species are of particular interest in the context of the present review. Burton et al.[68,69] investigated the relative uptake of radiolabeled microspheres in rats, rabbits (Table 2), and sheep. In each case, the ratio of arterially introduced microspheres lodging in tumor tissue compared with surrounding normal liver increased under the influence of angiotensin II. Thus, tumor in the liver, whether primary or metastatic, would appear to be a good candidate for vasoactive drug-modulated chemotherapy. The effectiveness of *cis*-DDP II and mitomycin C was markedly enhanced in several tumors by simultaneous intravenous administration of angiotensin II.[66,70-72]

There is also evidence that not only does angiotensin II produce a significant increase in tumor perfusion but it opens up vessels in regions, particularly the necrotic center where blood flow was entirely absent[68,69,73] or intermittent[74] before infusion. Unfortunately, this presentation of the available data probably oversimplifies what is really a much more complex picture. The relative timing of the administration of the angiotensin II and the marker substance is clearly important. It has been shown that the retention of marker (^{99m}Tc MDP) was relatively greater in liver tumor than in normal liver 1 min after angiotensin II administration, although the reverse was true after 90 min.[67] As a further complexity, these results were obtained only when the angiotensin II was given by injection directly into the hepatic artery; continuous intravenous infusion gave a tumor/liver ratio of 0.6 after 1 min. Not only is the timing and route of angiotensin II administration important,

TABLE 2
Ratio of Microspheres Lodged in the Central Portions of the Tumor Compared with Those in the Normal Liver Tissue in 13 Rabbit Tumors after Angiotensin II Administration

Tumor	Pressure elevation (%)	Ratio (central tumor/normal liver)		
		Before	After	% change
1	20	2.4	6.6	+175
2	25	15.4	103.3	+757
4	25	17.6	33.9	+93
5	25	66.9	100.5	+50
6	25	2.9	15.1	+421
7	30	3.2	4.7	+47
8	40	0.7	9.2	+1214
9	40	10.4	12.3	+18
10	50	2.9	8.7	+200
11	75	3.9	7.8	+100
12	100	4.6	12.7	+176
13	140	3.6	4.8	+33

From Burton, M. A., Gray, B. N., Self, G. W., Heggie, J. C., and Townsend, P. S., *Cancer Res.*, 45, 5390, 1985. With permission.

but the site of tumor growth influences the response. It has recently been shown[75] that a continuous intravenous infusion of angiotensin II increases relative perfusion in tumors growing in the skin and gut of mice but decreases it in tumors in fat and muscle (Figure 2). This is consistent with the increase in absolute blood flow by >200%, measured by laser doppler flowmetry in a subcutaneous mouse carcinoma.[74] These authors also showed that the effect of angiotensin II was mainly in reducing the amount of intermittent blood flow usually associated with the centers of larger tumors,[76] an observation that is consistent with the results of previous studies.[68,69]

The majority of studies in experimental animal tumors seem to indicate that angiotensin II gives a more reliable increase in relative tumor perfusion than other vasoconstrictors, such as norepinephrine, although there may be exceptions for tumors growing in some organs. Recent studies[77] have shown that the angiotensin receptors are mostly located in the smaller precapillary arterioles; thus, there should be a lower probability of the larger arteries that feed tumors constricting on exposure to the agent. The evidence also suggests that the small arterioles that would react are largely absent from most tumors and exist only where normal vasculature has been incorporated.

Measurements in human tumors are few. Sasaki et al.[78] first showed using [81m]Kr uptake that the blood flow to both primary and metastatic liver tumors was increased relative to normal liver by infusion of angiotensin II (Figure 3). It was also recently

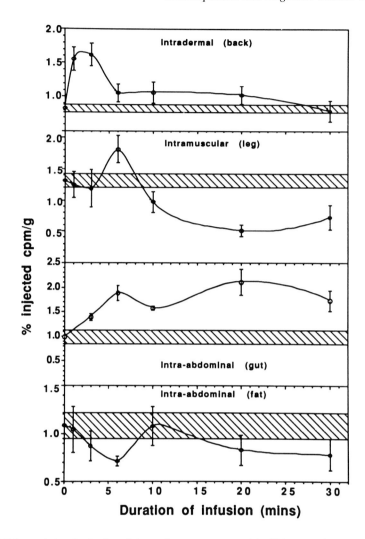

FIGURE 2.   Relative distribution of the cardiac output measured by ^{86}Rb uptake in mammary carcinomas growing in four sites in the CBA mouse, during infusion of angiotensin II (2 μg/kg/min). Hatched
area represents normal range. (Includes data from Hirst, D. G., Hirst, V. K., Shaffi, K. M., Prise, V.
E., and Joiner, B., *Int. J. Radiat. Biol.*, 60, 211, 1991. With permission.)

shown that the ratio of microsphere distribution to colorectal liver metastases[79-81]
and renal carcinomas[82] is markedly increased. There have also been clinical reports
of enhancement of the efficacy of chemotherapy by concomitant angiotensin II.
Mitsuhata et al.[83] combined intra-arterial angiotensin II with *cis*-platinum/doxorub-
icin chemotherapy of primary and metastatic bladder carcinoma and reported some
promising responses. Selective enhancement of tumor blood flow using [81m]Kr uptake
was also observed. A preliminary study of the combination of 5-fluorouracil with

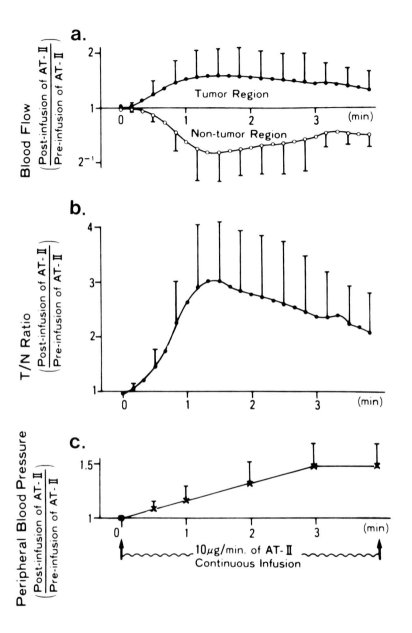

FIGURE 3. Effects in 14 patients with hepatic cancer of angiotensin II infusion (10 μg/min). (a) Blood flow in tumor and nontumor regions. (b) Ratio of tumor to local normal tissue blood flow. (c) Peripheral blood pressure. (From Sasaki, Y., Imaoka, S., Hasegawa, Y., Nakano, S., Ishikawa, O., Ohigashi, H., Taniguchi, K., Koyama, H., Iwanaga, T., and Terasawa, T., *Cancer,* 55, 311, 1985. With permission.)

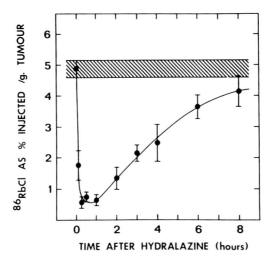

FIGURE 4. Changes in the relative distribution of the cardiac output (^{86}Rb uptake) to C3H/Tif mammary carcinomas with time after administration of 5 mg/kg hydralazine. Hatched area represents normal range. (From Horsman, M. R., Christensen, K. L., and Overgaard, J., *Int. J. Hyperthermia*, 5, 123, 1989. With permission.)

albumin microspheres and angiotensin II achieved results in colorectal metastases that were encouraging compared with historical controls,[84] although a carefully controlled trial will be necessary to establish the value of the combination.

2. Vasodilators

Some of the earliest experimental studies of tumor vasculature[42] showed that a large reduction in tumor blood flow could be produced by administering an arterial vasodilator, such as hydralazine. This effect was confirmed by numerous investigators over the following 30 years, but it was not until bioreductive cytotoxic drugs were tested as anticancer agents that the potential usefulness of vasodilators was recognized and the combination was considered as a therapeutic strategy. Many reports have since appeared in the literature describing the collapse of blood flow in a variety of subcutaneous rodent tumors after relatively large doses (5 mg/kg) of hydralazine.[85] An example is shown in Figure 4.

Clearly this effect could have important implications for the trapping of drugs within tumors, but it soon became apparent when hydralazine was tested on tumors in more clinically relevant sites that the effects were much smaller than for subcutaneous or intramuscular tumors (Figure 5).[75,86] Similar results were obtained in another study[36] of tumors growing in various sites in the rat (Table 3). Tumors in muscle were again most affected by hydralazine, although cecum tumors also showed a large flow reduction as measured by ^{125}I labeled microspheres. No significant reduction in flow was seen in liver tumors.

Also of concern are reports that most primary, radiation-induced skin tumors[87] and human tumor xenografts in nude mice did not show the collapse in blood flow

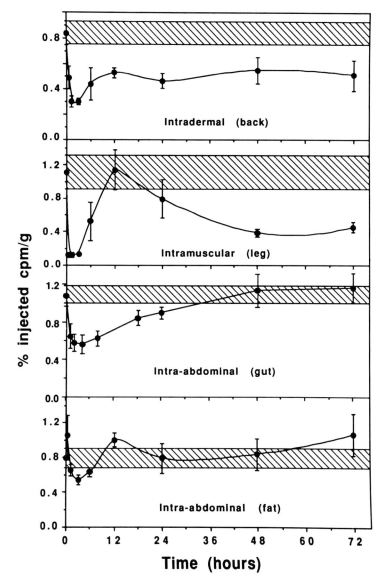

FIGURE 5. Relative distribution of the cardiac output measured by ^{86}Rb uptake in NT carcinomas growing in four sites in the CBA mouse, after an intraperitoneal injection of 5 mg/kg hydralazine. Hatched area represents normal range. (Includes data from Hirst, D. G., Hirst, V. K., Shaffi, K. M., Prise, V. E., and Joiner, B., *Int. J. Radiat. Biol.*, 60, 211, 1991. With permission.)

after hydralazine typical of subcutaneously transplanted mouse lines. More information is needed to determine whether this response is typical of all sites of growth or is peculiar to skin tumors. The crucial question must be whether the blood flow of human tumors can be effectively manipulated in this way. No clear result has

TABLE 3
The Effect of 5 mg/kg Hydralazine on Blood Flow (ml/min/100 g) in Tumor and Host Tissue

Tissue	Control		After 5 mg/kg hydralazine		Blood flow (hydralazine)/ blood flow (control)
	Blood flow[a] (ml/min/100 g)	Tumor/normal ratio	Blood flow[a] (ml/min/100 g)	Tumor/normal ratio	
Kidney	4.785 ± 0.095		3.758 ± 0.096		0.785
Tumor	0.400 ± 0.068	0.08	0.179 ± 0.024	0.05	0.448
Liver	1.263 ± 0.039		0.820 ± 0.031		0.649
Tumor	0.155 ± 0.024	0.12	0.145 ± 0.009	0.18	0.935
Intestine	3.455 ± 0.151		2.970 ± 0.114		0.860
Tumor	0.203 ± 0.061	0.06	0.109 ± 0.038	0.04	0.537
Mesentery	0.279 ± 0.015		0.184 ± 0.037		0.502
Tumor	0.217 ± 0.049	0.78	0.103 ± 0.019	0.56	0.475
Cecum	2.469 ± 0.141		1.327 ± 0.067		0.537
Tumor	0.375 ± 0.080	0.15	0.100 ± 0.020	0.08	0.266
Muscle	0.064 ± 0.004		0.167 ± 0.019		2.610
Tumor	0.154 ± 0.016	2.41	0.042 ± 0.006	0.25	0.272

[a] Values are mean ± SE.

Adapted from Hasegawa, T. and Song, C., *Int. J. Radiat. Oncol. Biol. Phys.*, 20, 1001, 1991. With permission.

yet emerged, and there is evidence for both increased and decreased blood flow in human tumors in several sites,[88] emphasizing that the use of this drug (and probably any other vasodilator with a similar mode of action, such as 5-hydroxytryptamine) cannot be relied upon. This presents a considerable problem for the use of vaso-dilators as a means of trapping drugs within tumors or creating a hypoxic environment where bioreductive agents will be activated, but this is probably not so important to the distribution of microspheres, which will become trapped within tumors without the need to induce any blood flow collapse. The problem would persist, however, if the microspheres are to be used as carriers for drugs requiring bioreductive activation, although it is possible that occlusion of blood vessels by embolized microspheres will itself induce hypoxia (see Chapter 5).

3. Calcium Channel Blockers

This class of drugs, which specifically block the entry of calcium into cells,[89] has been used in the treatment of angina, hypertension, and other cardiovascular disorders.[90] They may be divided into several categories based on their chemical structure[91] and their preferential site of action. The benzothiapine diltiazem is rather specific in its action, targeting mainly coronary vessels; the 1,4-dihydropyridine nifedipine causes relaxation of the larger blood vessels, whereas the diphenylpi-perizine flunarizine acts more peripherally. The phenylalkylamine verapamil is the least specific of these agents, acting on cardiac muscle, coronary vessels, and other large vessels.

As well as on smooth muscle cells some of these agents, particularly flunarizine, have effects on red blood cells that could be important for tissue oxygenation.[92,93] When red blood cells are exposed to a low pH environment, such as they encounter when they traverse poorly oxygenated regions of tumors, their metabolism is in-hibited so that they are unable to expel excess calcium ions.[94] One consequence of this is that their plasma membrane becomes stiffened and spherical, leading to a marked increase in blood viscosity. The inhibition of calcium entry by flunarizine prevents this stiffening process thus improving tumor tissue perfusion.[95]

The first application of the calcium entry blockers to the problem of the perfusion of malignant tumors was a study of the effects of verapamil.[96] Infusions of 100 to 200 mg/ml increased absolute blood flow, as measured by a microsphere technique in a rat adenocarcinoma, by about 50% in two implantation sites, muscle and mammary gland. There was no significant change in arterial blood pressure under these conditions. A subsequent study by the same group using the same systems showed that a bolus intravenous injection of flunarizine was equally effective.[97] Robinson et al.[98] studied the effect of both verapamil (10 mg/kg, intraperitoneally) and flunarizine (5 mg/kg, intraperitoneally) and found in each case that the fractional distribution of the cardiac output in a subcutaneous transplanted fibrosarcoma was unchanged. Verapamil also had no effect on a human melanoma xenograft.[98]

In a series of studies investigating the effects of flunarizine, cinnarizine, ni-fedipine, verapamil, and diltiazem, Wood and Hirst[99-102] reported the dose dependence of modification of blood flow (Figure 6) and radiosensitivity in two mouse tumors growing in two sites (skin and muscle). With the exception of flunarizine

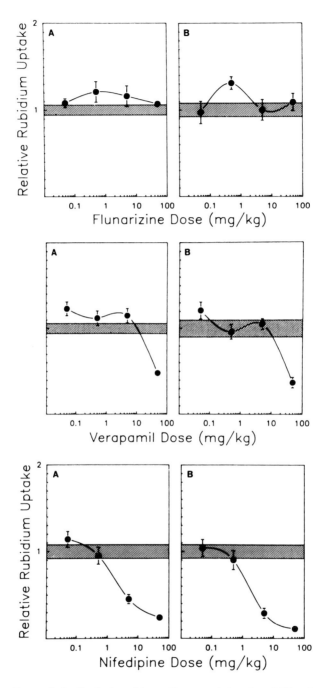

FIGURE 6. Changes in the distribution of the cardiac output in intradermal (A) or intramuscular (B) SCCVII/St carcinomas after a range of doses of four calcium channel blockers. Hatched area represents normal range. (Adapted from Wood, P. J. and Hirst, D. G., *Int. J. Radiat. Biol.*, 56, 355, 1989. With permission.)

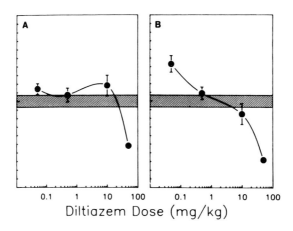

FIGURE 6 (Continued).

and cinnarizine, low doses of the drugs increased radiosensitivity and tended to increase relative tumor perfusion, whereas higher doses produced the opposite effects. Flunarizine produced radiosensitization at all doses from 0.05 to 100 mg/ kg; blood flow was also increased, although the effects were modest (~15 to 20%). This result is consistent with that reported by Vaupel and Menke,[103,104] in which 1 mg/kg intravenous flunarizine raised absolute tumor blood flow by up to 28% after 20 min, leading to an increase in oxygen availability by 20% (Figure 7). It is of interest that this change occurred in the absence of any alteration in systemic blood pressure, suggesting that reduced erythrocyte stiffening[95] could be the predominant mechanism.

Although we do not know exactly which of flunarizine's actions are important in radiosensitizing tumors, recent studies of tumor metabolism *in vivo* using magnetic resonance spectroscopy have shown a clear decrease in the ratio of inorganic phosphate (Pi) to total phosphate in cells,[105] indicating an improved metabolic status consistent with an increase in oxygen availability. Another potential therapeutic benefit of the calcium channel blockers may be their inhibitory effect on metastasis.[106,107] It has been suggested that increased blood flow may enhance the passage of tumor cells through tissues (liver) and delay the trapping of tumor cells in microvascular beds until they die in the bloodstream.[108]

4. Nicotinamide

Another compound that has been shown to be capable of sensitizing malignant tumors in animals to radiation is nicotinamide.[109-112] There is now clear evidence that its mode of action is through an increase in tumor oxygenation brought about by improved tumor perfusion.[113,114] A more detailed investigation of its effects[115] has recently shown that rather than increasing the overall perfusion of the tumor dramatically, nicotinamide prevents the intermittent closing off of blood vessels within tumors, thus producing greater uniformity of perfusion and oxygenation (Figure 8). The effect achieved is apparently similar to that produced by angiotensin

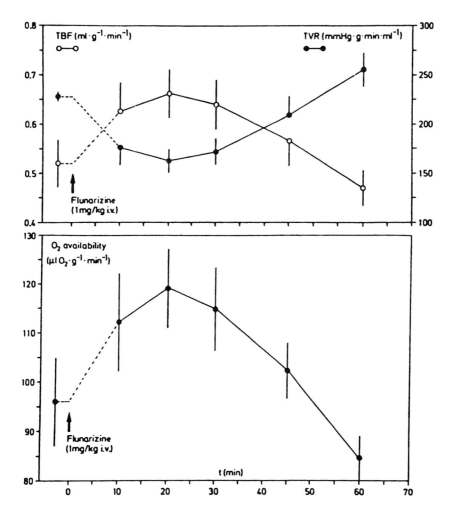

FIGURE 7.   The effect of flunarizine (1 mg/kg, intravenous) on tumor blood flow (TBF) in subcutaneous DS carcinosarcomas in the feet of rats measured using ^{85}Krypton clearance. Also shown are
tumor vascular resistance (TVR) from: TVR = mean arterial blood pressure/TBF (mmHg/ml · g^{-1} ·
min^{-1}) and oxygen availability from: O$_2$ availability = TBF × arterial [O$_2$] (µl O$_2$ · g^{-1} · min^{-1}).
(Adapted from Vaupel, P. and Menke, H., *Adv. Exp. Med. Biol.*, 215, 393, 1987. With permission.)

II, although the mechanisms must be different because at doses that give similar
increases in blood flow, angiotensin II elevates blood pressure by 50 to 100%,[66,78,71,74]
whereas nicotinamide reduces it by about 50%.[116] Nevertheless, the reduction of
temporal heterogeneity in tumor blood flow could have important implications for
the distribution of drugs or microspheres within tumors. There is also currently
considerable interest in nicotinamide as a tumor oxygenator and sensitizer in radiotherapy. Its proven efficacy when given with multiple small radiation fractions[112]
and low toxicity make it an attractive candidate for early clinical trials.

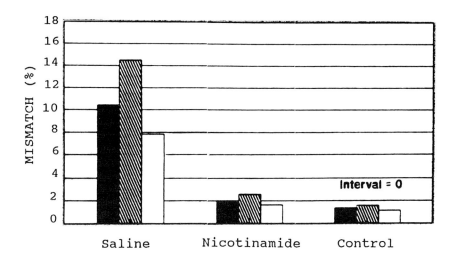

FIGURE 8. The "dye mismatch" technique used to determine the effect of 1000 mg/kg nicotinamide on intermittent opening and closing of blood vessels in central tumor regions (hatched bars), peripheral tumor regions (open bars), or whole SCCVII carcinomas in mice. Two fluorescent dyes, Hoechst 33342 and a carbocyanine, were administered intravenously 20 min apart and are taken up by tumor cells adjacent to blood vessels. Where only one dye is present in frozen sections of tumor, the blood vessel must have been closed at the time the other dye was given. The frequency of this occurrence is termed "mismatch". Reduced mismatch therefore implies more uniform perfusion. Control bars indicate "background" mismatch obtained when the two dyes were given at the same time (From Chaplin, D. J., Horsman, M. R., and Trotter, M. J., *J. Natl. Cancer Inst.*, 82, 672, 1990. With permission.)

5. Other Compounds

Vasoactive agents must constitute one of the most abundant classes of drugs. In addition, new, naturally occurring substances are continually being identified. Many of each type of agent have been tested for their effects on tumor blood flow,[41] although the majority of studies are much more superficial than those selected herein for special consideration. The problems associated with elucidating the vascular actions of drugs or natural peptides in tumor systems are much greater than in normal organs. Differences in tumor origin, size, histological type, implantation site, and host species introduce particularly difficult problems in making comparisons between different studies and recommendations for clinical application. Of the multitudes of vasoactive compounds available for investigation it is highly likely that many promising candidates will be missed. The ones selected herein are those for which there are sufficient data to draw meaningful conclusions, although others, both natural transmitters, including acetylcholine,[47,117] bradykinin,[118] histamine,[42,118] oxytocin,[58] prostaglandins,[119,120] and vasopressin,[55,58,121,122] and a variety of drugs[40,41] have been shown to produce effects on tumor vasculature in a limited number of studies.

There are also other interesting, recently discovered agents that have yet to be tested in tumor systems. The recent clarification of the mechanism of action of endothelium-derived relaxing factor[123] has led to a resurgence of interest in novel nitrovasodilators. Similarly, a vast literature has appeared in the last few years on endothelins, an extremely potent class of peptides with predominantly vasoconstricting action.[124-127] None of these agents has yet been studied in tumors.

III. CONCLUSIONS

There is now clear evidence from laboratory experiments that the perfusion of tumors can be modified over a wide range (-95% to $+200\%$) in relation to the perfusion of host normal tissues. There is, with some exceptions, rather poor reproducibility between systems; it is thus difficult to recommend specific drugs and doses that would be expected to achieve a given flow modification in a particular tumor. Conspicuously lacking in most of these studies are drug dose-response relationships. It has been shown for some of the calcium channel blockers, for example, that there are dose ranges over which these curves are steep, and it is likely that this could contribute to some apparently conflicting results.

As a general guiding principle, however, the concept that tumor vasculature is less reactive to many vasoactive agents is generally accurate, and steal effects, in which vasodilators produce a reduction in tumor perfusion and vasoconstrictors an increase, dominate the response to many agents at least for high doses in experimental animal systems. When attempting to apply these manipulations to human tumors for therapeutic benefit, the chances of success could be improved by obtaining preliminary information in the individual patient. The following approaches should be possible:

1. Evaluation of the systemic effects of the chosen agent on blood pressure and cardiac output and tailoring of the dose to achieve the maximal clinically acceptable changes in these parameters.
2. Assay from tumor biopsy material whether the blood vessels of a patient's tumor have receptors to the chosen agent. Tests for receptor binding by several agents are available.
3. Monitoring of the blood flow modification achieved, using one of a number of quantitative angiographic, nuclear magnetic resonance, and isotope-based methods.

The third of these approaches is clearly the most important and even to do that on each patient in a trial must add considerably to the work load. There is, however, a real risk with our present level of knowledge that the desired perfusion change will not be achieved in some patients' tumors or, worse still, that the effect will be the opposite of that intended. Even if a small fraction of the patients in a trial responded in this way, the potential benefit of the strategy could be concealed and a promising new therapeutic approach discarded.

REFERENCES

1. **Rubin, P. and Casarett, G.,** Microcirculation of tumors. I. Anatomy, function and necrosis, *Clin. Radiol.,* 17, 220, 1966.
2. **Falk, P.,** The vascular pattern of the spontaneous C3H mammary carcinoma and its significance in radiation response, *Eur. J. Cancer,* 26, 203, 1980.
3. **Falk, P.,** Differences in vascular pattern between the spontaneous and the transplanted C3H mammary carcinoma, *Eur. J. Cancer,* 18, 155, 1982.
4. **Shubik, P.,** Vascularization of tumors: a review, *J. Cancer Res. Clin. Oncol.,* 103, 211, 1982.
5. **Warren, B. A.,** Vascular morphology of tumors, in *Tumor Blood Circulation: Angiogenesis, Vascular Morphology and Blood Flow of Experimental and Human Tumors,* Petersson, H.-I., Ed., CRC Press, Boca Raton, FL, 1979, 1.
6. **Endrich, B., Intaglietta, M., Reinhold, H. S., and Gross, J. F.,** Hemodynamic characteristics in microcirculatory blood channels during early tumor growth, *Cancer Res.,* 39, 17, 1979.
7. **Asaishi, K., Endrich, B., and Gotz, J. F.,** Quantitative analysis of microvascular structure and function in the amelanotic melanoma A-Mel-3, *Cancer Res.,* 41, 1898, 1981.
8. **Vaupel, P.,** Hypoxia in neoplastic tissue, *Microvasc. Res.,* 13, 399, 1977.
9. **Jain, R. K.,** Determinants of tumor blood flow: a review, *Cancer Res.,* 48, 2641, 1988.
10. **Sevick, E. M. and Jain, R. K.,** Viscous resistance to blood flow in solid tumors: effect of haematocrit on intratumor blood viscosity, *Cancer Res.,* 49, 3513, 1989.
11. **Hirst, D. G., Denekamp, J., and Hobson, B.,** Proliferation studies of the endothelial and smooth muscle cells of the mouse mesentery after irradiation, *Cell Tissue Kinet.,* 13, 91, 1980.
12. **Hobson, B. and Denekamp, J.,** Endothelial proliferation in tumors and normal tissues: continuous labelling studies, *Br. J. Cancer,* 49, 405, 1984.
13. **Denekamp, J. and Hobson, B.,** Endothelial cell proliferation in experimental tumors, *Br. J. Cancer,* 46, 711, 1982.
14. **Jain, R. K.,** Transport of molecules in the interstitium: a review, *Cancer Res.,* 47, 3038, 1987.
15. **Rudolph, A. M. and Heymann, M. A.,** The circulation of the fetus *in utero:* methods for studying distribution of blood flow, cardiac output and organ blood flow, *Circ. Res.,* 21, 163, 1967.
16. **Buckberg, G. D., Luck, J. C., Payne, B., Hoffman, J. I., Archies, J. P., and Fixler, D. E.,** Some sources of error in measuring regional blood flow with radioactive microspheres, *J. Appl. Physiol.,* 31, 598, 1971.
17. **Utley, J., Carlson, E. L., Hoffman, J. I., Martinez, H. M., and Buckberg, G. D.,** Total and regional myocardial blood flow measurements with 25 micron, 15 micron, 9 micron and filtered 1–10 micron diameter microspheres and antipyrine in dogs and sheep, *Circ. Res.,* 34, 391, 1974.
18. **Hsu, C. H., Kurtz, T. W., Preuss, H. G., and Weller, J. M.,** Measurement of renal blood flow in the rat, *Proc. Soc. Exp. Biol. Med.,* 149, 470, 1975.
19. **Dickhoner, W. H., Bradley, B. R., and Harell, G. S.,** Diameter of arterial microvessels trapping 8–10 micron, 15 micron and 25 micron microspheres as determined by vital microscopy of the hamster cheek pouch, *Invest. Radiol.,* 13, 313, 1978.
20. **Hof, R. P., Wyler, F., and Stalder, G.,** Validation studies for the use of the microsphere method in cats and young minipigs, *Basic Res. Cardiol.,* 75, 747, 1980.
21. **Hof, R. P., Hof, A., Salzmann, R., and Wyler, F.,** Trapping and intramyocardial distribution of microspheres with different diameters in cat and rabbit hearts *in vitro, Basic Res. Cardiol.,* 76, 630, 1981.
22. **Hof, R. P. and Hof, A.,** A simple cutter for fresh tissue to facilitate the investigation of intramyocardial blood flow with tracer microspheres in cats and rabbits, *J. Pharmacol. Methods,* 7, 197, 1982.
23. **Consigny, P. M., Verrier, E. D., Payne, B. D., Edelist, G., Jester, J., Baer, R. W., Vlahakes, G. J., and Hoffman, J. I.,** Acute and chronic microsphere loss from canine left ventricular myocardium, *Am. J. Physiol.* 242, H392, 1982.

24. **Clausen, G., Tyssebotn, I., Kirkebo, A., Ofjord, E. S., and Aubland, K.,** Distribution of blood flow in the dog kidney. III. Local uptake of 10 μm and 15 μm microspheres during renal vasodilatation and constriction, *Acta Physiol. Scand.,* 113, 471, 1981.

25. **Utley, J. R., Marshall, W. G., Boatman, G. B., Dickerson, G., Ernst, G. B., and Daughtery, M. E.,** Trapping, non-trapping and release of nine and fifteen micron spheres in dog kidneys, *Surgery,* 87, 222, 1980.

26. **Maxwell, L. C., Shepherd, A. P., Riedel, G. L., and Morris, M. D.,** Effect of microsphere size on apparent intramural distribution of interstitial blood flow, *Am. J. Physiol.,* 241, H408, 1981.

27. **Maxwell, L. C., Shepherd, A. P., and McMahan, C. A.,** Microsphere passage through intestinal circulation: via shunts or capillaries?, *Am. J. Physiol.,* 248, 217, 1985.

28. **Path, M. G. and Meyer, M. W.,** Quantification of pulpal blood flow in developing teeth of dogs, *J. Dent. Res.,* 56, 1245, 1977.

29. **Triffit, P. D. and Gregg, P. J.,** Measurement of blood flow to the tibial diaphysis using 11-micron radioactive microspheres: a comparative study in the adult rabbit, *J. Orthop. Res.,* 8, 642, 1990.

30. **Jirtle, R. L., Klifton, K. H., and Rankin, J. H. G.,** Measurement of mammary tumor blood flow in unanesthetized rats, *J. Natl. Cancer Inst.,* 60, 811, 1978.

31. **Phibbs, R. H. and Dong, L.,** Nonuniform distribution of microspheres in blood flowing through a medium sized artery, *Can. J. Physiol. Pharmacol.,* 48, 415, 1970.

32. **Song, C. W., Rhee, J. G., and Levitt, S. H.,** Blood flow in normal tissues and tumors during hyperthermia, *J. Natl. Cancer Inst.,* 64, 119, 1980.

33. **Hilmas, D. E. and Gillette, E. L.,** Morphometric analysis of the microvasculature of tumors during growth and after X-irradiation, *Cancer,* 33, 103, 1974.

34. **Vogel, A. W.,** Intratumoral vascular changes with increased size of a mammary adenocarcinoma: new methods and results, *J. Natl. Cancer Inst.,* 34, 571, 1965.

35. **Meade, V. M., Burton, M. A., Gray, B. N., and Self, G. W.,** Distribution of different sized microspheres in experimental hepatic tumors, *Eur. J. Cancer Clin. Oncol.,* 23, 37, 1987.

36. **Hasegawa, T. and Song, C.,** Effect of hydralazine on the blood flow of tumors and normal tissues in rats, *Int. J. Radiat. Oncol. Biol. Phys.,* 20, 1001, 1991.

37. **Hennigan, T. W., Begent, R. H. J., and Allen-Mersh, T. G.,** Histamine, leukotriene C4 and interleukin-2 increase antibody uptake into a human carcinoma xenograft model, *Br. J. Cancer,* 64, 872, 1991.

38. **Tozer, G. M., Lewis, S., Michalowski, A., and Aber, V.,** The relationship between regional variations in blood flow and histology in a transplanted rat fibrosarcoma, *Br. J. Cancer,* 61, 250, 1990.

39. **Vaupel, P. and Frinak, S.,** Heterogeneous flow and oxygen distribution in microareas of malignant tumors, *Drug Res.,* 30, 2216, 1980.

40. **Jirtle, R. L.,** Chemical modification of tumor blood flow, *Int. J. Hyperthermia,* 4, 355, 1988.

41. **Hirst, D. G. and Wood, P. J.,** The control of tumor blood flow for therapeutic benefit, *BIR Rep.,* 19, 76, 1989.

42. **Algire, G., Legallais, F. Y., and Anderson, B. F.,** Vascular reactions of normal and malignant tissues *in vivo.* IV. The effect of peripheral hypotension on transplanted tumors, *J. Natl. Cancer Inst.,* 12, 399, 1951.

43. **Abrams, H. L.,** Altered drug response of tumor vessels in man, *Nature,* 201, 167, 1964.

44. **Kahn, P. C.,** Epinephrine effect in selective renal angiography, *Radiology,* 85, 301, 1965.

45. **Rockoff, S. D., Dopman, J., Block, J. B., and Ketcham, A.,** Variable response of tumor vessels to intra-arterial epinephrine, *Invest. Radiol.,* 1, 205, 1966.

46. **Edlich, R. F., Rogers, W., DeShazo, C. V., and Aust, J. B.,** Effect of vasoactive drugs on tissue blood flow in the hamster melanoma, *Cancer Res.,* 26, 1420, 1966.

47. **Gullino, P. M. and Grantham, F. H.,** Studies on the exchange of fluids between host and tumor. III. Regulation of blood flow in hepatomas and other rat tumors, *J. Natl. Cancer Inst.,* 28, 211, 1962.

48. **Young, S. W., Hollenberg, N. K., Kazam, E., Berkowitz, D. M., Hainen, R., Sandal, T., and Abrams, H. L.**, Resting host and tumor perfusion as determinants of tumor vascular responses to norepinephrine, *Cancer Res.*, 39, 1898, 1978.

49. **Grady, E.**, Internal radiation therapy of hepatic cancer, *Dis. Colon Rectum*, 22, 317, 1979.

50. **Grady, E. P., Auda, S. P., and Cheek, W. V.**, Vasoconstrictors to improve localization of radioactive microspheres in the treatment of liver cancer, *J. Med. Assoc. Ga.*, 70, 791, 1981.

51. **Mattson, J., Appelgren, L., Karlson, L., and Peterson, H.-I.**, Influence of vasoactive drugs and ischaemia on intra-tumor blood flow distribution, *Eur. J. Cancer*, 14, 761, 1978.

52. **Mattson, J., Alpsten, M., Appelgren, L., and Peterson, H.-I.**, Influence of noradrenaline on local tumor blood flow, *Eur. J. Cancer*, 16, 99, 1980.

53. **Mattson, J., Lilja, J., and Peterson, H.-I.**, Influence of vasoactive drugs on local tumor blood flow, *Eur. J. Cancer Clin. Oncol.*, 18, 677, 1982.

54. **Tveit, E., Weiss, L., and Hultborn, R.**, Blood flow reactivity to noradrenaline in induced and autotransplanted DMBA rat mammary neoplasia, *Eur. J. Cancer Clin. Oncol.*, 20, 253, 1984.

55. **Hafstrom, L., Nobin, A., Petersson, B., and Sundqvist, K.**, Effect of catecholamine on cardiovascular response and blood flow distribution in normal tissue and liver tumors in rats, *Cancer Res.*, 40, 481, 1980.

56. **Burton, M. A. and Gray, B. N.**, Redistribution of blood flow in experimental hepatic tumors with noradrenaline and propranolol, *Br. J. Cancer*, 56, 585, 1987.

57. **Miyuzaki, M.**, Intra-arterial infusion treatment for patients with malignant hepatic tumor: with special reference to hepatic pharmacokinetics and to combined use of vasoactive and antitumor drugs, *Jpn. J. Surg.*, 83, 359, 1981.

58. **Tvete, S., Gothlin, J., and Lekven, J.**, Effects of vasopressin, noradrenalin and oxytocin on blood flow distribution in rat kidney with neoplasia, *Acta Radiol. Oncol.*, 20, 253, 1981.

59. **Jirtle, R., Clifton, K. H., and Rankin, J. H. G.**, Effects of several vasoactive drugs on the vascular resistance of MT-W9B tumors in W/Fu rats, *Cancer Res.*, 38, 2385, 1978.

60. **Krylova, N. V.**, Characteristics of microcirculation in experimental tumors, *Bibl. Anat.*, 10, 301, 1969.

61. **Mattson, J., Appelgren, L., Hamberger, B., and Peterson, H.-I.**, Adrenergic innervation of tumor blood vessels, *Cancer Lett.*, 3, 347, 1977.

62. **Falk, P.**, The angioarchitecture of rat tumors, *Bibl. Anat.*, 15, 245, 1977.

63. **Eklund, L. and Lunderqvist, A.**, Pharmacoangiography with angiotensin, *Radiology*, 110, 533, 1974.

64. **Eklund, L., Laurin, S., and Lunderqvist, A.**, Comparison of a vasoconstrictor and a vasodilator in pharmacoangiography of bone and soft tissue tumors, *Radiology*, 122, 95, 1977.

65. **Kaplan, J. H. and Bookstein, J. J.**, Abdominal visceral pharmaco-angiography with angiotensin, *Radiology*, 103, 79, 1972.

66. **Suzuki, M., Hori, K., Abe, I., Saito, S., and Sato, H.**, A new approach to cancer chemotherapy: selective enhancement of tumor blood flow with angiotensin II, *J. Natl. Cancer Inst.*, 67, 663, 1981.

67. **Hemingway, D. M., Cooke, T. G., Chang, D., Grimes, S. J., and Jenkins, S. A.**, The effects of intra-arterial vasoconstrictors on the distribution of a radiolabeled low molecular weight marker in an experimental model of liver tumor, *Br. J. Cancer*, 63, 495, 1991.

68. **Burton, M. A., Gray, B. N., Self, G. W., Heggie, J. C., and Townsend, P. S.**, Manipulation of experimental rat and rabbit liver tumor blood flow with angiotensin II, *Cancer Res.*, 45, 5390, 1985.

69. **Burton, M. A., Gray, B. N., and Coletti, A.**, Effect of angiotensin II on blood flow in the transplanted sheep squamous cell carcinoma, *Eur. J. Cancer Clin. Oncol.*, 24, 1373, 1988.

70. **Wakui, A. and Suzuki, M.**, Cancer chemotherapy in combination with angiotensin-induced hypertension, *Jpn. J. Cancer Chemother.*, 10, 1577, 1983.

71. **Baba, T., Aoki, K., Kuroiwa, T., and Taniguchi, S.**, Some cardiotonics enhance the effectiveness of angiotensin II-induced hypertension cancer chemotherapy in mice, *Jpn. J. Cancer Res.*, 77, 432, 1986.

72. **Kuroiwa, T., Aoki, K., Tanigucki, S., Hasuda, K., and Baba, T.** Efficacy of "two route chemotherapy" using *cis*-diaminedichloroplatinum (II) and its antidote, sodium thiosulphate, in combination with angiotensin II in a rat hind limb tumor, *Cancer Res.,* 47, 3618, 1987.

73. **Hori, K., Suzuki, M., Abe, I., Saito, S., and Sato, H.,** Increase in tumor vascular area due to increased blood flow by angiotensin II in rats, *J. Natl. Cancer Inst.,* 71, 453, 1985.

74. **Trotter, M. J., Chaplin, D. J., and Olive, P. L.,** Effect of angiotensin II on intermittent tumor blood flow and acute hypoxia in the murine SCCVII carcinoma, *Eur. J. Cancer,* 27, 887, 1991.

75. **Hirst, D. G., Hirst, V. K., Shaffi, K. M., Prise, V. E., and Joiner, B.,** Influence of implantation site, time of day and vasoactive agents on tumor perfusion, *Int. J. Radiat. Biol.,* 60, 211, 1991.

76. **Brown, J. M.,** Evidence for acutely hypoxic cells in mouse tumors, and a possible mechanism of reoxygenation, *Br. J. Radiol.,* 52, 650, 1979.

77. **Grega, G. J. and Adamski, S. W.,** Patterns of constriction produced by vasoactive agents, *Fed. Proc.,* 46, 270, 1987.

78. **Sasaki, Y., Imaoka, S., Hasegawa, Y., Nakano, S., Ishikawa, O., Ohigashi, H., Taniguchi, K., Koyama, H., Iwanaga, T., and Terasawa, T.,** Changes in distribution of hepatic blood flow induced by intra-arterial infusion of angiotensin II in human hepatic cancer, *Cancer,* 55, 311, 1985.

79. **Goldberg, J. A., Kerr, D. J., Willmott, N., McArdle, C. S., Murry, T., and Hilditch, T.,** Increased uptake of radiolabeled microspheres with angiotensin II in colorectal hepatic metastases, *Eur. J. Surg. Oncol.,* 14, 715, 1988.

80. **Goldberg, J. A., Thomson, J. A. K., Bradman, M. S., Fenner, J., Bessent, R. G., McKillop, J. H., Kerr, D. J., and McArdle, C. S.,** Angiotensin II as a potential method of targeting cytotoxin-loaded microspheres in patients with colorectal metastases, *Br. J. Cancer,* 64, 114, 1991.

81. **Willmott, N., Goldberg, J., Anderson, J., Bessent, R., McKillop, J., and McArdle, C.,** Abnormal vasculature of solid tumors: significance for microsphere-based targeting strategies, *Int. J. Radiat. Biol.,* 60, 195, 1991.

82. **Anderson, J. H., Willmott, N., Bessent, R., Angerson, W. J., Kerr, D. J., and McArdle, C. S.,** Regional chemotherapy of inoperable renal carcinoma: a method of targeting therapeutic microspheres to tumor, *Br. J. Cancer,* 64, 365, 1991.

83. **Mitsuhata, N., Seki, M., Matsumura, Y., and Ohmori, H.,** Intra-arterial infusion chemotherapy in combination with angiotensin II for advanced bladder cancer, *J. Urol.,* 136, 580, 1986.

84. **Goldberg, J. A., Kerr, D. J., Willmott, N., McKillop, J. H., and McArdle, C. S.,** Regional chemotherapy for colorectal liver metastases: a phase II evaluation of targeted hepatic arterial 5-fluorouracil for colorectal liver metastases, *Br. J. Surg.,* 77, 1238, 1990.

85. **Chaplin, D. J., Peters, C. E., Horsman, M. R., and Trotter, M. J.,** Drug induced perturbations in tumor blood flow: therapeutic potential and possible limitations, *Radiother. Oncol.,* 20(Suppl.), 93, 1991.

86. **Hirst, D. G. and Hill, S. A.,** The control of tumor oxygenation in mice: the importance of tumor site, in *Selective Activation of Drugs by Redox Processes,* Adams, G. E., Breccia, A., Fielden, E. M., and Wardman, P., Eds., Plenum Press, NY, 1990, 223.

87. **Field, S. B., Needam, S., Burney, A. I., Maxwell, R. J., Coggle, J. E., and Griffiths, J. R.,** Differences in vascular response between primary and transplanted tumors, *Br. J. Cancer,* 63, 723, 1991.

88. **Rowell, N. P., Flower, M. A., McCready, V. R., Cronin, B., and Horwich, A.,** The effects of single dose oral hydralazine on blood flow through human tumors, *Radiother. Oncol.,* 18, 283, 1990.

89. **Greenberg, D. A.,** Calcium channels and calcium antagonists, *Ann. Neurol.,* 21, 317, 1987.

90. **Godfraind, T., Miller, R., and Wibo, M.,** Calcium antagonists and calcium entry blockade, *Pharmacol. Rev.,* 38, 321, 1986.

91. **Spedding, M.,** Calcium antagonist subgroups, *Trends Pharmacol. Sci.,* 6, 109, 1985.

92. **Scott, C. K., Persico, F. J., Carpenter, K., and Chasin, M.,** The effects of flunarizine, a new calcium antagonist, on human red blood cells *in vitro, Angiology,* 31, 320, 1980.

93. **DeClerck, F., Beerens, M., Thore, F., and Borgers, M.,** Effect of flunarizine on the human red cell shape changes and calcium deposition induced by A23187, *Thromb. Res.,* 24, 1, 1981.

94. **Weed, R. I., LaCelle, P. L., and Merrill, E. W.,** Metabolic dependence of red cell deformability, *J. Clin. Invest.,* 48, 795, 1969.

95. **Flameng, W., Verheyen, F., Borgers, M., DeClerck, F., and Brugmans, J.,** The effect of flunarizine treatment on human red blood cells, *Angiology,* 30, 516, 1979.

96. **Kaelin, W. G., Shrivastav, S., Shand, D. G., and Jirtle, R. L.,** Effect of verapamil on malignant tissue blood flow in SMT-2A tumor-bearing rats, *Cancer Res.,* 42, 3944, 1982.

97. **Kaelin, W. G., Shrivastav, S., and Jirtle, R. L.,** Blood flow to primary tumors and lymph node metastases in SMT-2A tumor-bearing rats following intravenous flunarizine, *Cancer Res.,* 44, 896, 1984.

98. **Robinson, D. A., Clutterbuck, J. L., Millar, J. L., and McElwain, T. J.,** Effects of verapamil and alcohol on blood flow, melphalan uptake and cytotoxicity, in murine fibrosarcoma and human melanoma xenografts, *Br. J. Cancer,* 53, 607, 1986.

99. **Wood, P. J. and Hirst, D. G.,** Cinnarizine and flunarizine as radiation sensitizers in two mouse tumors, *Br. J. Cancer,* 58, 742, 1988.

100. **Wood, P. J. and Hirst, D. G.,** Calcium antagonists as radiation modifiers: site specificity in relation to tumor response, *Int. J. Radiat. Oncol. Biol. Phys.,* 16, 1141, 1989.

101. **Wood, P. J. and Hirst, D. G.,** Modification of tumor response by calcium antagonists in the SCCVII/St tumor implanted at two different sites, *Int. J. Radiat. Biol.,* 56, 355, 1989.

102. **Wood, P. J. and Hirst, D. G.,** Cinnarizine and flunarizine improve the tumor radiosensitization induced by erythrocyte transfusion in anaemic mice, *Br. J. Cancer,* 60, 36, 1989.

103. **Vaupel, P. and Menke, H.,** Blood flow, vascular resistance and oxygen availability in malignant tumors upon intravenous flunarizine, *Adv. Exp. Med. Biol.,* 215, 393, 1987.

104. **Vaupel, P. and Menke, H.,** Effect of various calcium antagonists on blood flow and red blood cell flux in malignant tumors, *Prog. Appl. Microcirc.,* 14, 88, 1989.

105. **Wood, P. J., Counsell, C. J. R., Bremner, J. C. M., Horsman, M. R., and Adams, G. E.,** The measurement of radiosensitizer-induced changes in mouse tumor metabolism by ^{31}P magnetic resonance spectroscopy, *Int. J. Radiat. Oncol. Biol. Phys.,* 20, 291, 1991.

106. **Honn, K. V., Onoda, J. M., Diglio, C. A., and Sloane, B. F.,** Calcium channel blockers, potential antimetastatic agents, *Proc. Soc. Exp. Biol. Med.,* 174, 16, 1983.

107. **Tsuruo, T., Iida, H., Makishima, F., Yamori, T., Kawabata, H., and Tsukagoshi, S.,** Inhibition of spontaneous and experimental tumor metastasis by the calcium antagonist verapamil, *Cancer Chemother. Pharmacol.,* 14, 30, 1985.

108. **Blomqvist, G., Bagge, U., and Skolnik, G.,** Arterial occlusion reduces tumor cell lodgement in the rat liver, *Eur. J. Cancer Clin. Oncol.,* 24, 1573, 1988.

109. **Jonsson, G. G., Kjellen, E., Pero, R. W., and Cameron, R.,** Radiosensitization effects of nicotinamide on malignant and normal mouse tissues, *Cancer Res.,* 45, 3609, 1985.

110. **Horsman, M. R., Brown, D. M., Lemmon, M. J., Brown, J. M., and Lee, W. W.,** Preferential tumor radiosensitization by analogs of nicotinamide and benzamide, *Int. J. Radiat. Oncol. Biol. Phys.,* 12, 1307, 1986.

111. **Horsman, M. R., Chaplin, D. J., and Brown, J. M.,** Radiosensitization by nicotinamide *in vivo:* a greater enhancement of tumor damage compared with normal tissues, *Radiat. Res.,* 109, 479, 1987.

112. **Kjellen, E., Joiner, M. C., Collier, J. M., Johns, H., and Rojas, A.,** A therapeutic benefit from combining normobaric carbogen or oxygen with nicotinamide in fractionated X-ray treatments, *Radiother. Oncol.,* 22, 81, 1991.

113. **Horsman, M. R., Chaplin, D. J., and Brown, J. M.,** Tumor radiosensitization by nicotinamide: a result of improved blood perfusion and oxygenation, *Radiat. Res.,* 118, 139, 1989.

114. **Horsman, M. R., Brown, J. M., Hirst, V. K., Lemmon, M. J., Wood, P. J., Dunphy, E. P., and Overgaard, J.,** Mechanism of action of the selective tumor radiosensitizer nicotinamide, *Int. J. Radiat. Oncol. Biol. Phys.,* 15, 685, 1988.

115. **Chaplin, D. J., Horsman, M. R., and Trotter, M. J.,** Effect of nicotinamide on the microregional heterogeneity of oxygen delivery within a murine tumor, *J. Natl. Cancer Inst.,* 82, 672, 1990.

116. **Horsman, M. R., Christensen, K. L., and Overgaard, J.,** Hydralazine-induced enhancement of hyperthermic damage in a C3H mammary carcinoma, *Int. J. Hyperthermia,* 5, 123, 1989.

117. **Cater, D. B., Adair, H. M., and Grave, C. A.,** Effects of vasomotor drugs and mediators of the inflammatory reaction upon oxygen tension of tumors and tumor blood flow, *Br. J. Cancer,* 20, 504, 1966.

118. **Cater, D. B., Grigson, C. M. B., and Watkinson, D. A.,** Changes in oxygen tension in tumors induced by vasoconstrictor and vasodilator drugs, *Acta Radiol.,* 58, 401, 1962.

119. **Johnsson, K., Alonso de Santos, L., Wallace, S., and Anderson, J. H.,** Prostaglandin E_1 (PGE_1) in angiography of tumors of the extremities, *Am. J. Roentgenol.,* 130, 7, 1978.

120. **Rankin, J. H. G. and Phernetton, T.,** Effect of prostaglandin E_2 on blood flow in the V_2 carcinoma, *Fed. Proc. Fed. Am. Soc. Exp. Biol.,* 35, 297, 1976.

121. **Eklund, L., Gothlin, J., Jorsson, N., and Sjorgren, H. O.,** Pharmacoangiography in experimental tumors: evaluation of vasoactive drugs, *Acta Radiol. Diagn.,* 17, 329, 1976.

122. **Gothlin, J.,** Effect of vasopressin on human renal circulation investigated by angiography and a dye dilution technique, *Acta Radiol. Diagn.,* 17, 763, 1976.

123. **Palmer, R. M. J., Ferrige, A. G., and Moncada, S.,** Nitric oxide release accounts for the biological activity of endothelium derived relaxing factor, *Nature,* 327, 524, 1987.

124. **LeMonnier de Gouville, A. C., Mondot, S., Lippton, H., Hayman, A., and Cavero, I.,** Hemodynamic and pharmacological evaluation of the vasodilator and vasoconstrictor effects of endothelin-1 in rats, *J. Pharmacol. Exp. Ther.,* 252, 300, 1990.

125. **Luscher, T. F.,** Endothelium-derived vasoactive factors and regulation of vascular tone in human blood vessels, *Lung,* 168(Suppl.), 27, 1990.

126. **Luscher, T. F.,** Endothelial control of vascular tone and growth, *Clin. Exp. Hypertens.,* 12, 897, 1990.

127. **Luscher, T. F., Yang, Z., Tschudi, M., von Segesser, L., Stulz, P., Boulanger, C., Siebenmann, R., Turina, M., and Buhler, F. R.,** Interaction between endothelin-1 and endothelium-derived relaxing factor in human arteries and veins, *Circ. Res.,* 66, 1088, 1990.

Chapter 3

MICROPARTICULATE CARRIERS AS A THERAPEUTIC OPTION IN REGIONAL CANCER THERAPY: CLINICAL CONSIDERATIONS

J. H. Anderson, Colin S. McArdle, and T. G. Cooke

TABLE OF CONTENTS

I. RATIONALE FOR THERAPEUTIC STRATEGIES BASED ON EMBOLIZATION

Although surgery may afford effective palliation for patients with solid tumors, its failure to provide a cure must be conceded in many cases. Alternative therapeutic strategies have been explored and, among these, chemotherapy and radiotherapy have been foremost. However, there is a fine dividing line between doses of these modalities that are effective and those that are toxic. Only a small proportion of a systemically administered drug will reach a tumor while exposure of healthy tissues creates undesirable toxicity. Efforts have therefore been channelled into the development of methods for targeting therapy to tumors. Targeting may be obtained at three levels: first level targeting limits cytotoxic exposure to the tumor-bearing organ, second level targeting confines treatment to the tumor mass, and third level targeting selectively directs therapy to the malignant cells within the tumor mass.[1] The successful achievement of targeting should bring the dual benefits of enhanced tumor response and diminished systemic toxicity.

First level targeting of cytotoxic drugs employs administration via a regional artery. In 1950, Klopp reported the accidental infusion of methyl *bis*(β-chloroethyl) amine (nitrogen mustard) into a patient's brachial artery, instead of the antecubital vein, resulting in localized inflammation of the hand.[2] Over the past four decades the principle of intra-arterial chemotherapy has been applied to several organs, including the liver, stomach, and breast.[3-5] The liver is supplied by both the portal vein and the hepatic artery; however, it is generally accepted that liver tumors have a predominately arterial blood supply[6] (see also Chapter 7). Technical difficulties, due to the absence of a solitary end arterial blood supply, have prevented the application of these techniques to other organs, such as the esophagus. Intra-arterial delivery allows exposure of the target organ to the entire administered dose of drug on its first pass, and this advantage can greatly enhance tumor response.[5] The regional advantage (RA) following intra-arterial chemotherapy can be expressed as follows:

$$RA = 1 + Cl_s/Q_t$$

where Cl_s = systemic clearance and Q_t = target organ blood flow.[7]

Thus, it is predicted that organs with a high blood flow, such as liver and kidney, will achieve relatively little regional advantage unless the outflow of drug in the organ's venous system is reduced. Furthermore, drugs with rapid systemic clearance are preferable for targeted therapy. Clearly, a degree of uptake of the cytotoxic agent at its target site is required if systemic exposure is to be reduced. For example, it has been estimated from the change in serum drug concentrations in the hepatic artery and hepatic vein that 94 to 99% of 5-fluoro-2'-deoxyuridine and 19 to 51% of 5-fluorouracil (5-FU)(Chapter 6) is extracted on first pass through the liver after intrahepatic arterial administration.[8] Despite the high extraction efficiency, a hepatic arterial bolus of 5-FU provides comparable systemic exposure to that experienced with the same intravenous dose,[9] suggesting a saturable mechanism of liver clearance. This is confirmed by the finding that prolonged infusion increases target organ drug uptake: 24-h intra-arterial infusion of 5-FU reduced systemic exposure in comparison to equivalent doses delivered as an intra-arterial bolus.[9] Unfortunately, this method is inconvenient, entailing the protracted use of infusion devices.

First level targeting does not imply effective second level targeting of drug to the tumor rather than normal tissue. Indeed, it has been suggested that solid tumor tissue may be less effective than normal tissue at extracting low molecular weight compounds (such as drug molecules) from plasma[10,11] (see also Chapter 9). The concept of embolization has been introduced to address the problems described herein and enhance targeting of therapy. In brief, a given therapeutic agent is embodied in a particulate form, such as a microsphere or microcapsule. These particles are administered via a catheter, which has been positioned in the tumor-bearing organ's arterial blood supply. The particles are carried by blood flow to the arterioles and capillary bed where they embolize and gradually release their therapeutic payload. Furthermore, microvascular obstruction creates an area of infarction within the targeted tumor and retards blood flow, thus increasing tumor exposure to the drug.

Before embolization therapy may be attempted, patients must satisfy certain anatomical and pathological requirements. Access to the tumor-bearing organ must be obtainable via a surgically or percutaneously positioned arterial catheter (Chapter 7). Distribution studies must confirm that administered particles are confined to the tumor-bearing organ and that the entire tumor is exposed. These conditions may be demonstrated by infusing radioactive tracer microspheres and imaging patients with a gamma camera[12] (see also Chapter 8) or, more crudely, by infusing a dye.[13] It is preferable that the substances employed in these distribution studies are as similar as possible to the therapeutic particles because factors, such as particle size and concentration, may influence their distribution, which may not necessarily be in direct proportion to arterial blood flow.[14]

An understanding of the natural history of each tumor is a prerequisite to deciding whether chemoembolization is an appropriate therapeutic option. For instance, hepatic arterial therapy for patients with primary hepatocellular carcinoma may allow treatment of the patient's entire tumor burden. In contrast, it is possible that patients with liver metastases carry tumor deposits in other organs; therefore, regional therapy alone may control hepatic disease while extrahepatic metastases continue to progress. Another scenario involves slow-growing malignancies, such as the carcinoid tumor, in which embolization may offer effective palliation by chemically debulking the tumor mass even if all the metastatic sites are not treated.

Although embolization appears to be an attractive theoretical treatment option, critical assessment of its applications is necessary. Pharmacokinetic evidence of diminished systemic drug exposure is required and tumor concentrations of drugs and metabolites should be measured to ensure that the drugs have left their carrier particles. If systemic exposure to toxic substances can be reduced, side effects should be restricted. However, absence of local side effects due to damage to the tumor-bearing organ must be ensured. For example, the advantage of near-total hepatic uptake of regional 5-fluoro-2'-deoxyuridine is offset by the local complication of biliary sclerosis associated with this regimen. Finally, it should be established whether the attractive pharmacokinetic theory is translated into enhanced efficacy in terms of tumor response and patient survival.

Following a discussion of pharmaceutical considerations that our group has found to be of clinical importance, this chapter will describe clinical and relevant preclinical experience with individual microembolic systems with regard to pharmacokinetics, toxicity, and efficacy. It should be noted that only microembolic systems that incorporate active agents within the matrix are reviewed here.

II. PHARMACEUTICAL REQUIREMENTS FOR CLINICAL USE OF MICROEMBOLIC PARTICLES

The satisfactory design of therapeutic particles for clinical use requires that several factors are considered, including safety, size, resuspension characteristics, payload, and release profile of active agents.

A. SAFETY
The introduction of microspheres to clinical trials must be preceded by adequate *in vitro* and experimental animal model assessment. The absence of toxicity secondary to microencapsulating compounds must be established and particles must be in a sterile form prior to administration to humans.

B. PARTICLE SIZE
The indwelling catheters for regional chemotherapy used in our unit have an internal diameter of 0.6 mm. Particle diameter should therefore take this dimension into account. For example, in our experience, well-dispersed glass microspheres (mean diameter 20 μm) and albumin microspheres (mean diameter 40 μm) can be readily administered via an indwelling Infusaport® catheter (Shiley Infusaid Inc., Norwood, MA), whereas ethylcellulose microcapsules (mean diameter 250 μm) tend to form clumps that occlude such a narrow lumen. Administration to patients of ethylcellulose microcapsules was accomplished with some difficulty at laparotomy via a temporary, wide (inside diameter 1.2 mm) catheter, which was inserted into the hepatic artery.[15] However, it is not desirable to produce microspheres that are so small that they pass through the target organ's capillary bed and into the systemic circulation.[16] Particles in the 20 to 50 μm diameter range would therefore seem to be the best compromise.

C. DISPERSION OF PARTICLES IN AQUEOUS MEDIA
Because microsphere fate *in vivo* is influenced by suspension characteristics, ideally, a homogeneous suspension of individual particles in the aqueous injection fluid is necessary. Therefore, to achieve this, experimentation with various agents is necessary, taking into account the hydrophilic or hydrophobic properties of the microcapsule or microsphere surface. Particles that rapidly sediment in the infusion apparatus will almost certainly result in catheter occlusion. Other methods, such

as the addition of surfactants or resuspension in an ultrasonic bath, can aid administration.

D. DRUG PAYLOAD

The amount of particles that should be administered to a patient is equal to the desired dose of drug divided by the drug content of particles, usually expressed as micrograms of drug per milligram of particles. If an excessive amount of particles is administered, patients will complain of discomfort. For example, doses in excess of 300 mg of albumin microspheres delivered via the hepatic artery were associated with unacceptable right hypochondrial pain.[17] Furthermore, regional arterial flow may be totally occluded, resulting in flow reversal with consequent delivery of microspheres to tissues other than the target organ and undesirable side effects.

E. DRUG RELEASE

With the exception of radionuclides, therapeutic agents (e.g., cytotoxic drugs) incorporated into microparticles must be released following embolization to gain access to tumor cells. For the active agent to be largely incorporated within microparticle matrix at the point of administration, a delay or lag phase before extensive drug release occurs is required between suspension of dried particles in aqueous injection fluid and particle administration: 10 min is usually sufficient. *In vitro* and *in vivo* release rate studies are necessary to establish whether drug is released from the particles in a short "burst" or as a prolonged, slow release "infusion". Appropriate release characteristics are required for each drug. For example, the antimetabolite 5-FU may exhibit optimal efficacy when delivered as an infusion, thus allowing exposure of all the malignant cells as they pass through their growth and division cycle.[18] For novel drug delivery systems, such as microspheres, preclinical *in vivo* drug disposition studies in experimental animals are required because blood or tissue enzymes may promote particle breakdown. Finally, if a sterilization step is necessary prior to use in patients, its effect should be assessed because certain sterilization procedures alter release characteristics.[19]

In contrast to drug-loaded preparations, therapeutic radioactive particles should not release their radionuclide at all because systemic radiotherapy can lead to catastrophic myelosuppression. Initial experience with yttrium-90-loaded resin microspheres was hampered by this complication; therefore, new carriers were explored.[20] The introduction of glass microspheres provided a nondegradable carrier from which the radionuclide does not leach, and this has been reflected in the excellent safety profile of yttrium-90 glass microspheres in the regional treatment of patients with colorectal liver metastases.[21]

III. REVIEW OF MICROPARTICLE EMBOLIZATION OF SOLID TUMORS

A. LIVER

1. Ethylcellulose Microcapsules

In the 1970s Kato developed mitomycin-loaded ethylcellulose microcapsules.[22] These nonbiodegradable particles of approximately 250 μm diameter contained

TABLE 1
Embolization of Liver Tumors

Carrier	Agent	Tumor	N	Response (%)	Ref.
Ethylcellulose	Mitomycin C	Primary + secondary	4	0	23
Ethylcellulose	Mitomycin C	Hepatocellular	32	28	24
Ethylcellulose	Mitomycin C	Hepatocellular	20	38	25
Albumin	Mitomycin C	Primary + secondary	19	68	27
Polylactic acid	Aclarubicin	Hepatocellular	62	43	31
Ceramic	^{90}Y	Various secondary	37	32	32
Glass	^{90}Y	Colorectal secondary	12	0	34
Polystyrene	^{90}Y	Colorectal secondary	22	82	36
Plastic	^{90}Y	Primary + secondary	13	53	37
Glass	^{90}Y	Colorectal secondary	7	0	38

80% W/W of drug. Tumors of kidney, liver, bone, and pelvis were treated with 10 to 75 mg mitomycin C: despite a 65% overall response rate, with maximal efficacy observed 1 month post-treatment, activity against solid tumors of the liver was poor (Table 1). Systemic toxicity was mild, consisting of transient myelo-suppression in 30% of patients and this required no treatment.[23] Sugita et al.[24] reported a 28% response rate in 32 patients with hepatocellular carcinoma receiving mitomycin C incorporated in ethylcellulose microcapsules, and Ohnishi et al.[25] observed a 38% partial response rate in 20 patients with hepatocellular carcinoma with a survival of 8.4 ± 5.1 months (mean ± SD), an improvement compared with historical controls receiving nonencapsulated mitomycin C.

In our own unit, 15 patients with colorectal liver metastases have been treated with mitomycin C encapsulated in ethylcellulose.[15] Patients received doses of 20 mg (n = 6), 30 mg (n = 6), or 40 mg (n = 3). Pharmacokinetic studies on the six patients who received 20 mg of microencapsulated mitomycin C showed a significant reduction in systemic drug exposure after regional administration compared with bolus arterial delivery of free drug (Figure 1).[26] There was no evidence of myelosuppression, alopecia, or mucositis in any patient. However, two patients developed gastroduodenal ulceration and three patients experienced acute pancreatitis. Although response of the liver metastases to treatment was encouraging, median survival was only 4 months (range 1 to 18 months).

2. Albumin Microspheres

Fujimoto et al. reported the use of 45 μm bovine serum albumin microspheres incorporating 5% by weight of mitomycin C for embolization in patients with primary or secondary liver tumors.[27] Objective tumor response was achieved in 13 of 19 patients (68%). This trial was preceded by a cognate drug disposition study in the rat.[28] The microspheres were entrapped in the hepatic artery for at least 2 weeks and mitomycin C was detectable in the hepatic venous blood beyond 2 h after administration. More recently, human serum albumin microspheres (42 μm, 4.6% by weight of mitomycin C) were investigated by the same group. Greater

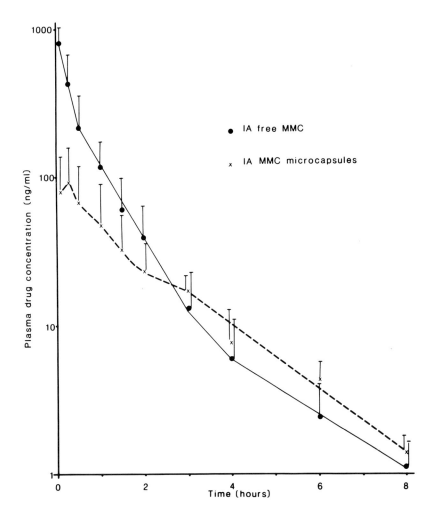

FIGURE 1. Pharmacokinetics of intrahepatic arterial mitomycin C (20 mg). Mean plasma concentration-time curves following administration of mitomycin C as drug in solution or microencapsulated in ethylcellulose (n = 6). (From Goldberg, J. A. et al., *Cancer*, 67, 952, 1991. With permission.)

control of solid tumor (AH272) deposits growing in the liver was achieved in rats receiving the drug-loaded microspheres than in those treated with regional saline or free mitomycin.[29]

In our own unit we have studied the efficacy of doxorubicin-loaded human albumin microspheres (20 to 40 μm, 3% by weight of doxorubicin) in an implanted Walker 256 rat liver tumor model.[30] Those animals treated with drug-loaded microspheres had significantly smaller tumors 4 days after treatment than those receiving saline, blank microspheres, or free doxorubicin. Fluorescent microscopy demonstrated intracellular doxorubicin in tumor and normal liver 4 days after treatment, whereas drug administered in solution was not detectable. This illustrates the potential of microspherical systems to prolong the duration of drug exposure (see Plate 1*).

3. Polylactic Acid Microspheres

Polylactic acid microspheres (mean diameter 200 μm) containing 10% by weight of aclarubicin were used for embolization following administration via the hepatic artery in 62 patients with hepatocellular carcinoma, resulting in a 42.6% partial response rate (<50% pretreatment tumor size) and 19.2% 3-year survival.[31] Side effects were transient and subsided with conservative treatment. Plasma pharmacokinetics of aclarubicin in dogs and humans indicated prolonged continuous drug release up to 72 h after administration; yet systemic exposure was significantly less than that experienced by patients receiving free drug in solution as a bolus by the same route.

In our unit, we recently began to evaluate poly(lactide-glycolide) copolymer microspheres (mean diameter 40 μm) loaded with mitomycin C (25%) in patients with colorectal liver metastases. These particles are small enough and suspend adequately to allow repeated administration via an indwelling hepatic artery catheter (internal diameter 0.6 mm). Furthermore, their relatively high drug content allows reasonable doses of mitomycin to be administered without undue discomfort secondary to overloading of the hepatic vasculature with embolic material. Unfortunately, batch variation has so far prevented accumulation of adequate data with this system.

4. Radioactive Glass, Resin, Ceramic, and Plastic Microspheres

Just as microspheres and microcapsules have been used in the delivery of cytotoxic drugs, similar principles have been applied to the delivery of radiation therapy. In an early study, a 32% response rate was reported following treatment of patients with liver metastases using ceramic yttrium-90 microspheres delivered into the aorta at the celiac axis origin.[32] Initial experience with resin yttrium-90 microspheres administered via a hepatic artery catheter was unsatisfactory because resin is a relatively unstable carrier and pancytopenia secondary to yttrium-90 leaching was reported.[20] In 1980 yttrium-90 microspheres were withdrawn by the U.S. Food and Drug Administration because of a batch of microspheres from which the radionuclide had eluted. However, the introduction of glass microspheres provided a carrier that neither leached nor degraded.[21] Studies in dogs demonstrated the safety of yttrium-90 microspheres, delivering a dose of 200 Gy to the liver after administration via the hepatic artery.[33] Human trials have failed to reveal hepatic toxicity following doses of up to 100 Gy.[34,35]

Another potential hazard of regional glass yttrium-90 microspheres therapy is the delivery of microspheres to extrahepatic organs via branches of the hepatic artery or through intrahepatic arteriovenous shunts. Herba et al. administered glass yttrium-90 microspheres via an angiographically positioned hepatic artery catheter, and although identifiable arterial branches to extrahepatic organs were occluded

---

* Color plate follows p. 70.

with coils, two patients developed gastroduodenal ulceration.[34] Although the methodology for delivery of radioactive microspheres has been intensively investigated, both in patients and animal experiments, phase II data are scarce. Only three trials quoted response data and one gave survival results. Herba et al. administered glass yttrium-90 microspheres in doses of up to 100 Gy to 12 patients with colorectal liver metastases; no patients responded and survival was not stated.[34] Gray et al.[36] treated 29 patients with colorectal liver metastases using yttrium-90 incorporated into resin microspheres via ion-exchange principles (see Chapter 1), with or without additional hepatic arterial infusion of 5-fluorouracil. Of 22 patients whose response was evaluated by serial CT scans, 18 showed some reduction in tumor volume and 10 greater than 50% reduction. In 1989 Blanchard et al.[37] reported on 13 patients treated with up to 2.7 GBq of yttrium-90 incorporated into plastic microspheres. More than half the patients responded and median survival was 15 months. There are no published phase III studies to date.

In our own unit, a phase I study has been undertaken to assess the potential for increasing the maximum tolerated dose of yttrium-90 glass microspheres in patients with colorectal liver metastases.[38] In seven patients microspheres were targeted to tumor by administration via the hepatic artery under the influence of an arterial infusion of angiotensin II (Chapter 8). Calculated absorbed dose was 100 Gy (n = 3), 125 Gy (n = 3), or 150 Gy (n = 1). There was no toxicity associated with this treatment. In particular, no patients experienced myelosuppression, pulmonary fibrosis, gastroduodenal ulceration, or hepatic failure. Although tumor shrinkage was not apparent, progression of hepatic metastases was delayed in six patients for a median duration of 6 months (range 4 to 25+ months). However, six patients developed extrahepatic metastases and these were diagnosed a median of 2 months (range 1 to 6 months) after treatment. Median survival was 11 months (range 5 to 25+ months). The results of clinical trials of embolic therapy for patients with liver tumors are summarized in Table 1.

B. KIDNEY

1. Ethylcellulose Microcapsules

Kato's initial studies of microencapsulated mitomycin C delivered into the renal artery of the dog demonstrated retention of drug for up to 6 h after administration. This was associated with extensive renal necrosis 5 days later.[39] Histological studies showed that microcapsules lodged in small arteries at the corticomedullary junction. Subsequent clinical trials confirmed the pharmacokinetic advantage in 33 patients with renal cell carcinoma. Furthermore, therapeutic response was enhanced in patients receiving a combination of gelatin sponge embolization and mitomycin microcapsules (78% of patients experiencing a decrease in tumor size; n = 14) compared with those treated with gelatin sponge plus nonencapsulated mitomycin.[40] This regimen was recommended for preoperative or palliative therapy.

2. Albumin Microspheres

Animal studies of regionally administered doxorubicin-loaded albumin microspheres have revealed a high renal entrapment (97%), with subsequent release of drug by diffusion and biodegradation of the albumin matrix over 48 h, resulting in reduced systemic exposure to the antineoplastic agent.[41] Tumor localization of microspheres under the influence of angiotensin II in a patient with an adenocarcinoma has been described (Chapter 8). Pilot studies have used these preparations for palliative treatment of two patients with renal tumors who were not fit for surgery. Symptomatic relief was satisfactory, but further clinical evaluation is required.

3. Radioactive Particles

An approach related to microsphere embolization for management of primary renal carcinoma involves transcatheter embolization of the kidney with radioactive pellets containing ^{125}I administered via the renal artery.[42] The low energy (27 to 35 keV) and long half-life (69.6 days) of this radionuclide allow sustained absorption of radiation close to the site of pellet deposition. Later studies combined this approach with interstitial ^{125}I implants for treatment of isolated bone metastases from the renal tumors to give a 2-year survival of 69% (9 of 13).[43]

C. BREAST

Intra-arterial chemotherapy, using cytotoxic drugs in solution infused via the subclavian artery, has provided effective local control of advanced breast cancer.[5] Subclavian artery perfusion allows perfusion of the entire breast and a temporary tourniquet prevents undesirable delivery of drug to the upper limb. Increased selectivity may be achieved by internal mammary artery cannulation, but this could prevent treatment of the lateral portion of the breast, which is supplied by the lateral thoracic artery. In a pilot study in our unit, doxorubicin-loaded human albumin microspheres (9 mg doxorubicin, 90 mg microspheres) were infused into the internal mammary artery via a percutaneous catheter in a patient with advanced inflammatory breast cancer. An excellent tumor response was obtained, but some microspheres migrated to the superior epigastric artery, resulting in necrosis of abdominal skin. The lack of a single identifiable artery perfusing the breast may limit the application of therapeutic strategies based on embolization in patients with breast cancer. Related to this, Cummings et al. (Chapter 6) found that distribution of microspheres is not optimal; thus, doxorubicin-loaded albumin microspheres administered regionally resulted in higher drug concentrations in normal tissue compared with breast tumor tissue.

D. LUNG

The lung, like the liver, has a dual blood supply. Lung tumors appear to be supplied by the bronchial arteries rather than the pulmonary artery.[44] Selective cannulation of bronchial arteries is a difficult technique; therefore, application of therapeutic strategies based on embolization of lung tumors is currently limited. However, Llaurado et al.[45] administered 10^6 ion-exchange resin microspheres (diameter 53 to 63 μm) labeled with 740 MBq of ^{32}P via lobar branches of the pulmonary artery of dogs and demonstrated organization and contraction of the treated lobe with minimal radioactivity in other tissues. There may be a place for "radioisotopic pulmonary lobectomy" in future human trials.

E. HEAD AND NECK

Okamoto et al. microencapsulated *cis*-platinum (60% by weight) in ethylcellulose.[46] The resultant particles (mean diameter 400 μm) were administered via the maxillary artery to five patients with carcinoma of the maxillary sinus or the oral cavity. A microencapsulated preparation incorporating 60 mg *cis*-platinum was associated with lower peak plasma concentrations (600 to 1,400 ng/ml at 1 to 2 days) compared with that found in patients treated with 20 mg *cis*-platinum administered in solution. Drug concentrations of *cis*-platinum in biopsied tumor tissue were markedly elevated over a period of 7 days when administered in microencapsulated form. Two of 14 patients treated with microencapsulated *cis*-platinum achieved a complete response and seven patients achieved a partial response.

IV. CONCLUSIONS

The pharmacokinetic principles underlying embolization have been confirmed in animal and human studies. Regional advantage is reflected in diminished systemic toxicity and encouraging tumor responses. There is little evidence of increased local toxicity in most studies, although target organs are subjected to intensified treatment compared with systemic therapy. Whether response rates are superior to those achievable with conventional systemic chemotherapy or external beam radiotherapy remains open to debate because there have been so few randomized controlled trials. Furthermore, it is not known if improved tumor response equates with prolonged survival. Lessons may be learned from experience with hepatic arterial chemotherapy for colorectal metastases in which the survival advantage is equivocal. Thus, in a prospective randomized trial (69 patients) to compare intra-arterial 5-fluoro-2'-deoxyuridine (floxuridine) with systemic 5-FU, despite a significantly higher response rate in the liver with regional chemotherapy (48% versus 21%), no survival advantage was seen.[47] However, in a similar study (166 patients), hepatic arterial chemotherapy with 5-fluoro-2'-deoxyuridine conferred a statistically significant survival advantage.[48]

Because the benefit of regional treatment will be blunted due to patients developing metastases outside the liver, a combination of chemoembolization or radioembolization and systemic therapy may be an effective treatment option. In summary, through intensification of therapy, embolization is a promising innovation in the management of identifiable but unresectable solid tumors at certain anatomical sites: final judgment of its utility must be reserved until controlled trial data on survival are available when used as sole therapy or in combination with systemic therapy.

REFERENCES

1. **Widder, K. J., Senyei, A. E., and Ranney, D. F.,** Magnetically responsive microspheres and other carriers for the biophysical targeting of antitumor agents, *Adv. Pharmacol. Chemother.,* 16, 213, 1979.
2. **Klopp, C. T., Alford, T. C., Bateman, J., Berry, G. N., and Winship, T.,** Fractionated intra-arterial cancer chemotherapy with methyl bis-amine hydrochloride; a preliminary report, *Ann. Surg.,* 132, 811, 1950.
3. **Sullivan, R. D., Norcross, J. W., and Watkins, E.,** Chemotherapy of metastatic liver cancer by prolonged hepatic artery infusion, *N. Engl. J. Med.,* 270, 321, 1964.
4. **Benthin, F. and Aigner, K. R.,** Intra-arterial chemotherapy for nonresectable and recurrent gastric cancer with a modified FAM–folinic acid regimen. Proc. 5th Int. Conf. Adv. Regional Cancer Treat., B2, Rosenheim, Germany, June 1991.
5. **Sainsbury, R.,** Intra-arterial chemotherapy for breast cancer, *Br. J. Surg.,* 78, 769, 1991.
6. **Breedis, C. and Young, G.,** The blood supply of neoplasms in the liver, *Am. J. Pathol.,* 30, 969, 1954.
7. **Daemen, M. J. A. P., Smits, J. F. M., Thijssen, H. H. W., and Struyker-Boudier, H. A. J.,** Pharmacokinetic considerations in target-organ directed drug delivery, *Trends Pharmacol. Sci.,* 9, 138, 1988.
8. **Ensminger, W. D., Rosowsky, A., Raso, V., Levin, D. C., Glode, M., Come, S., Steele, G., and Frei, E.,** A clinical-pharmacological evaluation of hepatic arterial infusions of 5-fluoro-2′-deoxyuridine and 5-fluorouracil, *Cancer Res.,* 38, 3784, 1978.
9. **Goldberg, J. A., Kerr, D. J., Watson, D. G., Willmott, N., Bates, C. D., McKillop, J. H., and McArdle, C. S.,** The pharmacokinetics of 5-fluorouracil administered by arterial infusion in advanced colorectal hepatic metastases, *Br. J. Cancer,* 61, 913, 1990.
10. **Jain, R. K.,** Transport of molecules across tumor vasculature, *Cancer Metastasis Rev.,* 6, 559, 1987.
11. **Ohkouchi, K., Imoto, H., Takakura, Y., Hashida, M., and Sezaki, H.,** Disposition of anticancer drugs after bolus arterial administration in a tissue-isolated tumor perfusion system, *Cancer Res.,* 50, 1640, 1990.
12. **Goldberg, J. A., Bradnam, M. S., Kerr, D. J., Haughton, D. M., McKillop, J. H., Bessent, R. G., Willmott, N., McArdle, C. S., and George, W. D.,** Arteriovenous shunting of microspheres in patients with colorectal liver metastases: errors in assessment due to free pertechnetate, and the effect of angiotensin II, *Nucl. Med. Commun.,* 8, 1033, 1987.
13. **Watkins, E., Khazei, A. M., and Nahra, K. S.,** Surgical basis for arterial infusion chemotherapy of disseminated carcinoma of the liver, *Surg. Gynecol. Obstet.,* 130, 581, 1970.
14. **Anderson, J. H., Angerson, W. J., Willmott, N., Kerr, D. J., McArdle, C. S., and Cooke T. G.,** Regional delivery of microspheres to liver metastases: the effects of particle size and concentration on intrahepatic distribution, *Br. J. Cancer,* 64, 1031, 1991.
15. **Anderson, J. H., Goldberg, J. A., Eley, J. G., Whateley, T. L., Kerr, D. J., Cooke, T. G., and McArdle, C. S.,** A phase I study of regionally administered mitomycin C microcapsules for patients with colorectal liver metastases, *Eur. J. Cancer,* 27, 1189, 1991.
16. **Goldberg, J. A., Thomson, J. A. K., McCurrach, G., Anderson, J. H., Willmott, N., Bessent, R. G., McKillop, J. H., and McArdle, C. S.,** Arteriovenous shunting in patients with colorectal liver metastases, *Br. J. Cancer,* 63, 466, 1991.
17. **Goldberg, J. A., Kerr, D. J., Willmott, N., McKillop, J. H., and McArdle, C. S.,** Pharmacokinetics and pharmacodynamics of locoregional 5-fluorouracil (5FU) in advanced colorectal liver metastases, *Br. J. Cancer,* 57, 186, 1988.
18. **Lokich, J. J., Ahlgren, J. D., Gullo, J. J., Philips, J. A., and Fryer, J. G.,** A prospective randomized comparison of continuous infusion fluorouracil with conventional bolus schedule in metastatic colorectal carcinoma: a Mid-Atlantic Oncology Program study, *J. Clin. Oncol.,* 7, 425, 1989.

19. **Spenlehauer, G., Vert, M., Benoit, J. P., and Boddaert, A.,** *In vitro* and *in vivo* degradation of poly(D,L lactide/glycolide) type microspheres made by solvent evaporation method, *Biomaterials,* 10, 557, 1989.

20. **Mantravadi, R. V. P., Spigos, D. G., Tan, W. S., and Felix, E. L.,** Intra-arterial yttrium-90 in the treatment of hepatic malignancy, *Radiology,* 142, 783, 1982.

21. **Ehrhardt, G. J. and Day, D. E.,** Therapeutic use of ^{90}Y microspheres, *Nucl. Med. Biol.,* 14, 233, 1987.

22. **Kato, T., Unno, K., and Goto, A.,** Ethylcellulose microcapsules for selective drug delivery, *Methods Enzymol.,* 112, 139, 1985.

23. **Kato, T., Nemoto, R., Mori, H., Takahashi, M., and Harada, M.,** Arterial chemoembolization with mitomycin C microcapsules in the treatment of primary or secondary carcinoma of the kidney, liver, bone and intrapelvic organs, *Cancer,* 48, 674, 1981.

24. **Sugita, S., Ohnishi, K., Hayasaka, A., Tsunoda, T., Tanaka, H., Nakada, H., Sato, S., Chin, N., Tanabe, Y., Saito, M., Terabyashi, H., Hatano, H., Saito, M., Nakayama, T., Iida, S., Nomura, F., Okuda, K., and Kondo, Y.,** Comparison of various therapeutic modalities with transcatheter arterial infusion of anticancer drugs in hepatocellular carcinoma, *Jpn. J. Gastroenterol.,* 83, 2375, 1986.

25. **Ohnishi, K., Tsuchiya, S., Nakayama, T., Hiyama, Y., Iwama, S., Soto, N., Takashi, M., Ohtsuki, T., Kono, K., Nakajima, Y., and Okuda, K.,** Arterial chemoembolization of hepatocellular carcinoma with mitomycin C microcapsules, *Radiology,* 152, 51, 1984.

26. **Goldberg, J. A., Kerr, D. J., Blackie, R., Whately, T. L., Pettit, L., Kato, T., and McArdle, C. S.,** Mitomycin C-loaded microcapsules in the treatment of colorectal liver metastases, *Cancer,* 67, 952, 1991.

27. **Fujimoto, S., Miyazaki, M., Endoh, F., Takahagi, O., Okui, K., and Morimoto, Y.,** Biodegradable mitomycin microspheres given intra-arterially for inoperable hepatic cancer, *Cancer,* 56, 2404, 1985.

28. **Fujimoto, S., Miyazaki, M., Endoh, F., Takahashi, O., Sherestha, R. D., Oku, K., Morimoto, Y., and Terao, K.,** Effects of intra-arterially infused biodegradable microspheres containing mitomycin C, *Cancer,* 55, 522, 1985.

29. **Morimoto, Y., Natsume, H., Sugibayashi, K., and Fujimoto, S.,** Effect of chemoembolization of albumin microspheres containing mitomycin C on AH 272 liver metastasis in rats, *Int. J. Pharm.,* 54, 27, 1989.

30. **Goldberg, J. A., Willmott, N., Kerr, D. J., Sutherland, C., and McArdle, C. S.,** An *in vivo* assessment of adriamycin-loaded albumin microspheres, *Br. J. Cancer,* 65, 393, 1992.

31. **Ichihara, T., Sakamoto, K., Mori, K., and Akagi, M.,** Transcatheter arterial chemoembolization therapy for hepatocellular carcinoma using polylactic acid microspheres containing aclarubicin hydrochloride, *Cancer Res.,* 49, 4357, 1989.

32. **Ariel, I. M. and Pack, G. T.,** Treatment of inoperable cancer of the liver by intra-arterial radioactive isotopes and chemotherapy, *Cancer,* 20, 793, 1967.

33. **Wollner, I., Knutsen, C., Smith, P., Prieskorn, D., Chrisp, C., Andrew, J., Juni, J., Warber, S., Klevering, J., Crudup, J., and Ensminger, W.,** Effects of hepatic arterial Y-90 glass microspheres in dogs, *Cancer,* 61, 1336, 1988.

34. **Herba, M. J., Illescas, F. F., Thirlwell, M. P., Boos, G. J., Rosenthall, L., Atri, M., and Bret, P. M.,** Hepatic malignancies: improved treatment with intra-arterial Y-90, *Radiology,* 169, 311, 1988.

35. **Houle, S., Yip, T. C. K., Shepherd, F. A., Rotstein, L. E., Sniderman, K. W., Theis, E., Cawthorn, R. H., and Richmond-Cox, K.,** Hepatocellular carcinoma: pilot trial of treatment with Y-90 microspheres, *Radiology,* 172, 857, 1989.

36. **Gray, B. N., Anderson, J. E., Burton, M. A., Van Hazel, G., Codde, J., Morgan, J., and Klemp, P.,** Regression of liver metastases following treatment with yttrium-90 microspheres, *Aust. NZ J. Surg.,* 62, 105, 1992.

37. **Blanchard, R. J. W., Morrow, I. M., and Sutherland, J. B.,** Treatment of liver tumors with yttrium-90 microspheres alone, *J. Can. Assoc. Radiol.,* 40, 206, 1989.

38. **Anderson, J. H., Goldberg, J. A., Bessent, R. G., Kerr, D. G., McKillop, J. H., Stewart, I., Cooke, T. G., and McArdle, C. S.,** Glass yttrium-90 microspheres for patients with colorectal liver metastases, *Radiother. Oncol.,* 25, 137, 1992.

39. **Kato, T., Nemoto, R., Mori, H., and Kumagai, I.,** Sustained release properties of microencapsulated mitomycin C with ethylcellulose infused into the renal artery of the dog, *Cancer,* 46, 14, 1980.

40. **Kato, T., Nemoto, R., Mori, H., Takahashi, M., and Tamakawa, Y.,** Transcatheter arterial chemoembolization of renal cell carcinoma with microencapsulated mitomycin C, *J. Urol.,* 125, 19, 1981.

41. **Kerr, D. J., Willmott, N., McKillop, J. H., Cummings, J., Lewi, H. J., and McArdle, C. S.,** Target organ disposition and plasma pharmacokinetics of doxorubicin incorporated into albumin microspheres after intrarenal arterial administration, *Cancer,* 62, 878, 1988.

42. **Lang, E. K.,** Superselective arterial catheterization of tumors of the urogenital tract: a modality used for perfusion with chemotherapeutic agents and infarction with radioactive pellets, *J. Urol.,* 104, 16, 1970.

43. **Lang, E. K. and Sullivan, J.,** Management of primary and metastatic renal cell carcinoma by transcatheter embolization with iodine-125, *Cancer,* 62, 274, 1988.

44. **Willmott, N.,** Drug delivery strategies in malignant disease of the lung, *Adv. Drug Delivery Rev.,* 5, 133, 1990.

45. **Llaurado, J. G., Brewer, L. A., Elam, D. A., Ing, S. J., Raiszadeh, M., Slater, J. M., Hirst, A. E., and Zielinski, F. W.,** Radioisotopic pulmonary lobectomy: feasibility study in dogs, *J. Nucl. Med.,* 31, 594, 1990.

46. **Okamoto, Y., Konno, A., Togawa, K., Kato, T., Tamakawa, Y., and Amano, Y.,** Arterial chemoembolization with cisplatin microcapsules, *Br. J. Cancer,* 53, 369, 1986.

47. **Martin, J. K., O'Connell, M. J., Wieand, H. S., Fitzgibbons, R. J., Mailliard, J. A., Rubin, J., Nagorney, D. M., Tschetter, L. K., and Krook, J. E.,** Intra-arterial floxuridine v systemic fluorouracil for hepatic metastases from colorectal cancer: a randomised trial, *Arch. Surg.,* 125, 1022, 1990.

48. **Rougier, P., Laplanche, A., Huguier, M., Hay, J. M., Ollivier, J. M., Escat, J., Salmon, R., Julien, M., Audy, J.-C., Gallot, D., Gouzi, J. L., Pailler, J. L., Elisa, D., Lacaine, F., Roos, S., Rotman, N., Luboinski, M., and Lasser, P.,** Hepatic arterial infusion of floxuridine in patients with liver metastases from colorectal carcinoma: long term results of a prospective, randomized trial, *J. Clin. Oncol.,* 10, 1112, 1992.

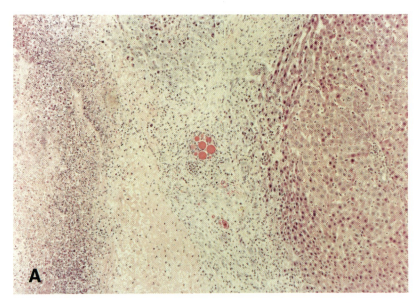

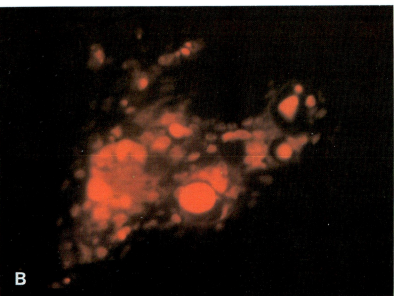

PLATE 1 (Chapter 3). (A) Histological section (hematoxylin-eosin) of Walker 256 hepatic tumor in a rat treated 4 days previously with doxorubicin-loaded albumin microspheres via the hepatic artery. Intra-arterial drug-loaded particles can be seen within viable tumor in the center of the field, necrotic tumor tissue is on the left, and normal liver is on the right. (B) Fluorescence photomicrograph of tumor tissue from a rat treated as in (A). Highly fluorescent intravascular fragments of drug-loaded particles can be seen as can lower intensity intracellular fluorescence. No fluorescence was detectable in tumors of animals treated with doxorubicin in solution. (From Goldberg, J.A., Willmott, N., Kerr, D.J., Sutherland, C., and McArdle, C.S., *Br. J. Cancer*, 65, 393, 1992. With permission.)

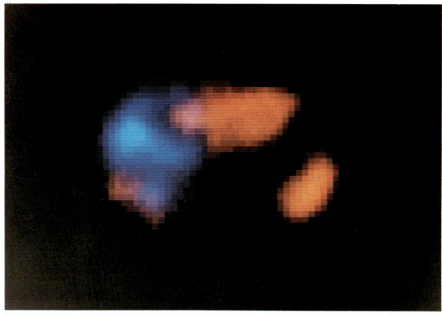

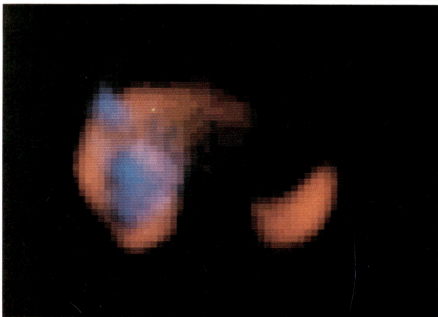

PLATE 2 (Chapter 8). Two examples of accurate tumor targeting with angiotensin II in patients with colorectal liver metastases. A slice from the ^{99m}Tc-colloid scan (orange) has been aligned with the corresponding slice from the study acquired after angiotensin II enhanced hepatic arterial perfusion scintigraphy with ^{99m}Tc-microspheres (blue).

Chapter 4

MAGNETICALLY CONTROLLED TARGETED CHEMOTHERAPY

P. K. Gupta and C. T. Hung

TABLE OF CONTENTS

0-8493-6952-5/94/$0.00 + $.50

I. INTRODUCTION

Theoretically, a diseased body compartment can be treated by administration of relevant drug into that biological unit; however, use of any conventional route of drug administration, e.g., intravenous (i.v.), intra-arterial (i.a.), or oral, does not allow drug to be concentrated in the area of interest without its comparable distribution to remaining healthy compartments of the body. This in turn requires administration of large amounts of drug, most of which is metabolized by normal tissues. In situations in which drug with low therapeutic index is prescribed, the amounts required for building up the effective concentrations in the diseased area may be too toxic for the remaining healthy tissues in the body. This is particularly true with all chemotherapeutic agents, which are an essential part of most cancer treatment schedules.[1,2] Hence, increased efforts have been made to confer regional or targeted drug delivery to diseased tissue or cells with reduced drug exposure to the normal cells.[2,3] It has been suggested that the therapeutic and toxic effects with cytotoxic agents are so closely balanced that even a slight change in drug distribution in favor of target tissue may be beneficial.[1] Hence, any approach that can improve tumor versus nontumor distribution of these agents is expected to increase their therapeutic efficacy. Attempts to improve therapeutic efficacy in cancer chemotherapy using modified dosage regimens, such as long-term low-dose infusion or short-term high-dose infusion of cytotoxic agents, have generally demonstrated limited benefit.[4-8] Hence, over the last two decades, several alternative drug delivery methods have been investigated for controlling the *in vivo* distribution of chemotherapeutic agents, including macromolecular drug conjugates[9] and a variety of particulate microcarrier systems with built-in specific characteristics, such as predetermined size, prolonged blood circulation time, responsiveness toward pH, temperature and magnetic field, reaction with target cell-specific epitopes, and controlled release of drug *in situ*.[10-14] Pharmacokinetic rationales of regional drug delivery have suggested the possibility of further improvement in chemotherapy following i.a. administration.[4,15] Among various regional drug delivery approaches, magnetically responsive systems have received considerable attention for targeted delivery of chemotherapeutic agents.[16,17] This chapter reviews the current status of this drug delivery method with particular emphasis on its application in the treatment

TABLE 1
Classification of Drug Targeting

Classification I
First-order
Second-order
Third-order
Classification II
Organ
Cellular
Subcellular
Classification III
Passive
Active
Physicochemical
Classification IV
Site-directed
Site-avoidance
Classification V
Biochemical
Biomechanical
Biophysical
Bioadhesive

of localized tumors. Following a brief discussion on the fundamentals and classification of drug targeting, the experiments conducted so far toward the development and evaluation of biodegradable and nonbiodegradable magnetically targeted drug delivery systems are summarized. Because magnetic albumin microspheres represent one of the most thoroughly investigated drug carriers for targeted chemotherapy,[16,17] detailed information on their methods of preparation, *in vitro* characterization, and efficacy in chemotherapeutic treatments is presented. Finally, the chapter outlines the future prospects and general limitations of magnetically controlled delivery systems in cancer chemotherapy.

II. DRUG TARGETING

Drug targeting is a phenomenon that maneuvers the distribution of drug in the body in such a manner that its major fraction interacts exclusively with the target tissue at cellular and/or subcellular level.[2] This is illustrated by the use of chemically modified chemotherapeutic agents and/or specialized drug delivery systems.[9-12] A specialized system could allow drug delivery to resistant cells, and sometimes also offer controlled, pulsed, and/or sustained-release properties, thus offering added benefit in terms of the frequency of parenteral dosing and overall improved patient compliance.[18]

Table 1 presents a list of various classifications of drug targeting. According to classification I, first-order drug targeting refers to the localization of drug at the capillary bed of the target site, organ, or tissue. Selective passage of the drug to tumor versus normal cells qualifies the phenomenon for second-order targeting, and the intracellular transport of drug due to cell fusion, endocytosis, or pinocytosis leads to the third-order drug targeting.[19] Implicitly, third-order targeting, which is also the most desirable level of drug delivery, is most difficult to accomplish because it requires solutions to the challenges of first- and second-order drug targeting.[19] This classification is analogous to classification II, i.e., organ, cellular, and subcellular targeting.[1,20] Whereas first-order targeting is determined mainly by the shape, size, and material properties of the carrier, and its route of administration, second- and third-order targeting are dependent upon a more specific interaction among the carrier, the drug, and the target cells.[1,19,20]

According to classification III, passive drug targeting utilizes natural *in vivo* deposition patterns of particulate material for drug delivery.[21,22] Effective drug targeting has been demonstrated by controlling the size of the drug carrier and its route of administration. For example, injection of drug-loaded particles ≥15 μm in diameter via the renal artery ensures efficient drug delivery to the kidneys. The targeted delivery of mitomycin C and 5-fluorouracil via albumin microspheres of 45 ± 8 μm in diameter has demonstrated promising results in the treatment of patients with inoperable hepatic cancer.[23] Active drug targeting requires guidance of drug, or drug carrier, to specific cells in a manner that differs from its normal disposition characteristics.[19] The carrier or technique designed for active targeting must possess characteristics that minimize drug removal by the normal cells of the body, particularly the phagocytes of the reticuloendothelial systems (RES). A good example of active drug targeting is the conjugation of drug to antibodies specific to the target cell antigens,[24] or its encapsulation in liposomes that release drug upon exposure to heat due to phase transition.[25] Physicochemical drug targeting refers to the use of carriers that release drug only in a specific environment, e.g., specific pH or enzyme, which is not available at any site other than the tumor tissue.[1] Indeed, pH- and temperature-sensitive liposomes have been explored for drug targeting.[25,26] As per classification IV, all the approaches that involve a passive, active, or physicochemical basis of drug delivery, and permit first-, second-, or third-order targeting, can be grouped under site-directed drug targeting. However, at times the use of a specific approach may not necessarily favor drug delivery to target cells; instead, it may reduce drug delivery to most vulnerable normal cells. This technique is regarded as site-avoidance drug targeting.[27,28] Application of cardiolipin liposomes to reduce the caridotoxicity of adriamycin is a good example of this type of drug delivery approach.[29]

Yet another way to classify drug targeting is based on the transport of carrier across the target tissue microvasculature.[27,28] Hence, according to classification V, biochemical targeting refers to extravascular transport due to specific interaction between target cell ligands and drug carrier, e.g., antigen-antibody binding. Biomechanical targeting refers to extravascular drug delivery due to transient, regional opening of endothelial junctions as a result of osmotic imbalance or anoxia following embolization. However, biophysical targeting refers to magnetic drag of responsive drug carrier through endothelium or use of temperature-sensitive drug carrier with concomitant regional hyperthermia. Bioadhesive targeting refers to a combination of biochemical and biophysical effects, e.g., a process in which specific binding of drug carrier to the endothelium is followed by transient alteration in the microvascular barrier, and it ultimately leads to the extravascular transfer of drug carrier.[27,28]

Absolute drug targeting requires use of an appropriate therapeutic system that allows interaction of near-total dose of the delivered drug exclusively with target cells. However, this is scarcely possible in routine practice. In most instances, complete eradication of the diseased target cells is not possible without some degree of destruction to normal healthy cells; thus, all therapeutic approaches currently available only allow partial drug targeting.[2] Nonetheless, irrespective of the type of therapeutic system and mechanism(s) used, and the level of specificity in cellular and/or subcellular drug delivery achieved, total eradication of the target cell population with no or minimal toxicity to nontarget cells is the single most critical factor that governs the ultimate success of targeted chemotherapy. Hence, absolute drug targeting not only requires altered *in vivo* kinetics of drug but also a significantly modified pharmacodynamic response in favor of the target cells.[2] It has been proposed that successful drug targeting should increase drug localization in target tissue by greater than or equal to half an order of magnitude, with drug levels in nontarget tissues increasing by $\leq 30\%$ of the increments achieved in the target tissue.[16]

III. MAGNETICALLY CONTROLLED DRUG TARGETING

A. PRINCIPLE

Magnetically controlled drug targeting is aimed at concentrating drug at a defined target site, generally away from the RES, with the aid of a magnetic field. Typically, the intended drug and a suitable magnetically active component, e.g., Fe_3O_4, are formulated into a pharmaceutically stable microcarrier system. It is then injected through the artery supplying the tumor tissue in the presence of an external magnet with sufficient field strength and gradient to retain the carrier at the target site. Prolonged retention of magnetic drug carrier at the target site impedes its RES clearance and facilitates extravascular uptake.

Historically, the concept of intravascular detection, estimation, and/or control of magnetically responsive materials with the aid of magnetic fields emerged in the 1960s, and later it was investigated for occlusion of intracerebral and renal aneurysms.[30-40] However, the problem of irreversible aggregation of native magnetic particles, in presence of a magnet, led researchers to investigate their coating and encapsulation in different polymeric systems.[41] Eventually, the technique was modified to incorporate drug in magnetic cells and microspheres, and tested for the possibility of magnetically controlled drug targeting.[42,43]

The process of drug localization using magnetic delivery systems is based on competition between forces exerted on the particles by the blood compartment and magnetic forces generated from the applied magnet. To effectively retain the magnetic drug carrier, the magnetic forces must exceed the linear blood flow rates in the tumor tissue vasculature, i.e., >10 cm/sec in arteries and >0.05 cm/sec in capillaries. It has been suggested that at the arteriocapillary blood flow rates of 0.05 to 0.1 cm/sec, an 8000 Gauss (G) magnet is sufficient to allow 100% localization of magnetic carrier containing 20% w/w of magnetite.[44] Ideally, the magnetic field is directed exclusively onto the tumor-bearing organ or tissue for a sufficient period to allow extravascular transfer of drug carrier. As will be discussed later, several factors influence the localization, extravascular transfer, and overall therapeutic outcome of magnetically controlled drug targeting. Recently, bioadhesion of delivery system to the endothelium of target tissue microvasculature, after its localization with the aid of an external magnet, has been proposed as a mechanism contributing toward specific drug delivery via magnetic carriers.[16]

One of the important characteristics of an ideal targetable drug delivery system is its ability to traverse the target tissue endothelium and release the included chemotherapeutic agent at cellular and/or subcellular level.[19,20] Indeed, it is also essential that the pharmacodynamic characteristics of the drug are not altered at any stage prior to reaching the target cells.[13] Although some studies have suggested the possibility of extravascular transport of submicron drug carriers through the vasculature of malignant tumor tissue due to their increased permeability,[45] from the therapeutic's standpoint, extremely small fractions of the administered dose of drug carrier ever reaches the target tissue interstitium. Even with monoclonal antibody-based delivery systems, the peak drug concentrations in tumor tissue are rarely 2- to 3-fold higher than the surrounding normal tissues.[46] In most instances the majority of carrier-delivered drug or macromolecular-conjugated drug is efficiently removed by the RES. Contrary to this standard *in vivo* deposition pattern, magnetic drug delivery systems offer unique characteristics in that they minimize drug carrier uptake by RES, facilitate its extravasation across the target tissue vasculature, and thus increase the probability of intracellular or third-order drug targeting.[19,43,45,47,48]

The rapid initial localization of magnetic drug carrier in the vascular bed of target tissue, in the presence of a magnetic field, is rarely affected by the biological differences that normally exist between healthy cells and diseased target cells, or by morphological differences that may exist in different regions of the same target tissue. However, once the carrier is retained, the biological differences (e.g., increased endothelial permeability or presence of specific endothelial determinants) in tumor tissue can accelerate carrier extravasation and hence drug delivery to the diseased cells. Controlled release of an encapsulated cytotoxic agent from the carrier localized at the cellular or subcellular level minimizes toxicity to normal tissues and injury to endothelium, which is normally observed following the systemic administration of chemotherapeutic agents.[49,50] It is therefore an attractive method of drug localization, provided that the target tissue has an abundant vascular supply and is accessible to magnetic fields. Investigations carried out using magnetic carriers have demonstrated a 5- to 50-fold increase in drug delivery to target tissue, and hence the therapeutic index of the delivered drug.[19,43,47,51-53] Similar levels of specificity in drug delivery and increase in the therapeutic index of chemotherapeutic agents have not been demonstrated so far with other targeted delivery systems.

B. INDICATIONS

Magnetic drug targeting allows localization of up to 70% of the administered dose in target tissue, with minimal interaction and toxicity to normal cells.[19,43] As will be shown later, this technique has demonstrated $\geq$8-fold increase in drug distribution to the target tissue at one third of the drug dose systemically administered as a solution, resulting in a relative increase in drug distribution to target tissue of 25-fold.[53] This dramatic change in drug distribution in favor of target tissue is believed to be due to multiple processes acting in harmony, i.e., effective transport of drug carrier to target tissue with minimal drug release in nontarget tissues during its transport, followed by local controlled release of drug in target tissue over an extended period of time with minimal flux of drug and/or drug carrier from target to nontarget tissues. These desirable characteristics, however, cannot be achieved in all experimental and clinical situations. The following general conditions have been suggested for the application of magnetically controlled drug targeting:[16]

1. When the exposure of blood components and nontarget tissues to the delivered agent is prohibitively toxic and unacceptable
2. When the drug is so unstable in biological fluids and tissues that it cannot be administered within practical guidelines of dosing volumes, and rate and/ or frequency of administration
3. When the drug is prohibitively expensive and does not allow $\geq$99% metabolic wastage in nontarget tissues
4. When the therapeutic outcome is dependent on selective *in vivo* localization of the delivered agent
5. When routine systemic treatments cannot be pursued or maintained due to life-threatening toxicities to vital body organs

C. LIMITATIONS

Magnetic drug targeting has generally demonstrated excellent therapeutic efficacy in various experimental animal models. However, this technique is not easy to pursue. There are several inherent limitations, including the following:

1. It requires a specialized drug carrier system and a magnet that fulfills the criteria of appropriate field strength, gradient, and geometry. These requirements make the technique expensive and rather scarce.
2. It is mainly applicable for the treatment of easily accessible tumors with well-defined blood supply and around which a magnet of appropriate size, strength, and geometry can be readily maneuvered.
3. Application of this technique for drug targeting to multiple body sites requires sequential treatment schedules.
4. It requires application of magnets with relatively constant field gradients to avoid focal overdosing of toxic compounds.

IV. CLASSIFICATION OF MAGNETICALLY CONTROLLED MICROCARRIER SYSTEMS

Over the last two decades several biodegradable and nonbiodegradable microcarrier systems have been explored for magnetically controlled drug targeting. Table

TABLE 2
Classification of Magnetically Controlled Targeted
Drug Delivery Systems

Class	Example	Ref.
Biodegradable		
Particulate carriers	Magnetic albumin microspheres	43, 45, 47, 48, 51, 52, 53, 118, 121
	Magnetic starch microspheres	56–58
	Magnetic poly(alkylcyanoacrylate) nanoparticles	59
Vesicular carriers	Magnetic emulsions	54,55
	Magnetic erythrocytes	78,87
	Magnetic liposomes	66,67
Nonbiodegradable		
Particulate carriers	Magnetic ethylcellulose microcapsules	76–79
	Magnetic polyglutaraldehyde nanoparticles	81

Modified from Gupta, P. K. and Hung, C. T., *Life Sci.*, 44, 175, 1989. With permission.

2 shows a general classification of these systems. The biodegradable magnetic drug carrier systems include emulsions, starch microspheres, poly(alkylcyanoacrylate) nanoparticles, erythrocytes, liposomes, neutrophils, and albumin microspheres. The nonbiodegradable magnetic drug carriers tested to date are limited to ethylcellulose microcapsules and polyglutaraldehyde nanoparticles. All these systems are briefly reviewed next. Details on the development and experimental evaluation of magnetic albumin microspheres for targeted chemotherapy are presented in Section V.

A. MAGNETIC EMULSIONS

Magnetic emulsions were among the early systems investigated for drug targeting. One group investigated the effect of magnetic field strength (0, 2000, 4000, or 6000 G) and field application time (10 or 60 min) on the localization of magnetic ethyloleate emulsion, containing ^{14}C-palmitic acid[54] or methyl-CCNU,[55] to the lung of rats. The results of these studies are summarized in Table 3. At 10 min after the tail vein administration of the magnetic emulsion containing ^{14}C-palmitic acid, the radioactivity in lungs was 1.78- to 2.3-fold higher in the presence of magnet compared with the control where no magnet was used. These levels in lung were 6 to 7 times higher than that in liver, spleen, kidney, and heart. However, at 60 min after administration, the radioactivity in lungs reduced appreciably with concurrent increase in the radioactivity in liver and heart. In addition, the increase in the magnet field strength did not demonstrate substantial increase in drug localization to the lung.[54] The evaluation of emulsion containing methyl-CCNU, however,

TABLE 3
Effect of Magnetic Field Strength and Field
Application Time on the Targeted Delivery of
Emulsions to the Lung of Rats

Magnetic field strength (Gauss)	^{14}C-Labeled emulsion (% injected radioactivity/g tissue)		Methyl-CCNU emulsion (μg/g tissue)
	10[a]	60 min[a]	10 min[a]
0	16.2	8.0	2.4
2000	28.9	10.5	5.2
4000	32.5	9.5	NE[b]
6000	37.2	10.5	15.1

[a] Refers to time for which the magnetic field was applied.
[b] Not evaluated.

Adapted from Morimoto, Y., Sugibayashi, K., and Akimoto, M., *Chem. Pharm. Bull.*, 31, 279, 1983, and Akimoto, M. and Morimoto, Y., *Biomaterials*, 4, 49, 1983. With permission.

demonstrated a remarkable increase in drug delivery to lung as a function of the magnetic field strength.[55] Unfortunately, these studies did not provide further information regarding the *in vivo* disposition of drug or magnetic emulsion as a function of time. Relatively low pharmaceutical stability, poor magnetic drag, and rapid drug release *in vivo* precluded their further development and testing for targeted drug delivery.

B. MAGNETIC STARCH MICROSPHERES

Limited work has been done toward the evaluation of magnetic starch microspheres for drug targeting.[56-58] This carrier system is typically prepared by adding heated (90°C) aqueous starch-magnetite slurry, with stirring, to toluene containing dissolved emulsifier at room temperature and then cooling the contents to 10°C. The stirring speed controls the size of the resulting microspheres.[56] They can be used to covalently couple compounds for drug targeting. In one case, the passage of ^{125}I-albumin or ^{14}C-ethanolamine coupled magnetic starch microspheres through the marginal ear vein of rabbits, in the presence of a 7000 G magnet applied for 10 min, demonstrated 4- to 8-fold increase in radioactivity in the target ear versus that recorded in the nontarget reference ear. However, immediately after removing the magnetic field, 80% of the injected radioactivity was detected in the lungs. The large size of the microspheres, 2 to 10 μm in diameter, accounted for this undesirable localization of the particles.[56]

Following i.v. administration of magnetic starch microspheres in the presence of a 5000 G electromagnet directed toward rabbit skulls, localization of microspheres in the superior part of brain was demonstrated histologically.[57] However, no further effort has been made to explore the full potential of this system in drug targeting.

C. MAGNETIC POLY(ALKYLCYANOACRYLATE) NANOPARTICLES

One study has investigated the application of magnetic poly(isobutylcyano-acrylate) nanoparticles in drug targeting.[59] Following i.v. administration to mice with their left kidney exposed to a 8500 G magnet for 10 min, the magnetic nanoparticle-adsorbed ^{3}H-dactinomycin was deposited 3 times more efficiently in the target kidney as opposed to the right kidney, which served as a control. When both kidneys of mice were exposed to 8500 G magnet for 10 min, the radioactivity in the kidneys was 3 times higher, and in liver one third lower, compared with the animals that were not exposed to magnetic field. However, no information was collected on distribution of radioactivity to other tissues.[59] Interestingly, the LD_{50} of these nanoparticles was found to be equivalent to nonmagnetic particles, i.e., 245 mg/kg.[59] Nonetheless, the chemical reactivity of the components used in the preparation of these particles appeared to complicate their regulatory approval for i.v. or i.a. drug delivery.

D. MAGNETIC ERYTHROCYTES

The clinical use of cell transfusions and the possibility of minimizing immunological complications by using a patient's own erythrocytes led to the investigation of magnetic erythrocytes for targeted drug delivery in cancer therapy.[42] According to one report, 10 to 20 nm magnetic particles can be easily incorporated in erythrocyte ghosts by applying an electric field intensity of 15 kV/cm and a pulse length of 50 μsec.[60] In addition, it has been suggested that the targeting efficiency of these carrier particles can be as high as 70% and their release profiles can be controlled by optimizing the stability of cell membranes.[60-62]

In a more recent study, application of a hypotonic dialysis technique allowed incorporation of 3 to 15% of the initially added magnetite in erythrocyte ghosts. The unincorporated magnetite was removed by using a 1200 G magnet for 5 min.[63] However, when tested *in vitro,* the magnetic erythrocytes lost their magnetic response with time. Cytotoxicity of high concentration magnetite to erythrocytes was suggested to cause cell damage and hence leakage of magnetite.[63] Application of magnetic erythrocytes for the localized delivery of acetyl salicylic acid to prevent platelet aggregation has also been investigated.[64] However, due to inadequate membrane stability, premature release of drug, and relatively poor efficiency of carrier particles to penetrate through tumor endothelium,[19,65] little effort has been made to further optimize this system for targeted chemotherapy.

E. MAGNETIC LIPOSOMES

Kiwada et al.[66] evaluated the feasibility of magnetically responsive liposomes for drug targeting. The liposomes were primarily composed of phosphatidylcholine, and they were prepared by evaporating a chloroform dispersion of lipid and magnetite and hydrating the lipid/magnetite crust with a buffer. The aggregated and/or unincorporated magnetite was removed by gel chromatography. Their study demonstrated a meager increase in the localization of ^{3}H-inulin delivered via this carrier in Yoshida sarcoma implanted in the foot pad of rats. It was suggested that increase in magnetic field strength may increase the tumor versus nontumor tissue distribution of drugs administered via this carrier.[66]

In another study, Ishii et al.[67] encapsulated magnetite and 5-fluorouracil in lipid vesicles composed of egg phosphatidylcholine and cholesterol. The vesicles were prepared by emulsifying an aqueous suspension of drug and magnetite in an ether solution of lipids. The resulting w/o emulsion was incorporated into aqueous hydrating media, with agitation, to obtain a w/o/w emulsion. Thereafter, the system was continuously stirred to evaporate ether and obtain lipid vesicles about 2 μm in diameter.[67] When injected into the upper artery of the ear of rabbits, >80% of the vesicles were found to be retained at the target site, suggesting good stability of the carrier system. However, no other *in vivo* information was collected in this study.

With respect to other classes of compounds, magnetic liposomes have demonstrated some success in the delivery of neuromuscular blocking agents.[68] However, despite the presence of magnetic field, the carrier particles were deposited in RES within a few hours after their administration.[68]

Liposomes traditionally possess relatively low stability *in vivo,* and it is believed that their stability would further decrease following the application of magnetic forces. For example, a static magnetic field $\geqslant 150$ G has been shown to increase passive transport of drug from phospholipid membrane bilayers near their phase transition temperature.[69] In addition, the preparation of magnetic liposomes with a reproducible response toward magnetic fields appears rather difficult.[19] For these reasons, this system has received limited attention for magnetically controlled drug targeting.

F. MAGNETIC ETHYLCELLULOSE MICROCAPSULES

Arterial chemoembolization is a relatively new technique that involves i.a. infusion of drug-loaded microcapsules into tumor tissue.[70-72] Due to their large size, typically 200 to 500 μm, these particles localize near the target site immediately after their administration. This, in turn, leads to ischemia and anoxia of tumor tissue. The sustained release of drug in high concentrations, from the localized carrier, increases its residence time in the tumor tissue.[70] Based on this principle, Kato et al. have extensively evaluated mitomycin C ethylcellulose microcapsules for the treatment of a variety of carcinomas.[70-75] Due to their physical characteristics, the microcapsules stay in the vascular compartment and are not transported to cellular or subcellular compartments. Although the intrinsic high permeability of tumor tissue and/or the increase in target tissue permeability due to anoxia is believed to assist in the transvascular transport of drug released from the microcapsules,[70] the observed high drug concentrations in the target tissue may not always guarantee equally high drug concentrations at intracellular target sites.

Drug-loaded ethylcellulose microcapsules have, however, demonstrated limited success in targeted drug delivery to carcinomas with arteriovenous fistula and complicated vascular supply.[70] To overcome these problems, ethylcellulose microcapsules with 16 to 50% w/w zinc ferrite and 30 to 50% w/w mitomycin C have

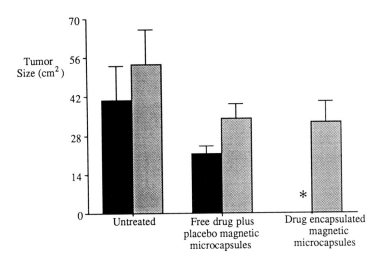

FIGURE 1.   Effect of presence (■) and absence (▨) of magnet along with various modes of treatment, on VX2 urinary bladder tumor size in rabbits at 14 days after transplantation and therapy. The treated groups received 10 mg mitomycin C physically mixed with placebo magnetic microcapsules or encapsulated in magnetic microcapsules. The microcapsules in the targeted therapy group were composed of 30% w/w drug, 50% w/w ferrite, and 20% w/w ethylcellulose. (*) Complete remission of tumor after therapy. The results are expressed as mean ± SD of four animals. (Adapted from Kato, T., Nemoto, R., Mori, H., Iwata, K., Sato, S., Unno, K., Murota, H., Echigo, M., Harada, M., and Homma, M., *J. Jpn. Soc. Cancer Ther.*, 15, 33, 1980. With permission.)

been developed for magnetic arterial chemoembolization.[76-80] In one study, the administration of 10 mg mitomycin C encapsulated in magnetic microcapsules in the presence of a 3500 G/cm magnet, to rabbits with VX2 bladder tumor demonstrated complete remission of tumor.[70,79] The untreated animals as well as the animals receiving a combination of placebo magnetic microcapsules plus drug solution in presence or absence of magnet did not respond to the therapy (Figure 1).[70,79] Similarly, the administration of 4 mg mitomycin C encapsulated in magnetic microcapsules to rabbits with VX2 tumors transplanted in their hind limb, in presence of a magnet applied for 30 min, led to complete tumor remission in 2 of 5 animals.[80] In addition, it controlled the growth of tumor in the remaining animals to ≤5 cm² over a period of 35 days. However, the control groups receiving either no treatment or an equivalent dose of drug solution demonstrated almost 13- and 6-fold greater tumor growth over the same period, respectively (Figure 2).[80]

G. MAGNETIC POLYGLUTARALDEHYDE NANOPARTICLES

Magnetic polyglutaraldehyde nanoparticles have been investigated *in vitro* for third-order active drug targeting.[81] This carrier system involves formulation of magnetic polyglutaraldehyde particles with free carboxyl groups, which are then covalently linked to a cytotoxic agent via a target cell-specific spacer.[81] The administration of this formulation in the presence of a magnet applied at the target tissue

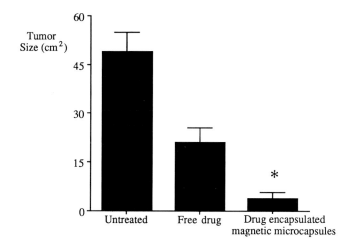

FIGURE 2. Effect of treatment type on VX2 tumor size transplanted in the hind limbs of rabbits. Different treatments were initiated on day 12 after transplantation, and outcome was measured on day 35 after transplantation. The treated groups received 4 mg mitomycin C alone or encapsulated in magnetic microcapsules. The microcapsule composition was as described in Figure 1. (*) 40% (2 of 5) tumor remission in the group receiving targeted chemotherapy. The results are expressed as mean ± SD of four or five animals. (Adapted from Kato, T., Nemoto, R., Mori, H., Abe, R., Unno, K., Goto, A., Murota, H., Harada, M., and Homma, M., *Appl. Biochem. Biotechnol.*, 10, 199, 1984. With permission.)

ensures carrier retention and perhaps its extravascular transfer to target cells. Use of an appropriate carrier material and spacer is expected to assist its intracellular uptake where the lysosomal enzymes trigger the release of drug. In a preliminary study, the incubation of polyglutaraldehyde nanoparticles ≤ 1 μm in diameter (encapsulating 8% w/w of magnetite and bearing up to 250×10^{-7} mol/g of surface carboxyl groups), in a buffer containing poly-L-lysine-methotrexate conjugate (256 μg drug/mg spacer), resulted in covalent linkage of 50% conjugate to the surface of the particles. The *in vivo* efficacy of this system for magnetically controlled drug targeting remains to be evaluated.

H. MAGNETIC NEUTROPHILS

Ranney and Huffaker[28] investigated the feasibility of targeting neutrophils containing ingested Fe_3O_4 to sites of severe infection. The magnetite particles were opsonized with human IgG to facilitate neutrophil binding and ingestion via Fc receptors. On a weight basis, the magnetite content of the neutrophils was between 0.8 to 2.2%. About 0.5 to 1×10^6 adherent cells were injected i.v. into neutropenic mice and a 5500 G magnet was applied perpendicular to the right chest wall for 20 min postdosing. At 40 min after dosing, the magnetic localization increased neutrophils in lung by 2.6-fold. Because neutrophil localization was apparent even in the absence of magnet (Figure 3), carrier bioadhesion to pulmonary vascular endothelium was suggested as an additional mechanism contributing toward their

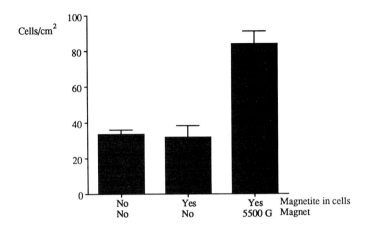

FIGURE 3. Localization of magnetic neutrophils in the lung of neutropenic mice at 40 min after their i.v. administration in the presence and absence of 5500 G magnet with gradient of 100 G/mm. The magnet was applied for 20 min after dose administration. (Adapted in part from Ranney, D. F. and Huffaker, H. H., *Ann. NY Acad. Sci.*, 507, 104, 1987. With permission.)

site-specific deposition and retention. This observation suggested bioadhesion as one of the possible mechanisms in magnetically controlled drug targeting.[27,28]

I. BIOADHESIVE MAGNETIC GRANULES

Ito et al.[82] proposed the application of bioadhesive magnetic granules for oral targeted chemotherapy of esophageal cancer. A variety of magnetic granules were prepared using combinations of different bioadhesive polymers, e.g., carboxymethylcellulose, hydroxypropylmethylcellulose, carbomer 934, tragacanth, carrageenan, and alginate. The *in vivo* studies in rabbits involved oral delivery of 5 mg granules containing 50% ferrite (γ-Fe_2O_3) and brilliant blue FCF, with 2 ml of 0.65% hydroxypropylcellulose H solution, in the presence of a 1900 G magnetic circuit applied around the esophagus. Although the magnetic field was applied for only 2 min after dosing, ~18% brilliant blue was detected in the target region of the esophagus at 2 h after administration of the granules. However, increase in the application time of magnet to 2 h did not improve localization of brilliant blue or ferrite.[82] The efficacy of this system in an appropriate cancer model remains to be investigated.

V. MAGNETIC ALBUMIN MICROSPHERES IN TARGETED CHEMOTHERAPY

A. BACKGROUND

Albumin microspheres are biodegradable colloidal particles, which can be readily formulated in the size range 1 to 200 μm.[83] Magnetic albumin microspheres, in general, share all the advantages of nonmagnetic microspheres. The information on their methods of preparation, physicochemical characterization, and evaluation for active drug targeting is reviewed next.

B. METHODS OF PREPARATION

The preparation of magnetic albumin microspheres involves the application of emulsion and suspension technologies (Figure 4).[84] Their routine synthesis utilizes an aqueous solution of albumin, a therapeutic agent dissolved or uniformly suspended in it, a magnetically active component, e.g., Fe_3O_4, suspended in the aqueous medium, and a suitable oil to form a w/o emulsion. The emulsification step requires ultrasonication to produce microspheres $\leqslant 1$ μm in diameter. Once a stable emulsion is formed, the albumin in the dispersed phase is cross-linked so as to form rigid particles, minimize their coalescence, and assist their isolation. Thereafter, excess oil is removed by washing the particles with a nonaqueous solvent, e.g., anhydrous ether, which does not interfere with the stability of drug and/or the microspheres. This step also assists in the removal of excess chemical cross-linking agent.[19] Thereafter, the unencapsulated magnetite is removed from the formulation by gel chromatography or application of a low strength magnet.[85]

Two methods are popular for the stabilization of magnetic albumin microspheres: (1) heat denaturation at temperatures between 90 to 180°C typically for $\leqslant 10$ min.[19,28,43,47,48,51-53,84] and (2) chemical stabilization using a suitable cross-linking agent, e.g., formaldehyde, glutaraldehyde, 2,3-butane-dione, or terephthaloyl dichloride.[19,86] The selection of the degree of microsphere stabilization is based on the intended biological half-life of these particles. The use of high temperatures for heat stabilization or concentrated aldehyde reagents for chemical cross-linking can allow fast yet efficient protein denaturation. However, unfavorable interactions between therapeutic agent and the process of stabilization may limit the choice of the processing technique. For example, adriamycin is heat-decomposed at temperatures >120°C,[87,88] formaldehyde interacts with epinephrine,[89] and glutaraldehyde interferes with methotrexate and salbutamol.[89]

Modifications of the aforementioned methods have been investigated for the preparation of albumin microspheres, e.g., using hydrophobic poly-(methylmethacrylate) or hydrophilic polyoxyethylene-polyoxypropylene block copolymer as dispersing agents,[90] a single-step heat denaturation of aerosolized solution,[91] interfacial polymerization technique,[92] and coacervation technique.[93] However, the feasibility of these methods to encapsulate magnetite and hence allow the formulation of magnetic albumin microspheres has not been reported.

C. PHYSICOCHEMICAL CHARACTERIZATION

In view of the fact that magnetic albumin microspheres are intended to be used parenterally, it is essential that these particles be rigorously characterized for their size and size distribution, drug encapsulation efficiency, magnetite encapsulation efficiency, drug release mechanism and release rates, stability of drug and carrier upon storage in a dry state and as a suspension in a suitable aqueous medium, and for any other parameter that may affect their application. Indeed, better understand-

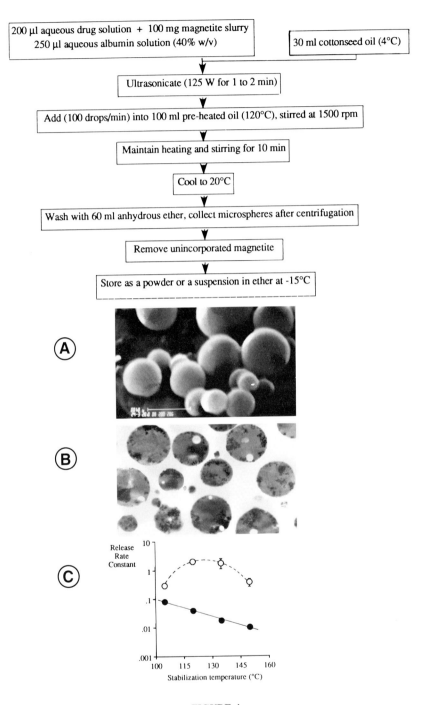

FIGURE 4.

ing of the physicochemical properties of drug encapsulated magnetic microspheres can be of value in gaining a better appreciation of their *in vivo* fate. The current information on the physicochemical characteristics of magnetic albumin microspheres for targeted chemotherapy is discussed next.

1. Particle Size and Hydration

The particle size of a drug carrier can generally affect the degree of drug entrapment, drug release profile, hydration characteristics, and distribution pattern and toxicity after *in vivo* administration.[2,12,13,21] Several studies have demonstrated that magnetic albumin microspheres can be readily prepared in the size range of 0.2 to 2 μm, with the major fraction ≤1 μm.[16,17,19] Factors that typically affect the size and size distribution of nonmagnetic albumin microspheres have been exhaustively evaluated;[83] however, all of these factors have not been investigated for magnetic microspheres. In our laboratory, we have found that for albumin microspheres prepared by heat stabilization between 105 to 150°C, the presence of 0.5 to 3% w/w adriamycin HCl and/or 16 to 22% w/w Fe_3O_4 does not influence their size and size distribution. In all cases, their mean diameter ranged between 0.68 ± 0.39 to 0.75 ± 0.44 μm.[84]

Magnetic albumin microspheres hydrate and swell in aqueous medium. For example, following incubation in saline at 37°C, microspheres prepared at 135°C swelled as a function of time at a rate of about 0.24 μm/h for 2 h; however, no detectable change in the particle diameter was noticed upon further hydration (Figure 5). Irrespective of their stabilization temperature, the size of the microspheres after 2 h of hydration in saline was significantly greater (40 to 80%) than those of the dry, unhydrated microspheres.[84] Also, after hydration for 2 h, the size of the adriamycin-encapsulated magnetic albumin microspheres stabilized at 105 or 120°C was significantly greater (~20%) than those stabilized at 135 or 150°C. This was attributed to greater tortuosity/lower porosity of microspheres stabilized at ≥135°C than those stabilized at ≤120°C.[84] Another interesting observation of this study was that the hydration and swelling of microspheres was associated with formation of pores and cavities, the extent of which increased with the increase in the incubation time.[84]

2. Drug Encapsulation

The higher the degree of drug encapsulation in a delivery system, the smaller the dose required for a specified pharmacological response. This in turn ensures

FIGURE 4. The steps involved in the preparation of magnetic albumin microspheres by heat denaturation. (A) Scanning electron photomicrograph of adriamycin-encapsulated magnetic albumin microspheres. (Original magnification ×7000.) Note the 1.0 μm line. (B) Transmission electron micrograph of adriamycin-encapsulated magnetic albumin microspheres after hydration in an aqueous medium for 2 h. (Original magnification ×7000.) (C) The effect of stabilization temperature on initial (○) and terminal (●) drug release rate constants (μg/mg/h). Note the log-linear relationship for the terminal release phase. (Adapted from Gupta, P. K., Hung, C. T., Lam, F. C., and Perrier, D. G., *Int. J. Pharm.*, 43, 167, 1988. With permission.)

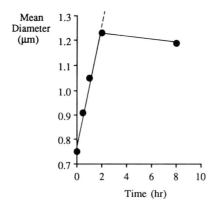

FIGURE 5. Typical change in the diameter of heat denatured magnetic albumin microspheres containing adriamycin HCl as a function of incubation time in saline at 37°C. This plot shows results of microspheres stabilized at 135 ± 5°C. The relationship between microsphere size (Y) and incubation time (X) up to 2 h can be expressed according to the relationship: $Y = 0.778 + 0.236 \, X$; $R^2 \geq 0.979$. (Adapted from Gupta, P. K., Hung, C. T., Lam, F. C., and Perrier, D. G., *Int. J. Pharm.*, 43, 167, 1988. With permission.)

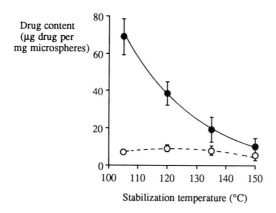

FIGURE 6. Effect of stabilization temperature and carrier washing on the adriamycin content of magnetic albumin microspheres: (●) fresh microspheres and (○) microspheres washed four times with normal saline. Note that the drug content of fresh microspheres represents efficiency in drug recovery, whereas the drug content of washed microspheres represents efficiency of drug entrapment. (Adapted from Gupta, P. K., Hung, C. T., Lam, F. C., and Perrier, D. G., *Int. J. Pharm.*, 43, 167, 1988. With permission.)

overall reduced toxicity due to carrier and/or other formulation components. Limited efforts have been made to optimize the encapsulation of drug in magnetic albumin microspheres (however, see Chapter 1). Investigation of the effect of temperature during heat stabilization has revealed that microspheres prepared at about 120°C allow better entrapment of adriamycin than those heat-stabilized at lower or higher temperatures (Figure 6). Although the use of temperatures ≤120°C allow higher overall recovery of adriamycin in the formulation, the majority of this drug is loosely bound on the surface of the particles and released immediately following suspension in an aqueous medium. At temperatures $>120°C$, adriamycin is heat-decomposed.[84,88] It is, however, possible that for heat-stable drugs the use of higher stabilization temperatures may improve their encapsulation efficiency in this delivery system. The presence of Fe_3O_4 in albumin microspheres has also been shown to reduce their drug encapsulation efficiency.[84]

Although variations in drug and polymer concentrations, use of chemical cross-linking methods, and control of the size of the microspheres could allow further improvements in drug encapsulation,[83] these parameters have not been thoroughly optimized for magnetic albumin microspheres.

3. Magnetite Encapsulation

The localization of magnetic microspheres at a given target site is governed by the magnetite content of the carrier and the magnitude of the applied magnetic field.[44,70,84] The relationship between force on particles (F), magnetic field gradient (∇H), and magnetic moment of particles (M) can be expressed according to the relationship:

$$F = M * \nabla H \tag{1}$$

It is therefore apparent that increase in the magnetic moment of particles can allow the use of smaller magnetic field gradients for the retention and extravascular transfer of drug magnetic carrier. However, a high degree of magnetite encapsulation can reduce the efficiency of drug entrapment.[61,84] Hence, it is important that the encapsulation of drug and magnetite be delicately balanced. In one study, the determination of microsphere Fe_3O_4 content using atomic absorption spectroscopy revealed that the carrier stabilization temperature has little effect on the encapsulation of magnetite; however, the presence of adriamycin increased its incorporation slightly and this increase was statistically significant ($p = 0.0014$).[84] In general, 18 to 23% w/w of Fe_3O_4 can be readily incorporated in albumin microspheres along with 0.5 to 5% w/w of adriamycin (Figure 7).[19,84,86] The transmission electron photomicrographs of adriamycin encapsulated magnetic albumin microspheres revealed that magnetite is distributed throughout the peripheral region (Figure 4B). Such a distribution of magnetite in microsphere matrix has been suggested to promote their magnetic response.[19,44]

4. Drug Release

The therapeutic efficacy of a delivery system is also dependent upon its drug release mechanism and drug release rate at the target site. Prolonged release of the incorporated drug in a controlled manner would minimize the frequency of dose administration and reduce toxic effects due to conventional burst release of drug. In the case of magnetic albumin microspheres, the drug release mechanism is dependent on the site(s) of location of drug in the carrier as well as on the properties of the microsphere matrix. Of the total drug incorporated in the formulation, typ-

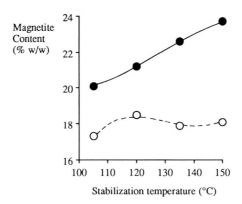

FIGURE 7.   Effect of stabilization temperature and presence of drug (adriamycin HCl) on the encapsulation of magnetite in albumin microspheres: (●) microspheres containing drug and (○) microspheres without drug. (Adapted from Gupta, P. K., Hung, C. T., Lam, F. C., and Perrier, D. G., *Int. J. Pharm.*, 43, 167, 1988. With permission.)

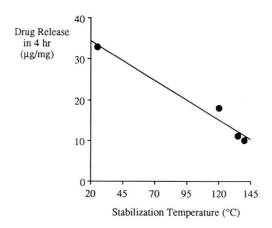

FIGURE 8.   Effect of stabilization temperature of magnetic albumin microspheres on the release of adriamycin in 4 h. In this study the drug release from microspheres was found to follow a first-order mechanism and the data could be described according to the relationship: Release (μg/mg) = 38.28 − 0.193*Stabilization temperature (°C), $R^2 \geqslant 0.966$. (Adapted from Widder, K. J., Senyei, A. E., and Scarpelli, D. G., *Proc. Soc. Exp. Biol. Med.*, 158, 141, 1978. With permission.)

ically a fraction is adsorbed on the particle surface and the remainder is encapsulated in the matrix. These factors collectively govern its release mechanism. Initially, the release of adriamycin from the magnetic albumin microspheres was suggested to follow a first-order mechanism, and the control of the matrix stabilization temperature resulted in formulations with drug release half-times varying between 0.25 to 8 h and release over 4 h varying between 10 to 33 μg/mg (Figure 8).[19,43,87] However, in our laboratory, magnetic albumin microspheres have been found to follow zero-order release of adriamycin according to the relationship:

$$dQ/dt = k_o \cdot C_m \qquad (2)$$

where dQ/dt is the rate of release of drug, k_o is the zero-order release rate constant, and C_m is the concentration of drug in the microspheres, which is taken to be constant.[95] Fresh, unwashed microspheres exhibited a triphasic release pattern; however, when the microspheres were tested for *in vitro* release after removing the loosely bound drug, they were found to follow biphasic drug release. The release rate of adriamycin depended upon the presence of magnetite as well as carrier stabilization temperature, and initial drug release rate was 40 to 100 times higher than the terminal release rate.[84] The initial drug release rate from the microspheres prepared at 120°C was higher than from the ones stabilized at lower or higher temperatures (Figure 4C). Interestingly, this correlates well with the maximal drug encapsulation in microspheres stabilized at 120°C (Figure 6). This, in turn, suggests that drug-loading efficiency may influence the initial release rate of drug. Once the initial drug release phase is complete, which takes between 2 to 8 h depending upon the stabilization temperature and hence upon the drug content, the terminal drug release phase lasts for ≥ 80 h. The regression analysis of the terminal drug release rate constant of microspheres as a function of their stabilization temperature demonstrated the following relationship (Figure 4C):[84]

$$\ln (\text{release rate constant}) = 2.41 - 0.047* (\text{stabilization temperature}) \qquad (3)$$

The decrease in terminal drug release rate with the increase in stabilization temperature of microspheres is probably a result of increased tortuosity and hydrophobicity and, hence, slow hydration of the particles.[84,96] Regardless of their stabilization temperature, the presence of magnetite was also found to decrease the terminal release rate of adriamycin from microspheres. This observation was attributed to comparatively lower drug content, and perhaps relatively greater hydrophobicity of magnetic microspheres.[84] Hence, it is possible that changes in the magnetite content of microspheres, without appreciably compromising their magnetic responsiveness, may allow an alternative means of controlling the release rate of drug.

5. Stability

It has been suggested that magnetic microspheres can be stored for 1 year at 22°C without loss of drug potency.[28] It has also been shown that adriamycin encapsulated albumin microspheres can be freeze-dried without loss of drug.[97] It is therefore possible that magnetic albumin microspheres could be stabilized for long-term use by application of this technique.

D. TISSUE DISTRIBUTION STUDIES

The first study on the *in vivo* efficacy of magnetic albumin microspheres for targeted chemotherapy was conducted by Widder et al.[43] The microspheres contained 9% w/w of adriamycin with 50% available for controlled release, and 20% w/w of Fe_3O_4. Rat tail was used as a target organ. It was demarcated into four

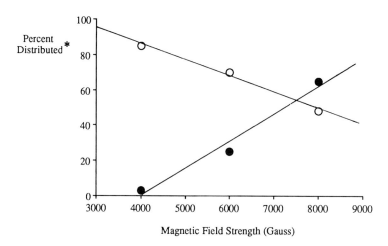

FIGURE 9.   Effect of magnetic field strength on the distribution of magnetic ^{125}I-albumin microspheres to the tail target site (●) and liver (○). For the target site, the relationship established was: % distributed = 0.0155* Magnetic strength − 62.0, R^2 > 0.973, and a similar relationship for the liver was percent distributed = 123.17 − 0.0093* Magnetic strength, R^2 > 0.988. (Adapted from Widder, K. J., Senyei, A. E., and Scarpelli, D. G., *Proc. Soc. Exp. Biol. Med.*, 158, 141, 1978. With permission.)

equal regions, 3.5 cm each, which were called T1, T2, T3, and T4, respectively, from the base of the tail. T1 was used for the i.a. administration of microspheres and T3 as the predetermined target site. In the first study, 0.5 mg of ^{125}I-magnetic albumin microspheres was administered at T1 in absence and presence of a 4000, 6000, or 8000 G magnet applied at T3 for 30 min. The results of this study are shown in Figure 9. The data collected at 30 min after dosing demonstrated a linear increase in radioactivity at the target site as a function of the magnetic field strength (r^2 = 0.973). Although application of the magnet could not prevent carrier distribution to the liver, the increase in magnetic strength generally reduced carrier distribution to this nontarget organ (r^2 = 0.988). Shunting by blood vessels around the target region was suggested as the possible cause of the undesirable microsphere distribution to the RES. Interestingly, even at 24 h after dose administration, high levels of radioactivity were detected at T3.[43] The extravascular transfer of carrier during magnetic field exposure was suggested to prevent its delocalization and redistribution after the magnet was removed.[43] This study also monitored drug concentrations at target site and in liver at 30 min after the administration of drug as a solution or via the microspheres. The i.a. administration of 0.05 mg/kg adriamycin via magnetic albumin microspheres in the presence of an 8000 G magnet was shown to deliver ~4 μg/g drug to the target site and <1 μg/g drug to the liver. When the drug was administered i.v. as a solution, a 5.0 mg/kg dose was required to achieve comparable drug concentrations at the target site, with drug levels in liver exceeding 15 μg/g (Figure 10). Hence, the administration of drug via magnetic albumin microspheres allowed a 100-fold reduction in dose along with ≥15-fold reduction in drug delivery to the general circulation. The estimation of

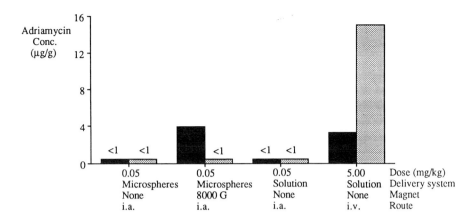

FIGURE 10. Effect of dose (0.05 vs. 5.0 mg/kg), dosage form (drug solution vs. magnetic microspheres) and route of administration (i.a. vs. i.v.) on drug concentrations at the target site (■) and liver (▧) at 30 min after administration. (Adapted in part from Widder, K. J., Senyei, A. E., and Scarpelli, D. G., *Proc. Soc. Exp. Biol. Med.*, 158, 141, 1978. With permission.)

targeting efficiency of the two drug delivery strategies, by comparing the ratio of drug concentration at target site versus liver, suggested almost 18-fold higher efficiency of magnetic microspheres at 100-fold smaller dose. This in turn highlights the extent of selectivity in drug delivery that could be achieved with magnetic microcarrier systems.

In subsequent experiments, these workers found that at 60 min after dosing, an i.a. dose of 0.05 mg/kg adriamycin via magnetic albumin microspheres, administered in presence of an 8000 G magnet, produced target site drug concentrations twice as high as that obtained with 5 mg/kg i.v. drug solution.[98] Also, the drug could not be detected in pooled nontarget organs following the administration of drug via microspheres; however, 8 μg/g drug was monitored in the pooled organs following the i.v. administration of 5 mg/kg drug solution, and these levels were 4-fold higher than that recorded at the target site.[98]

Ovadia et al.[99] evaluated the effect of the type of magnet on the targeting efficiency of magnetic albumin microspheres. A selected rat tail segment, the hind leg, and the head of animals were independently considered as target sites. In the rat tail model similar to that discussed above,[19,43] it was found that a 4200 G custom-made bar magnet, with a field gradient of 2700 G/cm at pole face, is as effective as a 7000 G horseshoe magnet with a gradient of 4000 G/cm. In either case, 30 to 50% of the injected dose could be localized at the target site. Hence, it was suggested that the magnetic responsiveness of the microspheres may achieve saturation at magnetic field strengths >4000 G.[99] In the hind leg model, only 18 to 25% of the dose could be localized at the target site. When targeted to the head, most of the microspheres were retained within the skin and in the soft tissues. Meager microsphere localization was obtained in the bone and no localization could be achieved in the brain. Alteration in the permeability of blood-brain barrier did not improve brain localization of the microspheres. This study therefore suggested that the complexity of target site vasculature and its depth and permeability may restrict wide application of magnetic albumin microspheres for targeted drug delivery.[99]

Morimoto et al.[100] reported the results of two sets of *in vivo* experiments with magnetic albumin microspheres. In the first experiment, 1 mg of 1 or 3 μm ^{125}I-magnetic albumin microspheres was administered i.v. to the lungs of mice in the presence of a 3000 G magnet. The microspheres contained about 50% magnetite by weight. At 10 min after dosing, the 1 μm microspheres administered in the presence of the magnet concentrated in the lungs 3 to 4 times more than those administered in absence of magnet. However, the magnetic field did not affect the distribution of 1 μm magnetic microspheres to liver, spleen, or kidney. The use of 3 μm microspheres substantially improved their lung versus liver distribution. The dose reaching the lung was at least 3-fold higher than that reaching the liver. Hence, microsphere size was suggested to be a critical factor influencing their localization in the lungs. However, this study did not evaluate the long-term *in vivo* fate of 1 or 3 μm microspheres.[100] In the second experiment, the right kidney of rats was used as the target organ and exposed to a 3000 G magnet. At 10 min after the administration of 1 mg microspheres, the presence of magnet increased the radioactivity in the target organ by 2.5-fold. The application of magnet for 60 min maintained the radioactivity levels in the target organ. However, once again, no information was collected regarding the long-term fate of microsphere distribution after removal of the magnet.[100]

In their subsequent study, Morimoto et al.[101] monitored the localization of micron-sized ^{125}I-magnetic albumin microspheres in the lungs and the left kidney of mice and rats, respectively. In both experiments 3000 G magnets were applied for 10 or 60 min postdosing and the radioactivity at the target site was monitored at 10 and 60 min after dosing. When the magnets were used throughout the experiment in mice, the lung radioactivity increased from 17% of the injected dose at 10 min to 28.2% at 60 min. However, when the magnet was applied for only 10 min, the radioactivity at 60 min decreased substantially compared with that at 10 min.[101] In the case of rats, when the magnet was applied to their left kidney throughout the experiment, no increase in the localization of radioactivity was noticed at 60 min compared with that at 10 min; however, when the magnet was applied only for 10 min, the radioactivity decreased from 56.4% of the injected dose at 10 min to 25.5% at 60 min. The reduction in radioactivity in the target kidney was associated with concurrent increase in the liver radioactivity levels. The redistribution of microspheres over a period of time after the removal of magnetic field was suggested as the cause of this observation. It was therefore hypothesized that an increase in magnetic field application time may improve microsphere retention at the target site.[101]

It is apparent that initial studies[43,98-101] demonstrated moderate to high levels of improvement in drug distribution to target organ as a result of its administration via magnetic microspheres compared with that observed with conventional delivery systems. None of these studies, however, evaluated quantitative changes in drug distribution due to magnetic microspheres, at target as well as nontarget sites, as

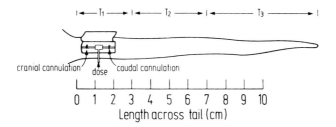

FIGURE 11. The tail target site and cannulation of ventral caudal artery. The dose was administered at T1. The middle segment T2 was considered as the target site and exposed to an 8000 G magnet in experiments involving administration of adriamycin magnetic microspheres in the presence of magnetic field.

a function of time. Hence, the studies conducted in our laboratory were specifically aimed at quantitatively comparing the disposition of adriamycin administered via magnetic albumin microspheres in the presence of a magnet versus drug administered as a solution or via magnetic microspheres in the absence of a magnet. In all experiments, a rat tail model similar to that discussed earlier, but with only three demarcated segments (T1, the pretarget site; T2, the target site; and T3, the post-target site), was used. The ventral caudal artery at T1 was used for dose administration (Figure 11).

Our initial attempts concentrated on the evaluation of the target as well as nontarget tissue disposition of 2 mg/kg adriamycin HCl infused i.a. over 1 min as a solution or via magnetic albumin microspheres suspended in saline. The magnetic microsphere formulation was infused in the presence of an 8000 G magnet applied at T2 for 30 min postdosing. After the drug administration as a solution or via microspheres, the animals were killed over a 48-h period, and various tissues analyzed for drug concentration using an HPLC method specific for adriamycin, its metabolites, and degradation products resulting from microsphere synthesis.[88,102] Details regarding animal preparation, tissue sample processing for drug extraction, and data analysis have been reported in original publications.[103,104]

Figure 12 shows mean drug concentrations over a period of 48 h in the target tissue, heart, and liver following administration of 2 mg/kg adriamycin HCl as a solution and via magnetic albumin microspheres. Drug levels at T2 were maintained at least 25 to 50% higher with the microspheres than those achieved with the drug solution. The microspheres increased the maximal drug concentration at T2 by a factor of 3. This resulted in an increase in target-tissue drug area under the curve (AUC) by almost 60%. In addition, the microspheres resulted in 50 to 100% reduction in drug levels in heart, with peak drug levels and AUC reducing by 70 and 65%, respectively (Figure 13). The adriamycin magnetic microspheres, however, increased drug levels in the liver by 25 to 50% (Figure 12) and its AUC by 100% (Figure 13). Hence, in this study the magnetic albumin microspheres were found to enhance drug delivery to the liver more readily than that to the target site.

The ability of magnetic microspheres to deliver drug preferentially to the liver is undesirable: the observation could be explained in terms of the saturation of

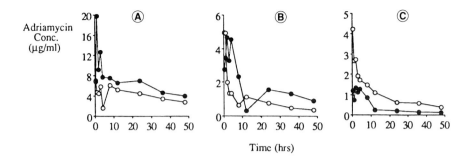

FIGURE 12. Adriamycin concentrations as a function of time in the target tissue (A) liver (B) and heart (C), following the i.a. administration of 2.0 mg/kg drug as a solution (○) and via magnetic albumin microspheres in presence of an 8000 G magnet applied for 30 min (●). Each point represents the mean of three rats. (Adapted from Gallo, J. M., Gupta, P. K., Hung, C. T., and Perrier, D. G., *J. Pharm. Sci.*, 78, 190, 1989. With permission.)

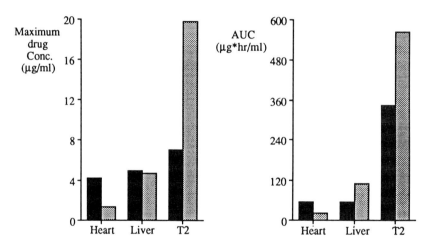

FIGURE 13. Maximal drug concentrations and AUC for heart, liver, and target tissue following the i.a. administration of 2.0 mg/kg drug as a solution (■) and via magnetic albumin microspheres in the presence of an 8000 G magnet applied for 30 min (▨). (Adapted in part from Gallo, J. M., Gupta, P. K., Hung, C. T., and Perrier, D. G., *J. Pharm. Sci.*, 78, 190, 1989. With permission.)

target tissue microvasculature. It is probable that at the dose of about 50 mg microspheres/250 g rat required to deliver 2.0 mg/kg adriamycin, the transport processes, including endocytosis and passage through the endothelial cell gaps, were saturated.[19] The rate and extent of extravascular transfer of microspheres through healthy endothelium are believed to be dependent on the characteristics of the applied magnet. The greater the magnetic field strength, the higher the initial rate of extravascular uptake, and the longer the magnetic field is applied, the greater the extent of extravascular transfer of magnetic microspheres. Once the magnetic field is removed, the microspheres in the vascular compartment would be expected

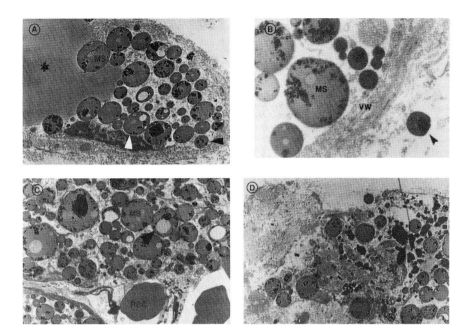

FIGURE 14. Transmission electron microscope photomicrographs of target tissue samples from rats dosed with adriamycin-loaded magnetic albumin microspheres in the presence of an 8000 G magnet and killed over a period of 72 h after dosing. (A) Target tissue samples collected at 0.5 h after dosing (Original magnification × 15,000.) Note the presence of microspheres (MS) within vascular compartment. The indentations on nuclei (white arrow) and the vessel wall (VW) (black arrow) are clear.* The lumen of the vessel contains plasma or serum. No RBC is seen in this section. (B) Target tissue samples collected at 2 h after dosing. (Original magnification × 30,000.) Most of the microspheres (MS) are seen within the vascular channels. One microsphere (solid arrow) is seen in the extravascular compartment. The blood vessel wall (VW) appears normal. (C) Target tissue samples collected at 8 h after dosing. (Original magnification × 10,000.) Large number of microspheres (MS) are present in tissue spaces along with RBC. Some microspheres show vacuolation and/or aggregation of magnetite particles (solid arrow). (D) Target tissue samples collected at 72 h after dosing. (Original magnification × 12,000.) The microspheres are seen in extravascular tissue spaces, and the advanced degenerative changes in the surrounding tissue is evidenced by its fragmentation and total loss of organization. (Adapted from Gupta, P. K., Hung, C. T., and Rao, N. S., *J. Pharm. Sci.*, 78, 290, 1989. With permission.)

compartment would be expected to be deposited in the RES. Hence, carrier dose and magnetic field characteristics appear to be the two most critical factors influencing the efficacy of magnetically controlled drug targeting.

To understand the mechanism for the modest increase in drug delivery to the target site and assess the probability of extravascular transfer of magnetic microspheres in healthy tissue, a group of animals given 2 mg/kg adriamycin via albumin magnetic microspheres, in presence of an 8000 G magnet applied at T2 for 30 min, were examined for the ultrastructural disposition of carrier at the target site.[48] Figure 14 displays sequential scanning electron photomicrographs of the transendothelial transfer of magnetic microspheres at the target site over a period of 72 h. At 0.5

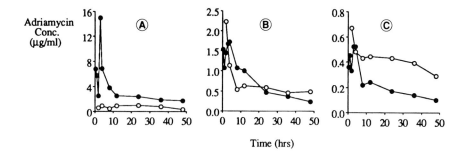

FIGURE 15. Adriamycin concentrations as a function of time in the target tissue (A), liver (B), and heart (C) following the i.a. administration of 0.4 mg/kg drug via magnetic albumin microspheres in the absence (○) and presence of an 8000 G magnet applied for 30 min (●). Each point represents the mean of three rats. (Adapted from Gupta, P. K. and Hung, C. T., *Life Sci.*, 46, 471, 1990. With permission.)

h after dosing, the microspheres were present in the vascular compartment causing indentations on vascular wall and nucleus (Figure 14A). However, the 2-h sample revealed extravascular transfer of magnetic carrier and suggested that the extravasation of carrier is probably size-dependent (Figure 14B). The phenomenon of microsphere extravasation could be explained as a series of activities occurring in harmony: (1) local injury to target tissue endothelium due to active cytotoxic drug released *in situ,* and (2) magnetic drag through the endothelium with increased permeability. The target tissue samples collected at later times demonstrated gradual loss of cellular components as a function of time, e.g., crenation of red blood cells, mitochondrial and endoplasmic reticulum swelling, disorganization of vessel wall, and advanced degeneration of the surrounding tissue (Figures 14C and 14D). This study, therefore, suggested that the pharmacodynamic characteristics of drug are not altered by its encapsulation and delivery via magnetic albumin microspheres. In addition, it confirmed that magnetically controlled delivery can allow transendothelial drug targeting across healthy target tissue vasculature.[48]

The evidence obtained from the ultrastructural study plus the need to assess the relationship between microsphere dose and target tissue drug uptake led us to evaluate the targeting potential of lower doses of drug delivered via magnetic albumin microspheres. Also, the previous study could not clarify whether the increase in targeted delivery of adriamycin was specifically due to individual or combined effects of i.a. drug administration, the use of a microcarrier system, and/ or the applied magnetic field. It was therefore important to assess the *in vivo* drug targeting efficacy of magnetic microspheres in the absence and presence of magnetic field.

In the second study, two groups of animals received 0.4 mg/kg adriamycin HCl via magnetic albumin microspheres in the presence and absence of an 8000 G magnet applied at T2 for 30 min. The animals were killed over a period of 48 h to determine tissue disposition of carrier-delivered drug.[52] Figure 15 shows the concentrations of adriamycin as a function of time at T2, heart, and liver of the two groups of animals. The microspheres administered in presence of magnet

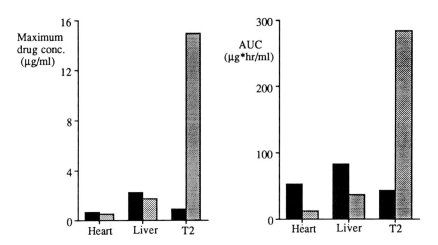

FIGURE 16. Maximal drug concentrations and AUC for heart, liver, and target tissue following the i.a. administration of 0.4 mg/kg drug via magnetic albumin microspheres in the absence (■) and presence of an 8000 G magnet applied for 30 min (▨). (Adapted from Gupta, P. K. and Hung, C. T., *Life Sci.*, 46, 471, 1990. With permission.)

sustained >2 μg/ml drug levels at T2 for up to 24 h and >1.7 μg/ml levels for up to 48 h. These concentrations were appreciably higher than the levels suggested for cytotoxic response.[105-107] Contrary to this, drug levels of 0.5 to 0.7 μg/ml were maintained in the group receiving microspheres in the absence of a magnet. Hence, the magnetic microspheres were able to maintain higher concentrations of adriamycin at the target site, for at least 48 h, even though the magnetic field was applied only for 30 min. This resulted in >6-fold increase in drug AUC at the target site (Figure 16). When the microspheres were administered in the absence of a magnet, drug delivery to T2 was less than or comparable to most nontarget tissues; however, the application of an 8000 G magnet enhanced drug delivery via magnetic microspheres to T2 by 5- to 20-fold compared with that observed in nontarget tissues.[52]

The maximal drug concentration in heart, after the administration of magnetic adriamycin microspheres in the presence of a magnet, was 23% less than that observed in the control animals (Figure 16). Between 8 to 48 h after dosing, the drug concentrations in heart, in the test group, were 2 to 3 times lower than in the control group (Figure 15). As a result of these lower drug levels, the microspheres administered in the presence of magnet reduced the drug AUC at heart by 76% (Figure 16). This in turn suggests that the delivery of adriamycin via magnetic microspheres, in the presence of a suitable magnet, may reduce dose-dependent irreversible cardiomyopathy associated with the administration of adriamycin solutions.[108,109]

Adriamycin is also known to cause toxicity to RES.[110] Therefore, it is desirable that in addition to allowing higher drug delivery to the target tissue, the delivery of adriamycin to RES be minimized. Following the delivery of 0.4 mg/kg adriamycin via magnetic microspheres in the presence of a magnet, uptake of microspheres by

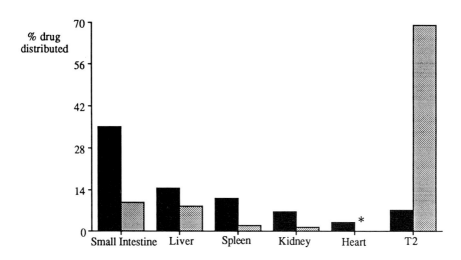

FIGURE 17. Distribution of drug to target site (T2) and several nontarget tissues (small intestine, liver, spleen, kidney, and heart) following the i.a. administration of 0.12 mg/kg adriamycin HCl as a solution (■) and 0.04 mg/kg adriamycin HCl via magnetic albumin microspheres delivered in the presence of an 8000 G magnet (▨). *Less than 0.1% drug distribution to heart with magnetic microspheres. (Adapted from Gupta, P. K. and Hung, C. T., *J. Microencap.*, 7, 85, 1990. With permission.)

the liver could not be totally prevented; however, the maximal drug concentration and the drug AUC in the liver were reduced by 23 and 55%, respectively, compared with those observed with microspheres administered in the absence of a magnet (Figure 16). It was suggested that the magnetic field application time of 30 min may not be sufficient to allow the extravascular transport of total carrier dose across the target tissue vasculature. Nonetheless, all nontarget tissues demonstrated lower drug levels as a result of its administration via magnetic microspheres in the presence of a magnet.[52]

Our next study evaluated the *in vivo* kinetics of a still lower dose (0.04 mg/kg) of adriamycin delivered via magnetic albumin microspheres in the presence of an 8000 G magnet applied at T2 for 30 min, and the data were compared with the kinetics of 0.12 mg/kg adriamycin administered as a solution.[53] With solution, the maximal drug delivery was observed for the small intestine. However, when magnetic microspheres were used, once again the maximal drug delivery was observed for the target site. Compared with the drug solution, one third the dose of microsphere-delivered drug resulted in almost 8 times higher drug AUC at the target site. If linear kinetics could be assumed, this would suggest that the drug delivered via magnetic microspheres resulted in almost 25-fold higher AUC at the target site than that estimated following administration of an equal dose (e.g., 0.04 mg/kg) of drug solution.[53] With microspheres, drug AUC at the target site was almost 10 times higher than that estimated for any other tissue in that group, and the AUC for the cardiac tissue was 10 to 100 times less compared with other tissues.[53]

Figure 17 compares the effect of the two delivery systems (solution and magnetic microspheres) on drug distribution to target site and major nontarget tissues. Following administration of magnetic microspheres in the presence of magnet, ~70% drug was distributed to the target site and <10% drug was distributed to any one given nontarget tissue. The most striking feature of the microsphere delivery system was distribution of <0.1% drug to the heart.[53] With solution, 35% drug was distributed to the small intestine. Drug distribution to all other nontarget tissues was also comparatively high, and the fraction distributed to the target site was 10-fold less than that observed with the microspheres.[53] Significant improvement in targeted drug delivery with magnetic microspheres may be attributed to the transport of a relatively large fraction of dose across the target tissue endothelium during the magnetic field application time, which in turn reduces the fraction of microsphere dose available for reticuloendothelial clearance and distribution to other tissues.

E. DOSE-DEPENDENT PHARMACOKINETICS

Figure 18 shows the effect of dose of drug administered via magnetic carrier in the presence of an 8000 G magnet on various pharmacokinetic parameters, i.e., AUC at target tissue, percentage drug distributed to target tissue and a major nontarget organ, liver, and relative exposure of target tissue versus liver to the administered drug. Nonlinear relationships were obtained between the carrier dose and the evaluated pharmacokinetic indices. This in turn suggested the existence of a "saturable mechanism" for the transport of administered drug carrier across the target tissue endothelium. In the past, dose-dependent kinetics have been observed following the i.v. administration of colloidal particles, e.g., gold and carbon.[111-113] Mechanistically, the i.v. administration of small particles, ~1 μm in diameter, results in deposition of ≥90% of the dose to the liver. However, above a certain dose, the particle uptake process by the liver is saturated. Administration of doses exceeding this saturating limit typically results in increased particle distribution to other tissues.[114] Dose-dependent pharmacokinetics of drugs delivered via liposomes have also been reported.[114-117]

From the viewpoint of efficacy of magnetically controlled drug targeting, the data displayed in Figure 18 and the information obtained from the ultrastructural studies (Figure 14) clearly suggest that the carrier size as well as its dose relative to the targeted tissue microvasculature must be carefully optimized.

F. EFFICACY STUDIES

The efficacy of magnetic albumin microspheres for targeted chemotherapy has been investigated in tumor-bearing animals.[47,51,118-121] In one study, at 6 to 8 days after the transplantation of Yoshida sarcoma at T3 region of rat tail, and when the tumor was 20 to 35 mm in size, the animals received a single i.a. dose of 0.5 mg/kg adriamycin encapsulated in magnetic albumin microspheres. A 5500 G magnet was applied onto the sarcoma for 30 min after the dose administration. The results were compared with the untreated animals and those receiving i.v. (5 mg/kg) or i.a. (0.5 or 5 mg/kg) adriamycin as a solution, drug-free magnetic albumin microspheres in presence of magnet, and drug-encapsulated magnetic albumin microspheres in the absence of magnet. Whereas 80 to 100% of animals in all the control groups died between 13 and 16 days after tumor transplantation due to

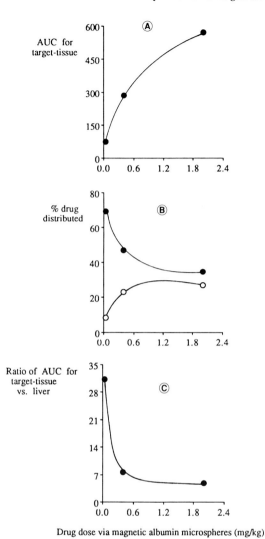

FIGURE 18. Effect of dose delivered via magnetic albumin microspheres in the presence of an 8000 G magnet applied at target site for 30 min on (A) drug AUC at target site, (B) percentage drug distributed to the target tissue (●) and liver (○), and (C) ratio of drug AUC for target tissue vs. liver. Note the dose dependency with all the estimated parameters.

widespread metastasis in the liver, kidneys, lungs, and heart, 100% of animals receiving 0.5 mg/kg adriamycin via magnetic carrier in the presence of a magnet survived for at least up to 30 days, 75% of animals (9 of 12) in this group exhibited complete remission of tumor and another 17% demonstrated definite tumor regression. One animal showed no change in tumor size over the 30-day observation period.[51]

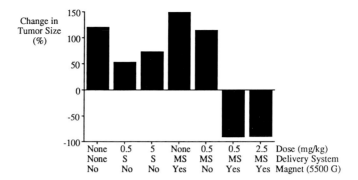

FIGURE 19.   Effect of drug dose (0, 0.5, 2.5, and 5 mg/kg), dosage form (drug solution vs. magnetic microspheres), and presence of 5500 G magnet on the size of Yoshida sarcoma transplanted in rat tail at 30 days after single i.a. treatments. Note the ~100% reduction in tumor size of animals receiving targeted chemotherapy via magnetic albumin microspheres in the presence of magnet. All other groups demonstrated 50 to 150% increase in their tumor size. (Adapted from Widder, K. J., Morris, R. M., Poore, G. A., Howard, D. P., and Senyei, A. E., *Eur. J. Cancer Clin. Oncol.*, 19, 135, 1983. With permission.)

These workers reported similar results in their next study.[118] All animals that did not receive any treatment or received a treatment other than adriamycin-encapsulated magnetic albumin microsphere administered in the presence of magnet demonstrated 50 to 100% increase in their tumor size over the study period of 30 days. However, when 0.5 or 2.5 mg/kg of adriamycin was delivered via magnetic microspheres in the presence of a 5500 G magnet, the mean reduction in tumor size approximated 90% (Figure 19).[118] All animals in these two treatment groups demonstrated regression of tumor and 80% demonstrated total tumor remission. Because no difference was observed between 0.5 and 2.5 mg/kg drug delivered via magnetic microspheres in the presence of a magnet, it was suggested that this technique may perhaps be efficacious at doses lower than 0.5 mg/kg.[118]

High efficacy of drug delivered via magnetic albumin microspheres in the presence of a magnet was explained on the basis of the results obtained from an ultrastructural carrier disposition study.[45] According to this study, the administration of drug-free magnetic albumin microspheres in the presence of a 5500 G magnet applied for 30 min, to rats bearing Yoshida sarcoma at T3, resulted in endocytosis of microspheres as early as 10 min after their dosing. At 30 min, the microspheres were found in the extravascular compartment adjacent to tumor cells. By 24 h, a small fraction of microspheres was endocytosed by tumor cells.[45] It was suggested that a magnetic drug carrier could confer cytotoxic activity by two mechanisms: (1) localized diffusion of drug from microspheres in the extravascular compartment resulting in exposure of numerous surrounding tumor cells to the cytotoxic agent in high concentrations, thus allowing multiple tumor cell kill per microsphere, and (2) internalization of the magnetic drug carrier by tumor cells and intracellular drug release, leading to direct cell damage. Hence, it was hypothesized that magnetically controlled drug delivery may allow intracellular activity of compounds to which cells are resistant due to poor transport across the cell membrane.[45]

Sugibayashi et al.[122] evaluated the efficacy of adriamycin-associated magnetic albumin microspheres, administered in the presence of a 6000 G magnet applied for 10 min, in rats bearing AH 7974 lung metastases. The microspheres contained 6 and 47% w/w of drug and magnetite, respectively. Compared with the untreated controls and the group receiving drug as a solution, drug delivery via magnetic albumin microspheres was shown to increase the survival of animals by 44% ($p <$ 0.001) and 11% ($p < 0.05$), respectively.[122]

Using magnetic albumin microspheres containing 10% w/w of vindesine sulfate, Morris et al.[119] demonstrated 85% total remission and almost 95% regression of Yoshida sarcoma in the rat tail. Once again, when delivered via magnetic microspheres, 0.5 and 2.5 mg/kg drug was found to be equally effective in the eradication of sarcoma. The control animals receiving either drug solution or nonmagnetic drug-loaded microspheres displayed widespread metastases and mortality.[119] Other studies[120,121] evaluated the effect of route of administration (i.a., i.v., and intra-medullary [i.m.]) on the localization of magnetic microspheres to various parts of a spontaneous canine osteosarcoma of dog limb. This animal model was suggested to possess histopathologic, cell kinetics, tumor volume, and biologic similarities to human neoplasms; therefore, a good preclinical model for evaluating the potential of magnetically controlled targeted chemotherapy.[121] Based on the vascular access studies, i.a. infusion of microspheres was recommended for drug delivery to tumors of soft tissues and the i.m. route was advised for tumors confined to bone. A combination of i.a. and i.m. drug delivery was suggested to be optimal for treating tumors consisting of osseous and extra-osseous components.[121] When ^{99m}Tc-labeled magnetic albumin microspheres were administered i.v. or i.m. to dogs with canine osteogenic sarcoma, the application of magnet did not improve microsphere distribution or retention in the tumor. However, when given i.a., application of the magnet slightly improved the distribution of magnetic microspheres and enhanced their retention in tumor by 50 to 100%.[121] The improvement in microsphere distribution and retention due to application of the magnet was confirmed using angiographic studies. The efficacy studies with adriamycin encapsulated in magnetic albumin microspheres in 27 dogs with spontaneous canine osteosarcoma demonstrated temporary improvement in 26% of the animals and measurable remission in 15% of the animals receiving microspheres via the i.a. route.[121]

G. TOXICITY AND BIOCOMPATIBILITY

Albumin microspheres have been extensively investigated for diagnostic and therapeutic applications,[123-130] and the results obtained from these studies can be of value in appreciating possible toxicity and biocompatibility of magnetic microspheres. Acute (7 day) and chronic (30 day) toxicity studies with albumin microspheres in mice have demonstrated no side effects at doses of 50 mg carrier per animal.[131] Detailed toxicity studies have revealed that the LD_{50} of albumin microspheres, about 10 μm in diameter, is 200 mg/kg.[123] In terms of number, the suggested LD_{50} of 28 $\pm$ 12 μm albumin microspheres is 30,000 particles/g body weight.[132]

Multiple intramuscular and subcutaneous injections of rabbit serum albumin microspheres, in rabbits, have been found to be free from inflammation or necrosis.[133] Experiments carried out using glutaraldehyde cross-linked albumin microspheres, 1 to 10 μm in diameter, have demonstrated good biocompatibility in the synovial tissues of rabbits.[134] With the exception of a few cases in which antigenic reactions with these particles in patients have been reported,[135,136] most studies have demonstrated their good acceptability in healthy as well as tumor-bearing patients.[124,137-145] In 1972, the U.S. Food and Drug Administration approved human serum albumin microspheres for clinical use (FDA New Drug Application No. 17, 382, Feb. 4, 1972). Due to these desirable properties, albumin microspheres have been clinically investigated for the delivery of encapsulated mitomycin C in patients with primary or metastatic liver cancer.[23] This study demonstrated $\geq 50\%$ reduction in the tumor load of 33% (5 of 15) patients and 30 to 50% reduction in the tumor load of another 33% of patients.[23,146]

Information is also available on the toxicity and biocompatibility of magnetic albumin microspheres. Acute (7 days) as well as chronic (90 days) toxicity studies in female BDF_1 mice have demonstrated negligible toxicity, and up to 400 mg/kg doses were tolerated without any histopathological changes in major organs.[43] The LD_{20} and LD_{50} of magnetic albumin microspheres have been reported to be 400 and 1250 mg/kg, respectively,[27,28] and the ratio between toxic versus effective dose of this carrier is believed to be ≥ 100.[28] Whenever any toxic symptoms have been observed, they have been attributed to pulmonary embolization, which typically occurs due to aggregation of microspheres (however, particle aggregation does not occur readily at low concentrations[19]). Hence, small microspheres are generally less toxic than the larger ones. According to Ibrahim et al.,[59] magnetite (i.e., Fe_3O_4) is nontoxic in mice up to doses of 1500 mg/kg.

VI. CURRENT AND FUTURE CONSIDERATIONS

The medical applications of magnetism have been known for 4 decades. In the 1960s magnetism was successfully applied for the detection of trace quantities of magnetically responsive materials in lung and liver,[35] detection of radiopaque ferromagnetic contrast materials,[36] determination of regional blood flow and arteriovenous malformations,[147] vascular catheterization,[148] moving selected tissues in the body,[38] cardiac pacing,[32] and treatment of aneurysms.[149] In the 1970s, the need to coat magnetic particles to minimize their aggregation and increased understanding of the role of encapsulation of therapeutic agents to control their release led to the concept of magnetically controlled drug targeting.[42,43] Based on the information reviewed in this chapter, it is apparent that magnetic drug targeting is the only technique that allows selective distribution of 25 to 90% drug dose to target tissue. The extravascular transfer of drug carrier, ~ 1 μm in diameter, occurs within 10 to 15 min of administration with minimal drug exposure to body fluids and tissues encountered during the deposition process. This rapid rate of drug delivery to target tissue is often 100- to 1000-fold superior than that achievable with conventional treatments as well as systems utilizing antibody drug conjugates.[46]

Despite encouraging data in small animal models, this system of drug targeting has not reached the stage of clinical testing. Initially, it was believed that the efficacy of magnetic drug targeting, at least in part, is due to the i.a. route of drug administration. However, tissue distribution as well as efficacy studies have clearly indicated little effect of i.a. administered drug solution even at doses 10-fold higher than that given in the magnetically targeted form.[51] Several other factors appear to be responsible for the lack of enthusiasm for this system:

1. Lack of data suggesting easy large-scale production of magnetic drug carrier
2. Lack of sufficient data supporting batch-to-batch reproducibility of the physicochemical characteristics of carrier
3. Hydrophobicity and aggregation of some magnetic carriers *in vivo*[19,94]
4. Need for magnets with constant field gradient[16]
5. Lack of convincing data to support its application for the treatment of clinically relevant tumors
6. Nonencouraging data obtained in some large animal models[120,121]
7. Concern regarding the long-term deposition of magnetite in the body
8. Overall cost of pursuing clinical trials
9. Regulatory approval
10. Economics of therapy

Nonetheless, it is believed that at least 50% of the newly developed recombinant biotechnological products possess limitations, e.g., extremely short half-life, and systemic toxicities due to undesirable biodistribution. Hence, successful applications of these and other similar products will undoubtedly require a microencapsulation technique for improved stability, biodistribution, and perhaps targeted delivery.[16]

Various factors that are known to affect the efficacy and overall outcome of magnetically controlled drug targeting, e.g., characteristics of the magnetic delivery system, the magnetic field, and tumor tissue, have been reviewed recently.[16,17] Careful optimization of these factors is essential for enhanced selectivity in chemotherapy and minimizing toxicities due to drug and/or carrier. It has been demonstrated by Kato et al.[70,80] that even in the presence of weak magnetic forces, the magnetic responsiveness of 200 to 300 μm magnetic ethylcellulose microcapsules in dog aorta, with a flow rate of 240 ml/min, can be as high as 89%. This is considerably higher than the 50% magnetic response estimated for 1 μm magnetic albumin microspheres in the presence of an 8000 G magnet in the caudal artery, where flow rates are only about 0.6 ml/min.[19,43,44] Therefore, it is possible that the increase in the size of magnetic drug carrier may allow the use of smaller magnetic fields. However, as mentioned earlier, magnetic albumin microspheres aggregate in the presence of a magnetic field.[19,94] It is generally believed that the larger the microsphere dose, the larger the size of aggregates. On the one hand, aggregation may assist particle retention by slowing the blood flow; on the other hand, aggregation may slow down the process of carrier extravasation through the capillary endothelium due to the increased diameter. Hence, carrier size is a good example of a parameter that plays an important role in controlling the efficacy in targeted therapy. However, its optimization is complex.

New information relevant to the optimization of magnetically controlled drug delivery is constantly emerging. For example, a mechanism for extravascular transfer of magnetic carrier in healthy target tissue has been proposed.[48] Noninvasive techniques involving nuclear magnetic resonance have been developed to monitor drug clearance from tissues of interest.[27,150] Some information is also available on differences in the endothelial antigens between target and nontarget tissue blood vessels, which could be exploited for achieving receptor-mediated drug targeting.[151] Ranney[27] was successful in achieving selective drug delivery to lungs by developing heparin-coated particles, which are complementary to pulmonary endothelial heparan sulfates. Rapid endothelial envelopment of such carrier particles results in their functional and anatomical extravasation and thus allows drug delivery at cellular and perhaps subcellular level.[27] Some other chemicals that bind specifically to pulmonary endothelial receptors include antibodies to endothelial factor VIII antigen, glycosylated albumin, and cationized ferritin.[27,152] In addition, *Ulex europaeus* I agglutinin, interleukin I, and antibodies against endothelial leukocyte adhesion molecule (ELAM, e.g., H4/18), Fc receptors, factor VIII antigen, glycoprotein IIb, and glycoprotein IIb/IIIa complex have been identified as substances that bind preferentially to activated and diseased endothelium.[152] It is therefore likely that a more thorough understanding of the relative roles of carrier particle size and surface characteristics specifically from the viewpoint of interaction with the surface determinants of the target tissue endothelium, and temporary control of blood flow may allow efficient magnetic drug targeting at low field strengths and gradient. Indeed, the type of coating used in the formulation of a magnetic drug carrier has been shown to influence its blood circulation time, e.g., dextran magnetic particles have a longer blood half-life than starch or albumin magnetic particles.[153]

As mentioned, successful magnetic drug targeting requires the use of magnets with constant field gradient. This property is not easily achieved with conventional magnets. It has been suggested that application of a magnet with a quadripolar field configuration may allow production of fields with less than 15% variation in gradient across the targeting volume.[28] It is also possible that the use of high energy magnet materials, e.g., rare earth, cobalt, or neodymium-iron-boron alloys, and optimization of magnetic field configurations may permit greater control of magnetic material over increased distances.

With regard to exposure to high strength magnetic fields, it is emphasized that magnetopharmaceuticals are routinely used for magnetic resonance imaging of body organs,[154] and the magnetic field in the environment ranges from earth's natural field of 0.3 G to between 1×10^5 and 1×10^6 G in the vicinity of superconducting cryogenic magnets.[155] Although some of the biological effects of electromagnetic fields may be short-term and reversible, areas, such as brain tissue, are likely to be more susceptible and sensitive than other organs.[155] It has been suggested, however, that even at strengths of 1×10^4 G, the interaction of magnetic field with brain tissue is minimal.[155] Another report suggested that a magnetic field strength of about 24×10^4 G is required to produce a 10% reduction in the conduction of nerve impulses.[156] It has also been shown that at normal body temperatures, static magnetic fields of about 1×10^4 G are required to produce significant alterations in enzyme conformation.[157] For those interested in more detailed discussion of the effects of magnetic field on the nervous system, a separate review on this topic is recommended.[158] Current understanding of the effect of magnetic field on hematological functions is rather controversial.[159-161] In the United States, FDA guidelines require adequate justification prior to the use of magnetic resonance imaging if the whole body or even part of it is exposed to static magnetic fields $\geq 2 \times 10^4$ G.[162] More recently, electromagnetically generated extracorporeal shock waves have been proposed for clinical gallstone lithotripsy.[163] In addition, extracorporeal magnetic configurations exist that produce constant field gradients over targeting gaps of 30 to 40 cm. These technological improvements should therefore allow targeting of magnetic microspheres to deep tumors in thoracic, abdominal, and cranial cavities. However, beyond and above all these facts, it should be appreciated that magnetically controlled drug targeting is likely to apply only for life-threatening diseases that do not respond to conventional drug delivery approaches. Consequently, the magnetic field hazards are unlikely to exceed the hazards due to disease and/or drug itself.

Despite recent developments and a better understanding of various factors related to magnetically targeted systems, there are several areas that need attention, e.g., determination of rate of extravascular transfer of specific magnetic drug carriers in target tissues with varying blood flow rates and endothelial barrier characteristics, and role of carrier and target tissue interaction in receptor-mediated drug delivery. Quantitative information is needed on the accumulation of magnetic drug carrier in anatomically and physiologically different subregions of target tissue and on the uptake of microspheres by tumor cells. Information is also needed on relative efficiency with which toxic compounds with varying physicochemical properties can be maintained in target tissue with the aid of different microcarrier systems. Indeed, more data is needed to support reproducible production of magnetic drug particles with acceptable within-batch and between-batch variations in terms of particle size, drug content, magnetite content, and drug release rates. It is obvious that variation in these parameters would not only influence retention and extravasation of drug carrier but would also affect its response toward tumor versus normal cells. Most clinical sarcomas have heterogeneous subregions with respect to their immune and chemotherapeutic response; thus it is important that methods be developed to monitor drug levels between extracellular and intracellular regions of target tissue, and in the subregions of lesional foci. Most work conducted to date has utilized magnetic fields enveloping normal as well as tumor tissue or target as well as nontarget sites within a given organ. However, ideal conditions warrant the development of magnets with field configurations such that only tumor tissue is exposed and focal overtreatment is avoided.

Finally, it can be said that magnetically controlled drug delivery is one of the few techniques that has allowed transendothelial delivery of potent compounds without toxicity to blood and endothelial tissue. It has allowed 50 to 80% localization of the administered drug and/or drug carrier in the intended target tissue, which otherwise would deposit at levels ≥95% in liver, spleen, kidney, and/or lung. In addition, it offers potential for the targeted delivery of potent and/or short-lived molecules, which normally cannot be tolerated by healthy tissues at equivalent concentrations.

ACKNOWLEDGMENTS

The permission granted by several authors and copyright owners for the use of their data and information in this chapter is gratefully acknowledged. The experimental work pursued by the authors and reported in this chapter was conducted at the Department of Pharmacy, University of Otago Medical School, Dunedin, New Zealand, and it was supported by the Medical Research Council of New Zealand. The authors are grateful to Drs. D. G. Perrier and J. M. Gallo for their advice and to Mrs. C. Morris for technical assistance during the course of the work.

REFERENCES

1. **Poste, G. and Kirsh, R.** Site specific (targeted) drug delivery in cancer therapy, *Biotechnology,* 10, 869, 1983.
2. **Gupta, P. K.,** Drug targeting in cancer chemotherapy: a clinical perspective, *J. Pharm. Sci.,* 79, 949, 1993.
3. **Gupta, P. K., Hung, C. T., and Lam, F. C.,** Application of particulate carriers in intra-tumoral drug delivery, in *Particulate Carriers: Clinical Applications,* Rolland, A., Ed., Marcel Dekker, New York, 1991.
4. **Collins, J. M.,** Pharmacologic rationale for regional drug delivery, *J. Clin. Oncol.,* 2, 498, 1984.
5. **Didolkar, M. S., Kanter, P. M., Baffi, R. R., Schwartz, H. S., Lopez, R., and Baez, N.,** Comparison of regional versus systemic chemotherapy with adriamycin, *Ann. Surg.,* 187, 332, 1978.
6. **El-Akkad, S., Amer, M., Bedikian, A., and Kerth, W.,** A multimodality approach with chemotherapy, surgery and radiotherapy to the treatment of esophageal cancer, *Proc. Am. Assoc. Cancer Res.,* 27, 186, 1986.
7. **Chiuten, D. F., Lu, K., Jeffries, D., Raber, M. N., Newman, R. A., and Neidhart, J. A.,** Comparative evaluation of continuous infusion (CI) vs. intermittent schedule (IS) cisplatin in solid tumors, *Proc. Am. Assoc. Cancer Res.,* 27, 187, 1986.
8. **Cocconi, G., Bisagni, G., Bacchi, M., DeLisi, V., Canaletti, R., Carpi, A., Buzzi, F., and Colozza, M. A.,** A comparison of continuation vs. late intensification followed by discontinuation of chemotherapy (CT) in advanced breast cancer (ABC), *Proc. Am. Assoc. Cancer Res.,* 27, 190, 1986.

9. **Sezaki, H. and Hashida, M.**, Macromolecule drug conjugates in targetted cancer chemotherapy, *CRC Crit. Rev. Ther. Drug Carrier Syst.*, 1, 1, 1984.
10. **Juliano R. L., Ed.**, *Drug Delivery Systems*, Oxford University Press, New York, 1980.
11. **Goldberg, E. P., Ed.**, *Targeted Drugs*, John Wiley, New York, 1983.
12. **Davis, S. S., Illum, L., McVie, J. G., and Tomlinson, E., Eds.**, *Microspheres and Drug Therapy: Pharmaceutical, Immunological and Medical Aspects*, Elsevier, New York, 1984.
13. **Poznansky, M. J. and Juliano, R. L.**, Biological approaches to the controlled delivery of drugs: a critical review, *Pharmacol. Rev.*, 36, 277, 1984.
14. **Poste, G.**, Drug targeting in cancer therapy, in *Receptor-Mediated Targeting of Drugs*, Gregoriadis, G., Poste, G., Senior, J., and Trouet, A., Eds., Plenum Press, New York, 1985, 427.
15. **Chen, H. S. G. and Gross, J. F.**, Intra-arterial infusion of anticancer drugs: theoretical aspects of drug delivery and review of responses, *Cancer Treat. Rep.*, 64, 31, 1980.
16. **Ranney, D. F.**, Magnetically controlled devices and biomodulation, in *Drug Delivery Devices: Fundamentals and Applications*, Tyle, P., Ed., Marcel Dekker, New York, 1988, 325.
17. **Gupta, P. K. and Hung, C. T.**, Magnetically controlled targeted micro-carrier systems, *Life Sci.*, 44, 175, 1989.
18. **Tomlinson, E.**, Theory and practice of site-specific drug delivery, *Adv. Drug Del. Rev.*, 1, 87, 1987.
19. **Widder, K. J., Senyei, A. E., and Ranney D. F.**, Magnetically responsive microspheres and other carriers for the biophysical targeting of antitumor agents, in *Advances in Pharmacology and Chemotherapy*, Vol. 16, Garattini, S., Goldin, A., Howking, F., Kopin, I. J., and Schnitzer, R. J., Eds., Academic Press, New York, 1979, 213.
20. **Florence, A. T. and Halbert, G. W.**, Drug delivery and targeting, *Phys. Technol.*, 16, 164, 1985.
21. **Illum, L. and Davis, S. S.**, The targeting of drugs parenterally by use of microspheres, *J. Parenter. Sci. Tech.*, 36, 242, 1982.
22. **Tomlinson, E.**, Passive and active vectoring with microparticles: localisation and drug release, *J. Controlled Release*, 2, 385, 1985.
23. **Fujimoto, S., Miyazaki, M., Endoh, F., Takahashi, O., Okui, K., and Morimoto, Y.**, Biodegradable mitomycin C microspheres given intra-arterially for inoperable hepatic cancer with particular reference to a comparison with continuous infusion of mitomycin C and 5-fluorouracil, *Cancer*, 56, 2404, 1985.
24. **Ford, C. H. J. and Casson, A. G.**, Antibody-mediated targeting in the treatment and diagnosis of cancer: an overview, *Cancer Chemother. Pharmacol.*, 17, 197, 1986.
25. **Magin, R. L. and Weinstein, J. N.**, Tumor delivery of methotrexate in temperature-sensitive liposomes, *Proc. Am. Assoc. Cancer Res.*, 23, 178, 1982.
26. **Liu, D. and Huang, L.**, pH-sensitive, plasma-stable liposomes with relatively prolonged residence time in circulation, *Biochim. Biophys. Acta*, 1022, 348, 1990.
27. **Ranney, D. F.**, Drug targeting to the lungs, *Biochem. Pharmacol.*, 35, 1063, 1986.
28. **Ranney, D. F. and Huffaker, H. H.**, Magnetic microspheres for the targeted controlled release of drugs and diagnostic agents, *Ann. NY Acad. Sci.*, 507, 104, 1987.
29. **Rahman, A. and Schein, P. S.**, Use of liposomes in cancer chemotherapy, in *Liposomes as Drug Carriers: Recent Trends and Progress*, Gregoriadis, G., Ed., John Wiley, New York, 1988, 381.
30. **McCarthy, H. H., Hovnanian, H. R., Brennan, T. A., and Gegner, P. L.**, Magnetic intubation, *Surgery*, 50, 740, 1961.
31. **Meyers, P. H., Cronic, F., and Nice, C. M. Jr.**, Experimental approach in the use and magnetic control of metallic iron particles in the lymphatic and vascular system of dogs as a contrast and isotopic agent, *Am. J. Roentgenol. Radium Ther. Nucl. Med.*, 90, 1068, 1963.
32. **Weinman, J.**, Incorporation of a magnetic switch into an implanted pacemaker, *J. Thorac. Cardiovasc. Surg.*, 48, 690, 1964.
33. **Alksne, J. F., Fingerhut, A., and Rand, R.**, Magnetically controlled metallic thrombosis of intracranial aneurysms, *Surgery*, 60, 212, 1966.

34. **Rosomoff, H. L.,** Stereomagnetic occlusion of intracranial aneurysms, *Trans. Am. Neurol. Assoc.,* 330, 1966.
35. **Bauman, J. H. and Hoffman, R. W.,** Magnetic susceptibility meter for *in vivo* estimation of hepatic iron stores, *IEEE Trans. Biomed. Eng.,* 14, 239, 1967.
36. **Frei, E. H., Gunders, E., Pajewsky, M., and Alkan, W. J.,** Ferrites as contrast material for medical x-ray diagnosis, *J. Appl. Physiol.,* 39, 999, 1968.
37. **Yodh, S. B., Pierce, N. T., Weggel, R. J., and Montgomery, D. B.,** A new magnet system for intravascular navigation, *Med. Biol. Eng.,* 6, 143, 1968.
38. **Grob, D. and Stein, P.,** Magnetically induced function of heart and bladder, *J. Appl. Physiol.,* 40, 1042, 1969.
39. **Roth, D. A.,** Occlusion of intracranial aneurysms by ferromagnetic thrombi, *J. Appl. Physiol.,* 40, 1044, 1969.
40. **Hilal, S. K., Michelsen, W. J., Driller, J., and Leonard, E.,** Magnetically guided devices for vascular exploration and treatment, *Radiology,* 113, 529, 1974.
41. **Nakamura, T., Konno, K., Morone, T., Tsuya, N., and Hatawo, M.,** Magneto-medicine: biological aspects of ferromagnetic fine particles, *J. Appl. Physiol.,* 42, 1320, 1971.
42. **Zimmermann, U. and Pilwat, G.,** Organ specific application of drugs by means of cellular capsule systems, *Z. Naturforsch.,* 31, 732, 1976.
43. **Widder, K. J., Senyei, A. E., and Scarpelli, D. G.,** Magnetic microspheres: a model system for site specific delivery, *Proc. Soc. Exp. Biol. Med.,* 158, 141, 1978.
44. **Senyei, A., Widder, K., and Czerlinski, G.,** Magnetic guidance of drug carrying microspheres, *J. Appl. Physiol.,* 49, 3578, 1978.
45. **Widder, K. J., Marino, P. A., Morris, R. M., Howard, D. P., Poore, G. A., and Senyei, A. E.,** Selective targeting of magnetic albumin microspheres to the Yoshida sarcoma: ultrastructural evaluation of microsphere disposition, *Eur. J. Cancer Clin. Oncol.,* 19, 141, 1983.
46. **Pimm, M. V. and Baldwin, R. W.,** Quantitative evaluation of the localization of a monoclonal antibody (791T/36) in human osteogenic sarcoma xenografts, *Eur. J. Clin. Oncol.,* 20, 515, 1984.
47. **Ranney, D. F.,** Targeted modulation of acute inflammation, *Science,* 227, 182, 1985.
48. **Gupta, P. K., Hung, C. T., and Rao, N. S.,** Ultrastructural disposition of adriamycin-associated magnetic albumin microspheres in rats, *J. Pharm. Sci.,* 78, 290, 1989.
49. **Lazo, J. S.,** Endothelial injury caused by antineoplastic agents, *Biochem. Pharmacol.,* 35, 1919, 1986.
50. **Gerlowski, L. E. and Jain, R. K.,** Microvascular permeability of normal and neoplastic tissues, *Microvasc. Res.,* 31, 288, 1986.
51. **Widder, K. J., Morris, R. M., Poore, G., Howard, D. P. Jr., and Senyei, A. E.,** Tumor remission in Yoshida sarcoma-bearing rats by selective targeting of magnetic albumin microspheres containing doxorubicin, *Proc. Natl. Acad. Sci. USA,* 78, 579, 1981.
52. **Gupta, P. K. and Hung, C. T.,** Comparative disposition of adriamycin delivered via magnetic albumin microspheres in presence and absence of magnetic field in rats, *Life Sci.,* 46, 471, 1990.
53. **Gupta, P. K. and Hung, C. T.,** Targeted delivery of low dose doxorubicin hydrochloride administered via magnetic albumin microspheres in rats, *J. Microencap.,* 7, 85, 1990.
54. **Morimoto, Y., Sugibayashi, K., and Akimoto, M.,** Magnetic guidance of ferro-colloid entrapped emulsion for site-specific drug delivery, *Chem. Pharm. Bull.,* 31, 279, 1983.
55. **Akimoto, M. and Morimoto, Y.,** Use of magnetic emulsions as a novel drug carrier for chemotherapeutic agents, *Biomaterials,* 4, 49, 1983.
56. **Mosbach, K. and Schroder, U.,** Preparation and application of magnetic polymers for targeting of drugs, *FEBS Lett.,* 102, 112, 1979.
57. **Mosbach, K. and Schroder, U.,** Magnetic microspheres for targeting of drugs, *Enz. Eng.,* 5, 239, 1981.
58. **Schroder, U. and Mosbach, K.,** Magnetic microspheres for targeting of drugs, *Appl. Biochem. Biotechnol.,* 7, 63, 1982.

59. **Ibrahim, A., Couvreur, P., Roland, M., and Speiser, P.,** New magnetic drug carrier, *J. Pharm. Pharmacol.,* 35, 59, 1983.

60. **Zimmermann, U., Pilwat, G., and Esser, B.,** The effect of encapsulation in red blood cells on the distribution of methotrexate in mice, *J. Clin. Chem. Clin. Biochem.,* 16, 135, 1978.

61. **Zimmermann, U.,** Cellular drug-carrier systems and their possible targeting, in *Targeted Drugs,* Goldberg, E. P., Ed., John Wiley, New York, 1983, 153.

62. **Zimmermann, U.,** Electrical breakdown electropermeabilization and electrofusion, *Rev. Physiol. Biochem. Pharmacol.,* 105, 175, 1986.

63. **Sprandel, U., Lanz, D.-J., and von Horsten, W.,** Magnetically responsive erythrocyte ghosts, *Methods Enzymol.,* 149, 301, 1987.

64. **Samokhin, B. P. and Domogatsky, S. P.,** Drug targeting with erythrocytes, *Zh. Vses. Khim. Ova.,* 32, 527, 1987.

65. **Gregoriadis, G.,** Targeting of drugs, *Nature,* 265, 407, 1977.

66. **Kiwada, H., Sato, J., Yamada, S., and Kato, Y.,** Feasibility of magnetic liposomes as a targeting device for drugs, *Chem. Pharm. Bull.,* 34, 4253, 1986.

67. **Ishii, F., Takamura, A., and Ishigami, Y.,** Preparation and characterization of lipid vesicles containing magnetite and an anticancer drug, *J. Disp. Sci. Technol.,* 11, 581, 1990.

68. **Kharkevich, D. A., Alyautdin, R. N., and Filippov, V. I.,** Employment of magnet-susceptible microparticles for the targeting of drugs, *J. Pharm. Pharmacol.,* 41, 286, 1989.

69. **Liburdy, R. P., Tenforde, T. S., Magin, R. L., and Niesman, M.,** Magnetic field-induced drug permeability in liposome vesicles, *Biophys. J.,* 49, 515, 1986.

70. **Kato, T.,** Encapsulated drugs in targeted cancer therapy, in *Controlled Drug Delivery,* Vol. 2, Bruck, S. D., Ed., CRC Press, Boca Raton, FL, 1982, 189.

71. **Whateley, T. L., Goldberg, J. A., Kerr, D. J., McArdle, C. S., Anderson, J., Eley, J. G., and Kato, T.,** Microencapsulated mitomycin C for intra-arterial targeting of hepatic metastases, *Proc. Int. Symp. Control Rel. Bioact. Mater.,* 17, 458, 1990.

72. **Audisio, R. A., Doci, R., Mazzaferro, V., Bellegotti, L., Tommasini, M., Montalto, F., Machiano, A., Piva, A., DeFazio, C., Damascelli, B., Gerranri, L., and van Thiel, D. H.,** Hepatic arterial embolization with microencapsulated mitomycin C for unresectable hepatocellular carcinoma in cirrhosis, *Cancer,* 66, 228, 1990.

73. **Kato, T., Nemoto, R., Mori, H., and Kumagai, I.,** Microencapsulated mitomycin C therapy in renal cell carcinoma, *Lancet,* 2, 479, 1979.

74. **Kato, T., Nemoto, R., Mori, H., Takahashi, M., and Harada, M.,** Arterial chemoembolization with mitomycin C microcapsules in the treatment of primary and secondary carcinoma of the kidney, liver, bone and intrapelvic organs, *Cancer,* 48, 674, 1981.

75. **Kato, T., Nemoto, R., Mori, H., Takahashi, M., Tamakawa, Y., and Harada, M.,** Arterial chemoembolization with microencapsulated anticancer drug: an approach to selective cancer chemotherapy with sustained effects, *JAMA,* 245, 1123, 1981.

76. **Kato, T., Nemoto, R., Mori, H., Sato, S., Unno, K., Homma, M., Okada, M., and Minowa, T.,** Magnetic control of ferromagnetic mitomycin C microcapsules in the artery and urinary bladder, *IRCS Med. Sci.,* 7, 621, 1979.

77. **Kato, T., Nemoto, R., Mori, H., Unno, K., Goto, A., Harada, M., and Homma, M.,** Preparation and characterization of ferromagnetic mitomycin C microcapsules as a means of magnetic control of anticancer drugs, *Proc. Jpn. Acad.,* 55, 470, 1979.

78. **Kato, T., Nemoto, R., Mori, H., Unno, K., Goto, A., and Homma, M.,** An approach to magnetically controlled cancer chemotherapy: I, preparation and properties of ferromagnetic mitomycin C microcapsules, *J. Jpn. Soc. Cancer Ther.,* 15, 58, 1980.

79. **Kato, T., Nemoto, R., Mori, H., Iwata, K., Sato, S., Unno, K., Murota, H., Echigo, M., Harada, M., and Homma, M.,** An approach to magnetically controlled cancer chemotherapy. IV. Magnetically controlled intravesicle instillation of ferromagnetic mitomycin C microcapsules for bladder tumor of the rabbit, *J. Jpn. Soc. Cancer Ther.,* 15, 33, 1980.

80. **Kato, T, Nemoto, R., Mori, H., Abe, R., Unno, K., Goto, A., Murota, H., Harada, M., and Homma, M.,** Magnetic microcapsules for targeted delivery of anticancer drugs, *Appl. Biochem. Biotechnol.,* 10, 199, 1984.

81. **Hung, C. T., McLeod, A. D., and Gupta, P. K.,** Formulation and characterization of magnetic polyglutaraldehyde nanoparticles as carriers for poly-l-lysine-methotrexate, *Drug Dev. Ind. Pharm.,* 16, 509, 1990.

82. **Ito, R., Machida, Y., Sannan, T. and Nagai, T.,** Magnetic granules: a novel system for specific drug delivery to esophageal mucosa on oral administration, *Int. J. Pharm.,* 61, 109, 1990.

83. **Gupta, P. K. and Hung, C. T.,** Albumin microspheres. I. A review of its physico-chemical characteristics, *J. Microencap.,* 6, 427, 1989.

84. **Gupta, P. K., Hung, C. T., Lam, F. C., and Perrier, D. G.,** Albumin microspheres. III. Formulation and characterization of microspheres containing magnetite and adriamycin, *Int. J. Pharm.,* 43, 167, 1988.

85. **Gupta, P. K.,** Magnetite as a tracer for the estimation of bio-distribution of microspheres: a critical consideration, *Int. J. Pharm.,* 52, 87, 1989.

86. **Widder, K. J., Flouret, G., and Senyei, A. E.,** Magnetic microspheres: synthesis of a novel parenteral drug carrier, *J. Pharm. Sci.,* 68, 79, 1979.

87. **Widder, K. J., Senyei, A. E., and Ranney, D. F.,** *In vitro* release of biologically active adriamycin by magnetically responsive albumin microspheres, *Cancer Res.,* 40, 3512, 1980.

88. **Gupta, P. K., Gallo, J. M., Hung, C. T., and Perrier, D. G.,** Influence of stabilization temperature on the entrapment of adriamycin in albumin microspheres, *Drug Dev. Ind. Pharm.,* 13, 1471, 1987.

89. **Yapel, A. F. Jr.,** Albumin medicament carrier systems, U.S. Patent 4,147,767, 1979.

90. **Longo, W. E., Iwato, H., Lindheimer, T. A., and Goldberg, E. P.,** Preparation of hydrophilic albumin microspheres using polymeric dispersing agents, *J. Pharm. Sci.,* 71, 1323, 1982.

91. **Przyborowski, M., Lachnik, E., Wiza, J., and Licinska, I.,** Preparation of HSA microspheres in a one step thermal denaturation of protein aerosol carried in gas medium, *Eur. J. Nucl. Med.,* 7, 71, 1982.

92. **Benita, S., Fickat, R., Benoit, J. P., Bonnemain, B., Samaille, J. P., and Modoule, P.,** Biodegradable cross-linked albumin microcapsules for embolization, *J. Microencap.,* 1, 317, 1984.

93. **Ishizaka, T., Ariizumi, T., Nakamura, T., and Koishi, M.,** Preparation of serum albumin microcapsules, *J. Pharm. Sci.,* 74, 342, 1985.

94. **Driscoll, C. F., Morris, R. M., Senyei, A. E., Widder, K. J., and Heller, G. S.,** Magnetic targeting of microspheres in blood flow, *Microvasc. Res.,* 27, 353, 1984.

95. **Gupta, P. K., Hung, C. T., and Perrier, D. G.,** Albumin microspheres. I. Release characteristics of adriamycin, *Int. J. Pharm.,* 33, 137, 1986.

96. **Gallo, J. M., Hung, C. T., and Perrier, D. G.,** Analysis of albumin microsphere preparation, *Int. J. Pharm.,* 22, 63, 1984.

97. **Willmott, N. and Harrison, P. J.,** Characterization of freeze-dried albumin microspheres containing the anti-cancer drug adriamycin, *Int. J. Pharm.,* 43, 161, 1988.

98. **Senyei, A. E., Reich, S. D., Gonczy, C., and Widder, K. J.,** *In vivo* kinetics of magnetically targeted low-dose doxorubicin, *J. Pharm. Sci.,* 70, 389, 1981.

99. **Ovadia, H., Paterson, P. Y., and Hale, J. R.,** Magnetic microspheres as drug carriers: factors influencing localisation at different anatomical sites in rats. *Isr. J. Med. Sci.,* 19, 631, 1983.

100. **Morimoto, Y., Sugibayashi, K., Okumura, M., and Kato, Y.,** Biomedical applications of magnetic fluids. I. Magnetic guidance of ferro colloid entrapped albumin microsphere for site specific drug delivery *in vivo, J. Pharm. Dyn.,* 3, 264, 1980.

101. **Morimoto, Y., Okumura, M., Sugibayashi, K., and Kato, Y.,** Biomedical applications of magnetic fluids. II. Preparation and magnetic guidance of magnetic albumin microspheres for site specific drug delivery *in vivo, J. Pharm. Dyn.,* 4, 624, 1981.

102. **Gallo, J. M., Hung, C. T., and Perrier, D. G.,** Reversed-phase ion-pair HPLC of adriamycin and adriamycinol in rat serum and tissues, *J. Pharm. Biomed. Anal.,* 4, 483, 1986.

103. **Gallo, J. M., Gupta, P. K., Hung, C. T., and Perrier, D. G.,** Evaluation of drug delivery following the administration of magnetic albumin microspheres containing adriamycin to the rat, *J. Pharm. Sci.,* 78, 190, 1989.

104. **Gallo, J. M., Hung, C. T., Gupta, P. K., and Perrier, D. G.,** Physiological pharmacokinetic model of adriamycin delivered via magnetic albumin microspheres in the rat, *J. Pharmacokinet. Biopharm.,* 17, 305, 1989.
105. **Cummings, J. and McArdle, C. S.,** Studies on the *in vivo* disposition of adriamycin in human tumors which exhibit different responses to the drug, *Br. J. Cancer,* 53, 835, 1986.
106. **Peterson, C., Gunven, P., and Theve, N. O.,** Comparative pharmacokinetics of doxorubicin and epirubicin in patients with gastrointestinal cancer, *Cancer Treat. Rep.,* 70, 947, 1986.
107. **Wassermann, K. and Rasmussen, S. N.,** Comparative responsiveness and pharmacokinetics of doxorubicin in human tumor xenografts, *Eur. J. Cancer Clin. Oncol.,* 23, 303, 1987.
108. **Rinehart, J. J., Lewis, R. P., and Balcerzak, S. P.,** Adriamycin cardiotoxicity in man, *Ann. Intern. Med.,* 81, 475, 1974.
109. **Buzdar, A. U., Marcus, C., Smith, T. L., and Blumenschein, G. R.,** Early and delayed clinical cardiotoxicity of doxorubicin, *Cancer,* 55, 2761, 1985.
110. **Aviles, A., Herrera, J., Ramose, E., Ambriz, R., Aguirre, J., and Pizzuto, J.,** Hepatic injury during doxorubicin therapy, *Arch. Pathol. Lab. Med.,* 188, 912, 1984.
111. **Bioozi, G., Bennacerraf, B., and Halpern, B. N.,** Quantitative study of the granulopectic activity of the reticuloendothelial system. II. A study of the kinetics of the granulopectic activity of RES in relation to the dose of carbon injected, relationship between the weight of the organs and their activity, *Br. J. Exp. Pathol.,* 34, 441, 1953.
112. **Baillif, B.,** Reaction patterns of the reticuloendothelial systems under stimulation, *Ann. NY Acad. Sci.,* 88, 3, 1960.
113. **Saba, T. M.,** Physiology and physiopathology of the reticuloendothelial system, *Arch. Intern. Med.,* 126, 1031, 1970.
114. **Abra, R. M., Bosworth, M. E., and Hunt, C. A.,** Liposome disposition *in vivo:* effects of pre-dosing with liposomes, *Res. Commun. Chem. Pathol. Pharmacol.,* 29, 349, 1980.
115. **Gregoriadis, G. Nerrunjun, D. E., and Hunt, R.,** Fate of liposome-associated agent injected into normal and tumor-bearing rodents: attempts to improve localization in tumor tissue, *Life Sci.,* 21, 357, 1977.
116. **Bosworth, M. E. and Hunt, C. A.,** Liposome disposition *in vivo.* II. Dose dependency, *J. Pharm. Sci.,* 71, 100, 1982.
117. **Sato, Y., Kiwada, H., and Kato, Y.,** Effects of dose and vesicle size on the pharmacokinetics of liposomes, *Chem. Pharm. Bull.,* 34, 4244, 1986.
118. **Widder, K. J., Morris, R. M., Poore, G. A., Howard, D. P., and Senyei, A. E.,** Selective targeting of magnetic albumin microspheres containing low-dose doxorubicin: total remission in Yoshida sarcoma-bearing rats, *Eur. J. Cancer Clin. Oncol.,* 19, 135, 1983.
119. **Morris, R. M., Poore, G. A., Howard, D. P., and Sefranka, J. A.,** Selective targeting of magnetic albumin microspheres containing vindesine sulphate: total remission in Yoshida sarcoma-bearing rats, in *Microspheres and Drug Therapy: Pharmaceutical, Immunological and Medical Aspects,* Davis, S. S., Illum, L., McVie, J. G., and Tomlinson, E., Eds., Elsevier, New York, 1984, 439.
120. **Bartlett, J. M., Richardson, R. C., Elliot, G. S., and Blevins, W. E.,** Localization of magnetic microspheres in 36 canine osteogenic sarcomas, in *Microspheres and Drug Therapy: Pharmaceutical, Immunological and Medical Aspects,* Davis, S. S., Illum, L., McVie, J. G., and Tomlinson, E., Eds., Elsevier, New York, 1984, 413.
121. **Richardson, R. C., Elliot, G. S., Bartlett, J. M., Blevins, W. E., Janas, W., Hale, J. R., and Silver, R. L.,** Magnetic drug-containing microspheres, *Dev. Oncol.,* 26, 227, 1984.
122. **Sugibayashi, K., Okumura, M., and Morimoto, Y.,** Biomedical applications of magnetic fluids. III. Antitumor effect of magnetic albumin microsphere-entrapped adriamycin on lung metastasis of AH 7974 in rats, *Biomaterials,* 3, 181, 1982.
123. **Rhodes, B. A., Zolle, I., Buchanan, J. W., and Wagner, H. N.,** Radioactive albumin microspheres for studies of the pulmonary circulation, *Radiology,* 92, 1453, 1969.
124. **Wagner, H. N. Jr., Rhodes, B. A., Sasaki, Y., and Ryan, J. P.,** Studies of the circulation with radioactive microspheres, *Invest. Radiol.,* 4, 374, 1969.

125. **Zolle, I., Hosain, F., Rhodes, B. A., and Wagner, H. N. Jr.,** Human serum albumin microspheres for studies of the reticuloendothelial system, *J. Nucl. Med.,* 11, 379, 1970.

126. **Zolle, I., Rhodes, B. A., and Wagner, H. N. Jr.,** Preparation of metabolizable radioactive human serum albumin microspheres for studies of the circulation, *Int. J. Appl. Radiat. Isotopes,* 21, 155, 1970.

127. **Kramer, P. A. and Burnstein, T.,** Phagocytosis of microspheres containing an anticancer agent by tumor cells *in vitro, Life Sci.,* 19, 515, 1976.

128. **Lee, T. K., Sokoloski, T. D., and Royer, G. P.,** Serum albumin beads: an injectable, biodegradable system for the sustained release of drugs, *Science,* 213, 233, 1981.

129. **Willmott, N., Cummings, J., Stuart, J. F. B., and Florence, A. T.,** Adriamycin-loaded albumin microspheres: preparation, *in vivo* distribution and release in the rat, *Biopharm. Drug Dispos.,* 6, 91, 1985.

130. **Noteborn, H. P. J. M., Varossieau, F., Blanken, G., Burger, J. J., and McVie, J. G.,** Clinical pharmacokinetics of cisplatin in intra-arterial carrier-mediated delivery in treatment of metastatic liver cancer, *Proc. Int. Symp. Control. Rel. Bioact. Mater.,* 15, 127, 1988.

131. **Sugibayashi, K., Akimoto, M., Morimoto, Y., Nadai, T., and Kato, Y.,** Drug-carrier property of albumin microspheres in chemotherapy. III. Effect of microsphere-entrapped 5-fluorouracil on Ehrlich ascites carcinoma in mice, *J. Pharm. Dyn.,* 2, 350, 1979.

132. **Davis, M. A. and Taube, R. A.,** Pulmonary perfusion imaging: acute toxicity and safety factors as a function of particle size, *J. Nucl. Med.,* 19, 1209, 1978.

133. **Royer, G. P., Lee, T. K., and Sokoloski, T. D.,** Entrapment of bioactive compounds within albumin beads, *J. Parenter. Sci. Technol.,* 37, 34, 1983.

134. **Ratcliffe, J. H., Hunneyball, I. M., Smith, A., Wilson, C. G., and Davis, S. S.,** Preparation and evaluation of biodegradable polymeric systems for the intra-articular delivery of drugs, *J. Pharm. Pharmacol.,* 36, 431, 1984.

135. **Littenberg, R. L.,** Anaphylactoid reaction to human albumin microspheres, *J. Nucl. Med.,* 16, 236, 1975.

136. **Ford, L., Shroff, A., Benson, W., Atkins, H., and Rhodes, B. A.,** SNM drug problem reporting system, *J. Nucl. Med.,* 19, 116, 1978.

137. **Taplin, G. V., Dore, E. K., and Johnson, D. E.,** Hepatic blood flow and reticuloendothelial system studies with radiocolloids, in *Clinical Dynamic Studies with Radioisotopes,* Symposium Series 3, Kniseley, R. M. and Tauxe, W. N., Eds., Oak Ridge, USAEC, TID, 1964, 285.

138. **Taplin, G. V., Johnson, D. E., Dore, E. K., and Kaplan, H. S.,** Suspensions of radioalbumin aggregates for photoscanning of the liver, spleen, lung and other organs, *J. Nucl. Med.,* 5, 259, 1964.

139. **Rhodes, B. A., Zolle, I., and Wagner, H. N.,** Properties and uses of radioactive albumin microspheres, *Clin. Res.,* 16, 245, 1968.

140. **Palmer, D. R., Rifkind, D., and Brown, D. W.,** ^{131}I-labelled colloidal human serum albumin in the study of reticuloendothelial system function. II. Phagocytosis and catabolism of test colloid in normal subjects, *J. Infect. Dis.,* 123, 457, 1971.

141. **Bouveng, R., Schildt, B., and Sjoqvist, J.,** Estimation of RES phagocytosis and catabolism in man by the use of ^{125}I-labeled microaggregates of human serum albumin, *J. Reticuloendothel. Soc.,* 18, 151, 1975.

142. **Gates, G. F. and Goris, M. L.,** Stability of radiopharmaceuticals for determining right-to-left shunting, *J. Nucl. Med.,* 18, 255, 1977.

143. **Pujara, S. S. and Russell, C. D.,** Evaluation of peritoneo-venous shunt, *J. Nucl. Med.,* 20, 72, 1979.

144. **Reske, S. N., Vyska, K., and Feinendegen, L. E.,** Kinetics of phagocytosis and proteolytic metabolism in liver macrophages in normal persons and tumor patients, *J. Nucl. Med.,* 20, 606, 1979.

145. **Reske, S. N., Vyska, K., and Feinendegen, L. E.,** *In vivo* assessment of phagocytic properties of Kupffer cells, *J. Nucl. Med.,* 22, 405, 1981.

146. **Morimoto, Y. and Fujimoto, S.,** Albumin microspheres as drug carriers, *CRC Crit. Rev. Ther. Drug Carrier Syst.,* 2, 19, 1985.

147. **Rosenzweig, R. E. and Neuringer, T.,** Ferrohydrodynamics, *Phys. Fluids,* 7, 1964, 1964.
148. **Frei, E. H., Driller, J., Neufeld, H. N., Barr, I., Bleiden, L., and Askenazy, H. M.,** The POD and its applications, *Med. Res. Eng.,* 5, 11, 1966.
149. **Driller, J. and Frei, E. H.,** A review of medical applications of magnet attraction and detection, *J. Med. Eng. Technol.,* 11, 271, 1987.
150. **El-Tahtawy, A. and Wolf, W.,** Differential tumor pharmacokinetics of 5-fluorouracil (5-FU) in rats using noninvasive 19F NMR spectroscopy (NMRS) with and without pretreatment with methotrexate, *Proc. Am. Assoc. Cancer Res.,* 32, 344, 1991.
151. **Fidler, I. J. and Kripke, M. L.,** Metastasis results from preexisting variant cells within a malignant tumor, *Science,* 197, 893, 1977.
152. **Ranney, D. F.,** Endothelial envelopment drug carriers, U.S. Patent 4,925,678, 1990.
153. **Papisov, M. I., Savelyev, V. Y., Sergienko, V. B., and Torchilin, V. P.,** Magnetic drug targeting. I. *In vivo* kinetics of radiolabeled magnetic drug carriers, *Int. J. Pharm.,* 40, 201, 1987.
154. **Wesbey, G. E.,** Magnetopharmaceuticals, in *Biomedical Magnetic Resonance Imaging: Principles, Methodology and Application,* Wehrli, F. W., Shaw, D., and Kneeland, J. B., Eds., VCH, New York, 1988, 157.
155. **Adey, W. R.,** Tissue interactions with nonionizing electromagnetic fields, *Physiol. Rev.,* 61, 435, 1981.
156. **Wiksow, J. P. Jr. and Barach, J. P.,** An estimate of the steady magnetic field strength required to influence nerve conduction, *IEEE Trans. Biomed. Eng.,* 27, 722, 1980.
157. **Atkins, P. W.,** Magnetic field effects, *Chem. Br.,* 12, 214, 1976.
158. **Kholodov, Y.,** Effects of magnetic fields on the nervous system, in *Influence of Magnetic Fields on Biological Objects,* Kholodov, Y., Ed., Moscow Science, Moscow, 1971.
159. **Barnothy, M. F.,** Hematological changes in mice, in *Biological Effects of Magnetic Fields,* Vol. 1, Barnothy, M. F., Ed., Plenum Press, New York, 1964, 109.
160. **Vardanyan, V. A.,** Effect of magnetic field on blood flow, *Biofizika,* 18, 491, 1973.
161. **Okazaki, M., Maeda, N., and Shiga, T.,** Effects of an inhomogeneous magnetic field on flowing erythrocytes, *Eur. Biophys. J.,* 14, 139, 1987.
162. Department of Health and Human Services, Food and Drug Administration Public Health Services, Guidelines for evaluating electromagnetic exposure risk for trials of clinical NMR systems, Villforth, J. C., Ed., 1982.
163. **Staritz, M., Rambow, A., Mildenberger, P., Goebel, M., Scherfe, Th., Grosse, A., Junginger, Th., Hohenfellner, R., Thelen, M., and Meyer Zum Buschebfelde, K.-H.,** *Eur. J. Clin. Invest.,* 19, 142, 1989.

Chapter 5

AGENTS FOR MICROSPHERE INCORPORATION: PHYSICOCHEMICAL CONSIDERATIONS AND PHYSIOLOGICAL CONSEQUENCES OF PARTICLE EMBOLIZATION

Neville Willmott

TABLE OF CONTENTS

I. INTRODUCTION

An implicit assumption in drug delivery research is that the carrier is no more than a passive instrument in changing native drug disposition in a quantitative way, more here, less there. Viewed from this standpoint it follows that the mechanism of drug action will be the same irrespective of the mode of delivery. Consequently, little attention is paid to how the carrier system employed may influence factors, such as mode of drug incorporation, *in vivo* drug metabolism, and mechanism of drug action.

The drug-delivery system axis is one aspect of the complex interrelationship (Figure 1) among the disease it is desired to treat, the therapeutic agent used, the delivery system employed, and the destination at which the drug should arrive. This is illustrated by the finding that there is an optimal particle diameter for microsphere localization in solid tumors, particles of 40 μm mean diameter being superior to smaller particles[1] or to soluble drug molecules requiring extraction from plasma.[2] Other contributors to this volume will discuss the clinical and experimental data on the use of microspherical systems in relation to disease state and destination. It is the purpose of this chapter to focus on the drug-delivery system axis and illustrate how (1) the mode of incorporation of agents within microspherical delivery systems can affect subsequent *in vivo* fate and (2) the physiological consequences of microsphere administration can influence the way active agents are handled by tumor tissue. Fundamental to this discussion are the implications for activity of incorporated agents.

II. INCORPORATION OF THERAPEUTIC AGENTS IN MICROSPHERES

A. COVALENT COUPLING OF DRUGS TO MATRIX
1. Nature of the Chemical Bond in Relation to Regeneration of Active Drug
The rationale for covalently coupling drugs to microspheres depends on the aims of individual investigators. For example, in the case of Tritton and colleagues,[3,4] it was a means of confining drug-cell interaction to the plasma membrane and thereby investigating whether, in the putative absence of drug-DNA interaction, the drug was still cytotoxic. With regard to anthracyclines this was found to be the case. Alternatively, drug immobilization within microspheres may be for a more pragmatic reason. Thus, we have attempted to utilize covalent binding of drug to biodegradable microsphere matrices to overcome the initial rapid release of loosely bound native drug (burst effect) that is invariably seen with low molecular weight water-soluble agents incorporated within matrices, such as protein[5-7] or polylactic acid.[8] As opposed to the work of Tritton and colleagues,[3,4] this type of system utilizes the process of covalent binding of drug to microsphere matrix, in conjunction with particle biodegradation, to control availability of incorporated agents. The subject of release of drugs incorporated within microspheres in diffusible form, i.e., not covalently bound to the matrix, is discussed in Chapter 1.

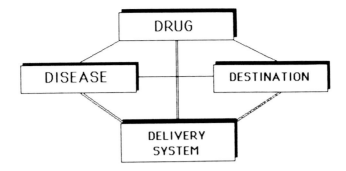

FIGURE 1. Interrelationships important in drug delivery.

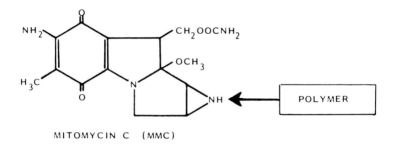

MITOMYCIN C (MMC)

FIGURE 2. Structure of mitomycin C and proposed site of covalent linkage to polymer.

Attachment to matrix polymers is facilitated if the drug possesses either a primary (doxorubicin) or secondary amine (mitomycin C), which is the reason these compounds figure prominently in this context; the chemistry of attachment is shown in Figure 2 and 3 and Table 1. It is clear that conjugation of these drugs in this way does not abrogate activity. Thus, when assessed by growth inhibition of tumor cells *in vitro*, mitomycin C conjugated to polylysine[10] and dextran[16] retained activity comparable to native drug. In these studies highest growth inhibition was found when mitomycin C was conjugated to high molecular weight cationic polymers. Thus, both positive charge and high molecular weight may contribute to efficient absorption to the cell membrane.

With mitomycin C conjugated directly to polymers through nonbiodegradable saturated hydrocarbon spacers, it has been suggested that native drug will be regenerated extracellularly by chemical hydrolysis rather than enzymically within the lysosomal compartment.[17] Indeed, this appears the most likely mechanism when it is considered that mitomycin C will be activated under the acidic conditions prevailing in lysosomes: because the locus of drug action is considered to be cellular DNA,[18] drug activation is unlikely to be beneficial if confined to this cellular organelle. Further evidence consistent with the importance of regeneration of native mitomycin C is that under conditions of continuous drug exposure *in vitro*, polymeric

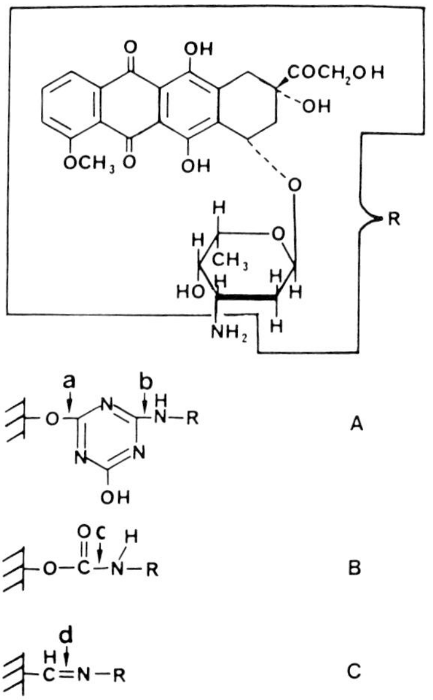

FIGURE 3. Structure of doxorubicin and proposed sites of covalent linkage to polymers. (A) Via cyanuric chloride to cross-linked polyvinyl alcohol. (B) Via 1,1'-carbonyldi-imidazole activated agarose. (C) Free aldehyde group. Sites of potential cleavage are shown as a, b, c, and d. R represents the nonamino portion of doxorubicin. (From Wingard, L. B. and Narasinhan, K., *Appl. Biochem. Biotechnol.*, 19, 117, 1988. With permission.)

systems that regenerated native mitomycin C most rapidly exhibited greatest activity, that is, were similar to unconjugated native drug with regard to cytotoxicity.[16,17] Incorporation of water-soluble macromolecular conjugates of mitomycin C within microspheres suitable for embolization resulted in efficient drug localization and retention in tissue.[19] The situation with doxorubicin bound to microspheres is more intriguing because there is evidence consistent not only with carrier matrix sustaining drug release and prolonging duration of exposure, but also with retention of activity by immobilized drug incapable of diffusion to intracellular sites of action.[3]

Anthracyclines bound to microspherical systems (Table 1) as well as both synthetic[20] and natural[21] water-soluble polymers retain activity. From Table 1 retention of activity appears independent of matrix polymer, chemical nature of linkage, or even orientation of anthracycline in relation to the target cell. Thus, anthracyclines immobilized either via the daunosamine sugar residue or via the planar ring structure exhibit comparable cytotoxic activity.[4] However, although doxorubicin covalently conjugated to microspherical drug delivery systems retains activity, it is not axiomatic that activity is mediated through the same mechanisms as drug conventially formulated or will involve precisely the same chemical entity.

The data demonstrating that doxorubicin immobilized on the microsphere surface, in the absence of detectable native drug,[3,14] implicate the plasma membrane as the locus of drug action. The lack of specificity with regard to chemical linkage

TABLE 1
Linkage of Drugs to Actual and Potential Microsphere Matrices

Conjugation reagent	Functional group on matrix polymer	Functional group on drug	Linkage	Example	Ref.
1-(3-Dimethylaminopropyl)-3-ethyl carbodi-imide	$-CO_2H$	$-NH_2$ or $>NH$	Amide (see Figure 2)	Mitomycin C-albumin	9
				Mitomycin C-polyamino acids	10
Cyanuric chloride	$-OH$	$-NH_2$	See Figure 3A	Doxorubicin-polyvinyl alcohol	11
1,1′-Carbonyldi-imidazole	$-OH$	$-NH_2$	Carbamate (see Figure 3B)	Doxorubicin-agarose	3
				Primaquine-starch	12
Glutaraldehyde	$-CHO$	$-NH_2$	Azomethine/Schiff's base (see Figure 3C)	Doxorubicin-albumin	13, this chapter
				Doxorubicin-polyglutaraldehyde	14
None	$-CO_2H$	Alkyl bromide	Ester	Doxorubicin-polyaspartic acid	15
	$-NH_2$		C-N	Doxorubicin-polylysine	15

and drug orientation relative to the target cell appears to rule out a specific receptor on the cell surface and suggests an effect on a generalized property of the cell membrane, such as fluidity. The microspherical systems described herein are designated to be nonbiodegradable, whereas systems designed for clinical use should be biodegradable.[22,23] Here the question arises of whether drugs covalently bound to protein macromolecules are regenerated in native form or as drug covalently bound to peptide fragments.

In vitro observations suggest that amine-containing compounds coupled via peptide spacer chains to polymers[24,25] can be regenerated in native form when exposed to the appropriate enzymes (endopeptidase, aminopeptidase). Regeneration of native drug is dependent on both length and amino acid composition of peptide spacer, with the absence of amino acid spacers yielding no regeneration of native drug. Considering water-soluble polymers coupled to anthracyclines, antitumor activity is critically dependent on the sensitivity of the peptide spacer to enzymic digestion and therefore presumably to regeneration of native drug.[20,24] Interestingly, although efficient enzymic regeneration of chromatographically pure native drug from soluble drug-peptide[12] or drug-peptide-polymer[24] conjugates is observed, regeneration from drug-spacer-microsphere systems was much less efficient,[12] even with a pentapeptide spacer. This may be due to steric hindrance of protease enzyme action by microspheres.

2. Tumor Disposition and Activity of Doxorubicin in Protein Microspheres

In the course of work with doxorubicin-loaded protein microspheres chemically stabilized with glutaraldehyde, we found that by no means was all drug incorporated in native form. Thus, a proportion remained associated with the protein matrix and so was not detected in *in vitro* release assays. Moreover, when microsphere matrix was digested and solubilized by trypsin two doxorubicin species were separated by thin layer chromatography, native doxorubicin and a form coeluting in association with matrix components.[26] An analogous separation was achieved with high performance liquid chromatography (HPLC).[13] Accurate quantitation of each form of drug incorporated within microspheres was possible with ^{14}C-doxorubicin (Tables 2 and 3).

It is instructive to compare the pattern of drug loading using albumin/polyaspartic acid as microsphere matrix (100% native drug) with systems using albumin alone as matrix material (15 to 50% native drug, remainder covalently bound). On the basis of this comparison it is proposed that all doxorubicin in protein microspheres is not in native form due to formation of a drug-protein conjugate with the bifunctional aldehyde, glutaraldehyde, linking amine groups of drug and protein (Figure 4A). In the presence of polyaspartic acid, the amine group of doxorubicin is not available for reaction with glutaraldehyde due to formation of an ionic complex with the polyanion (Figure 4B).

The state of doxorubicin within the microsphere matrix (i.e., native and diffusible or covalently bound and immobilized) will influence tissue pharmacokinetics, dictate drug-tumor cell interactions, and so determine activity. Therefore, an investigation of relationships between drug disposition and activity in these two

TABLE 2
Quantitation of Doxorubicin in Protein
Microspheres: Albumin

Glutaraldehyde concentration (mg/100 mg protein)	Doxorubicin content of albumin microspheres (µg/mg)		
	Total	Native	Covalently bound[a]
4	21.6	10.8	10.8
5	25.1	7.9	17.2
7.5	26.2	6.4	19.8
10	31.3	4.7	26.6

Note: ^{14}C-Doxorubicin-loaded albumin microspheres, prepared using the glutaraldehyde concentrations shown, were digested and solubilized in 0.4% trypsin for determination of drug content by HPLC (native drug) and β-scintillation counting (total drug). Higher concentrations of glutaraldehyde resulted in microspheres that were resistant to trypsin digestion.

[a] Computed by subtracting native (measured by HPLC) from total drug content (measured using ^{14}C-doxorubicin).

TABLE 3
Quantitation of Doxorubicin in Protein
Microspheres: Other Proteins

Protein (mg/100 mg)	Doxorubicin content of microspheres (µg/mg)		
	Total	Native	Covalently bound[a]
Casein (10)	30.9	3.2	27.7
Transferrin (5)	26.4	6.5	19.9
Albumin/PAA[b] (5)	34.3	34.3	0

Note: ^{14}C-Doxorubicin-loaded protein microspheres, prepared using the matrix materials shown, were digested and solubilized in 0.4% trypsin for determination of drug content by HPLC (native drug) and β-scintillation counting (total drug).

[a] Doxorubicin incorporated via covalent binding to protein matrix = total drug content minus native drug content.
[b] Microsphere matrix was mixture of 195 mg albumin and 5 mg polyaspartic acid (PAA).

microspherical systems that differ only in mode of doxorubicin incorporation might define factors important for optimal drug activity.

The animal model employed was the subcutaneously growing Sp107 mammary carcinoma:[27] drug disposition, metabolism, and activity were assessed following intratumoral injection of known amounts of doxorubicin in solution or in micros-

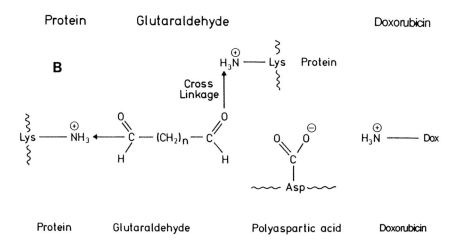

FIGURE 4.   (A) Proposed mechanism of incorporation of doxorubicin within albumin microspheres in native form and covalently linked to matrix. (B) Proposed mechanism of incorporation of doxorubicin within albumin/polyaspartic acid microspheres in native form only.

pherical form. Following administration of ^{14}C-doxorubicin in solution drug was measured both by ^{14}C-activity and HPLC. These measurements are analogous to those in Tables 2 and 3 showing drug content of microspherical systems where ^{14}C-activity measures total drug concentration (μg/g) and HPLC measures native drug concentration (μg/g) in tumor tissue.

It can be seen from Figure 5A that when administered in solution at no point were drug concentration-time profiles significantly different. Thus, doxorubicin in tumor tissue was present essentially in native form: if any drug metabolism or covalent binding to cellular macromolecules had occurred, it accounted for only a small proportion of drug.

Following administration of doxorubicin in microspherical form the situation is markedly different (Figure 5B). Thus, at all time points native doxorubicin

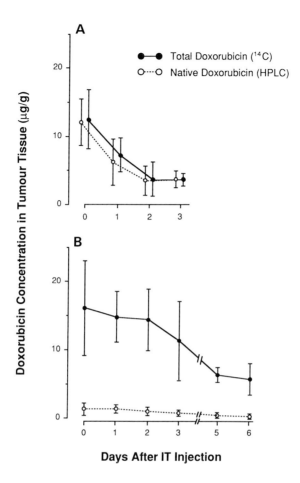

FIGURE 5. Doxorubicin disposition in solid tumor tissue. ^{14}C-Doxorubicin administered intratumorally (Sp 107 mammary carcinoma growing subcutaneously in Wab/Not rats) and at intervals tissue concentrations of drug assessed both by ^{14}C-activity (total doxorubicin concentration) and HPLC (native doxorubicin concentration); 4 rats per group. Error bars represent mean and 95% confidence interval. (A) Doxorubicin in solution. (B) Doxorubicin in microspherical form.

concentration as measured by HPLC was significantly lower than the total drug concentration as measured by ^{14}C-activity. It is considered that the major doxorubicin species present in tumor tissue is covalently bound to microsphere protein matrix and therefore not detectable by HPLC. Metabolism, either hydrolytic to 7-hydroxyaglycones or reductive to 7-deoxyaglycones, was not prominent with this microspherical system incorporating a low proportion of native drug.

The question of antitumor activity was also addressed; 100 μg of doxorubicin, either in microspherical form or in solution, was administered intratumorally and growth delay measured by standard methods.[28] It should be noted, in contrast to a previous work[28,29] that considered only native drug content of microspheres, these

TABLE 4
In Vivo Antitumor Activity of Doxorubicin-Loaded Protein Microspheres

Experiment	Form of doxorubicin[a]	Growth delay[b] (days)
1	Solution	9.1
	Albumin microspheres (biodegradable[c])	12.0
2	Solution	5.6
	Albumin microspheres (biodegradable[c])	6.8
	Albumin microspheres (nonbiodegradable[d])	3.5
3	Solution	10.0
	Casein microspheres (biodegradable[c])	12.0
4	Solution	6.4
	Albumin/PAA[e] microspheres	4.0

[a] 100 μg doxorubicin in microspherical form or in solution injected intratumorally.

[b] Growth delay defined as time taken for treated tumors to reach 10 g minus time taken for untreated tumors to reach 10 g.

[c] Susceptible to digestion and solubilization by trypsin. Total drug content obtained after solubilization of microspheres in 0.4% trypsin.

[d] Not susceptible to digestion and solubilization by trypsin. Total drug content obtained after solubilization of microspheres in 1 M NaOH.

[e] Albumin/polyaspartic acid.

studies compared a defined amount of doxorubicin in solution with the same total dose of drug in microspherical form (i.e., derived from measurements of ^{14}C-doxorubicin activity). The group of animals treated with 100 μg doxorubicin in solution included in each experiment served to control for interexperimental variation.

Biodegradable protein microspheres, containing doxorubicin predominantly present in a form covalently bound to microsphere matrix (Tables 2 and 3), reproducibly exhibited higher growth delay than drug in solution (Table 4, Experiments 1 to 3). It should be noted, however, that the growth curves were not significantly different when compared by regression analysis. The tendency with microspherical systems resistant to protease digestion and albumin/polyaspartic acid systems incorporating doxorubicin in native form only (Table 3) was toward reduced activity relative to drug in solution (Table 4, Experiments 2 and 4, respectively). Again, the growth curves were not significantly different.

In the case of the albumin/polyaspartic acid system we have previously examined doxorubicin disposition after intratumoral injection. Marked biotransformation to 7-deoxyaglycones, rapid elimination of parent drug, and no detectable complexed

TABLE 5
Doxorubicin-Loaded Microspheres: Summary of Drug-Loading Characteristics and Drug Fate *In Vivo*

Formulation	Drug loading		Drug fate	
	Covalently bound	Native	Clearance[a]	Metabolism[b]
Native doxorubicin in solution	None	All	Rapid	Low
Doxorubicin in albumin/PAA microspheres[c]	None	All	Rapid	High
Doxorubicin in albumin microspheres	Major	Minor	Slow	Low

[a]   Clearance of drug from tumor tissue.
[b]   Metabolism to 7-deoxyaglycones in tumor tissue.
[c]   Albumin/polyaspartic acid microspheres.

doxorubicin were observed.[13] This is in marked contrast to the more active systems in which (because doxorubicin is predominantly in complexed form) little metabolism and slow elimination of complexed drug were observed in tumor tissue (Figure 5B).

As yet it is uncertain how doxorubicin initially complexed to microspheres exerts antitumor activity. It is of interest that doxorubicin, bound to nonbiodegradable microspheres incapable of entering cells, retains activity;[3,4] however, in our model it is the biodegradable systems incorporating covalently bound drug that show highest activity, suggesting the importance of this process in drug availability. The paucity of native doxorubicin in tumor tissue (Figure 5B) suggests that this system does not regenerate native drug *in vivo* as is thought to be the case with soluble carriers.[12,24]

The detection of doxorubicin covalently bound to fragments of microsphere matrix following *in vitro* protease digestion of drug-loaded particles[13] may be analogous to the *in vivo* situation in tumor tissue. Hence, protease enzymes could release doxorubicin covalently bound to protein fragments within the tumor milieu. It should be noted that the HPLC analysis performed in Figure 5B would not detect such species because an extraction step was involved. If the hypothesis is correct, a prodrug of doxorubicin of the type discussed elsewhere[30] will have been fashioned by accident. However this may be, Table 5 summarizes the salient findings with doxorubicin-loaded protein microspheres, which will inform the choice of chemotherapeutic agents for incorporation within these systems.

B. THERAPEUTIC RADIONUCLIDES AND MICROSPHERES

The use of radionuclides in cancer therapy has long been an attractive proposition. However, although sealed sources are widely used, the hopes for unsealed sources have not been fulfilled with regard to therapy of the common, solid epithelial tumors. Essentially, the problems are twofold: (1) to rapidly and precisely deliver the radionuclide to the target site and (2) to retain the radionuclide at the site of

TABLE 6
β-Emitting Radionuclides Used in Radioembolization

Radionuclide	Half-life (days)	E_β (max)[a] (keV)	Range[b] (max) (mm)	Microsphere matrix	Ref.
[131]I[c]	8.0	610	2.4	Albumin	33
[186]Re[c]	3.8	1070	5.0	Isobutyl cyanoacrylate	34
[32]P	14.3	1710	8.7	Ion-exchange resin	35
[90]Y	2.7	2280	12.0	Ion-exchange resin	36
[90]Y	2.7	2280	12.0	Glass	37

[a] Energy of β-emission: E_β (average) $\sim^1/_3$ E_β (maximum).
[b] Penetration of radiation through tissue.
[c] Emit γ-radiation useful for monitoring particle distribution *in vivo*.

Physical data adapted from Adelstein, S. J. and Kassis, A. I., *Nucl. Med. Biol.*, 14, 165, 1987.

action until emission of radiation has decayed to nontoxic levels. These requirements for maximal targeting efficiency of a radionuclide/carrier combination can be formally stated in terms of temporal variables of radionuclide and carrier:

Half-life of radionuclide $\gg$ Time for carrier/radionuclide localization

Half-life of radionuclide $\ll$ Time for radionuclide release from carrier

Although for a given system the physical half-life of the radionuclide is fixed, it is possible to control the carrier-related variables by choice of appropriate carrier system and matrix material. Thus, by careful attention to the radiological and chemical properties of the radionuclide as well as the chemical properties and *in vivo* fate of the carrier, it is possible to go some way to fulfilling these conditions and thereby maximize the carrier-bound radiation dose delivered to the tumor and minimize that to normal tissue.

The first condition is readily fulfilled for radionuclides incorporated within microspheres suitable for embolization because the time interval between intra-arterial administration and localization is only a few seconds. This is in marked contrast to antibody localization in which accumulation in solid tumor tissue takes place over a period of days with consequent dose-limiting bone marrow exposure recorded in animals[31] and patients.[32] Table 6 shows various radionuclide/microsphere combinations used for radioembolization.

An approach to fulfilling the second condition is incorporation of radionuclide as an integral component[37] or covalently bound[2,33] to microsphere matrix (Table 6). In this way it is possible to confine the radiation dose to the area where the particles embolize, and so, prevent systemic toxicity from premature release of radionuclide into the circulation. ^{90}Y-yttrium oxide has been incorporated into nonbiodegradable glass microspheres with minimal leaching of radionuclide. Another advantage of ^{90}Y is that it can be incorporated as the oxide of nonradioactive [89]Y, which can

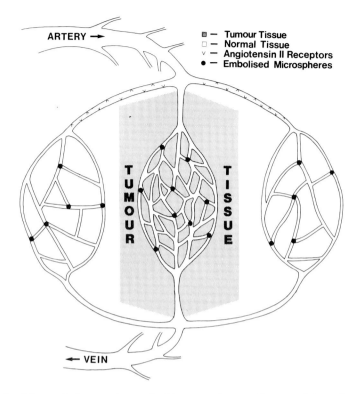

FIGURE 6. Schema of microvasculature of solid tumor and surrounding normal tissue. Localization of microspheres administered intra-arterially.

then be activated to ^{90}Y by neutron bombardment, provided a suitable nuclear reactor is available.[37] (See Chapter 1 for details of the development of ^{90}Y-based systems.)

Iodine in the form of iodide can be covalently coupled to protein; this technique has been used to prepare ^{131}I-albumin microspheres.[2] However, in patients the median biological half-life when embolized in solid tumor tissue is 2.4 days,[33] which appears suboptimal for use with the radionuclides listed in Table 6. In addition, dehalogenation may be a problem with this system. An alternative microspherical system for radioembolization incorporates either ^{32}P or ^{90}Y via ionic bonds to a microspherical ion-exchange resin;[35,36] this author is not aware of data on leaching of radionuclide.

III. PHYSIOLOGICAL CONSEQUENCES OF MICROSPHERE ADMINISTRATION: SIGNIFICANCE FOR CHOICE OF ACTIVE AGENTS

A. HYPOXIA-SELECTIVE CYTOTOXINS IN CONJUNCTION WITH MICROSPHERES

Figure 6 shows in schematic form the microvasculature of a solid tumor and surrounding tissue: it also illustrates the concepts involved in regional drug delivery with microspherical systems of suitable size for embolization in capillaries. Chapters 3, 7, and 8 consider strategies for localization of microspheres (and incorporated active agent) in solid tumor deposits of target organs; another consideration is that these delivery systems, through retention and biodegradation in tumor capillaries, might overcome the low extraction of drugs from plasma by solid tumors relative to surrounding normal tissue[38-40] (see Chapter 2).

A less obvious point is the way in which carrier-induced conditions might modify drug fate and activity. Intra-arterial administration of microspheres (40 μm) has been shown to elicit tissue ischemia as measured by reduction of blood flow, oxygen tension, and concentrations of high energy phosphates. This is consistent with the finding that perfusion is the major determinant of tumor hypoxia.[41] The onset of tissue ischemia following microsphere administration is rapid and its duration depends on biodegradation of particles, lasting longer than 5 days for non-biodegradable microspheres.[42,43] Indeed, with regard to liver metastases, it is predicted that microsphere-induced ischemia will be greater than in surrounding normal liver because the latter has an alternative blood supply, the portal vein, whereas the tumor does not.[44]

From the aforementioned analysis it is clear that there is a complementarity between the ischemia-inducing properties of microspheres and the class of compounds known to be preferentially cytotoxic to hypoxic cells. Under optimal conditions *in vitro* such compounds require from 10- to 100-fold lower concentrations for equivalent cytotoxicity toward hypoxic cells compared with their aerobic counterparts.[45] Although therapeutic approaches based on this class of compounds are novel, their locus of action is still considered to be DNA.[45,46] A factor limiting their use as single agents is that hypoxic cells are generally a minority of the clonogenic cells of a solid tumor and the remaining aerobic cells are resistant. One approach to this problem is the combination of hypoxia-selective cytotoxins with treatments that, by rendering the tumor ischemic, increase the proportion of sensitive hypoxic tumor cells. Indeed, it has been concluded on theoretical grounds that, provided an efficient hypoxia-selective cytotoxin is available, the more hypoxia, the better.[47]

A recent study compared ischemia induced pharmacologically (using hydralazine) with that induced physically (arterial occlusion by clamping) in augmentation of activity of different classes of hypoxia-selective cytotoxin.[48] The dual-function nitroheterocyclic RSU 1069 was markedly superior to other agents tested in conjunction with arterial occlusion. However, it is also of significance that, although both methods induce close to 100% radiobiological hypoxia, the ischemic response induced in tumors pharmacologically was markedly inferior to that induced by arterial occlusion in potentiation of RSU 1069 activity (Table 7). In this respect it should be recalled that the ischemic response elicited by arterial clamping is comparable with that elicited by arterial administration of microspheres.[42]

Our group has directly investigated, in a rat model of liver metastasis, the reduction in blood flow following embolization with albumin microspheres (radiolabeled with ^{125}I to compute tumor/normal tissue [T/N] ratio) administered via the hepatic artery. The results in Table 8 show that for both normal and tumor tissue

TABLE 7
Specific Growth Delay[a] Following Treatment with Bioreductive Drugs and Induction of Tumor Hypoxia

Induction of tumor hypoxia	Bioreductive drug		
	None	Mitomycin C	RSU 1069
None	0	-0.21 ± 0.19	0.07 ± 0.20
Clamping[b]	0.37 ± 0.31	$2.45 \pm 0.67^{c,d}$	$7.65 \pm 0.86^{c,d}$
Hydralazine[b]	0.33 ± 0.27	1.32 ± 0.41	0.30 ± 0.25

[a] Specific growth delay = $T_t - T_c/VDT$, where T_t = time for treated tumors to reach 4 × initial treatment volume, T_c = time for control tumors to reach 4 × initial volume, and VDT = volume doubling time of untreated control tumors.
[b] Both regimens produced a radiobiological hypoxic fraction close to 100%.
[c] Significantly different compared with bioreductive drug alone ($p < 0.001$).
[d] Drugs administered intraperitoneally at maximal tolerated dose.

From Bremner, J. C. M., Stratford, I. J., Bowler, J., and Adams, G. E., *Br. J. Cancer*, 61, 717, 1990. With permission.

TABLE 8
Tumor and Hepatic Blood Flow after Embolization with Albumin Microspheres

		Saline (n = 5)	Microspheres (n = 6)
Normal liver flow	Preinjection	23.2 ± 6.4	16.1 ± 3.8
(ml/100 g/min)	Postinjection[a]	22.7 ± 4.9	7.1 ± 1.9^b
Tumor flow	Preinjection	22.0 ± 8.3	21.2 ± 7.6
(ml/100 g/min)	Postinjection[a]	24.9 ± 8.5	1.6 ± 0.6^b

Note: Values are mean ± SE. Solid tumor deposits (HSN sarcoma) were induced in the livers of rats by an inoculation of cells. The dual-reference microsphere technique was used to measure blood flow to tumor and normal liver before and after a hepatic arterial injection of ^{125}I-labeled albumin microspheres (2×10^5 particles, 40 μm mean diameter) or saline.

[a] Tumor to normal (T/N) ratio for embolization of intrahepatic arterial albumin microspheres was 3.9.
[b] Postembolization (T = 5 min) blood flow was significantly different ($p < 0.05$ Student's paired t test) from preembolization.

there were no significant differences between blood flow measurements recorded before and after the control hepatic arterial infusion of saline. However, albumin microspheres administered via the same route resulted in significant reduction in flow to both normal liver and tumor tissue. In the latter case the reduction in mean values was by more than 90%. It is of interest that "partitioning" of albumin

TABLE 9
Comparison of Hypoxia-Selective Cytotoxicity of
Mitomycin C and Doxorubicin

Experimental system	Mitomycin C	Doxorubicin	Ref.
Electron affinity	Cytotoxicity reduced by artificial electron acceptors	Cytotoxicity not affected by artificial electron acceptors	52
Cytotoxicity *in vitro*	Cytotoxicity increased under nitrogen	Cytotoxicity not affected by oxygen tension	53
Cytotoxicity *in vivo*	Cytotoxicity greatest in cells distant from blood vessels (i.e., hypoxic cells)	Cytotoxicity greatest in cells closest to blood vessels (i.e., euoxic cells)	54

microspheres between tumor and liver (T/N = 3.9) was not determined solely by pretreatment baseline flow to these tissues, which were similar (Table 8). The higher concentration of albumin microspheres in tumor tissue may account for the greater decrease in blood flow relative to normal liver.

The important initiating step common to all hypoxia-selective cytotoxins is activation by metabolic reduction. Our results[13,28,49] and those reported in Chapter 6 with doxorubicin incorporated within albumin microspheres show that, at least with regard to quinones, microsphere-induced ischemia is adequate for reductive drug metabolism (to the stable end products 7-deoxyaglycones). However, we have also demonstrated using the analogue 4'-deoxydoxorubicin that antitumor activity of doxorubicin in microspherical form could be dissociated from reductive drug metabolism by tumor tissue; therefore, activity and reductive metabolism were not causally related in this system.[49]

Although considerable support exists for the importance of electrophilic intermediates, generated by bioreductive activation, in the biological activity of mitomycin C,[50,51] there is no experimental evidence of a similar role for reductive drug metabolism in the antitumor activity of doxorubicin. Thus, when mitomycin C and doxorubicin have been directly compared, it has been found that mitomycin C, in contrast to doxorubicin, behaves as an electron acceptor and is preferentially cytotoxic to hypoxic cells both *in vitro* and *in vivo*. The experimental observations leading to these conclusions are shown in Table 9.

Because both mitomycin C (Figure 2) and doxorubicin (Figure 3) are quinones at first sight, there appears to be an anomaly between the redox dependence of mitomycin C cytotoxicity and the finding that doxorubicin cytotoxicity is independent of drug bioreduction. An explanation may lie in the innately weak electrophilic character of the intermediate (quinone methide or semiquinone) generated from doxorubicin under anaerobic conditions and/or instability of the adduct formed with cellular nucleophiles, such as DNA. In addition, although mitomycin C can form the *bis*-adduct necessary for DNA cross-linking, this is unlikely to be the case with anthracyclines.[55] The molecular pharmacology of these drugs is discussed in greater detail in Chapter 6.

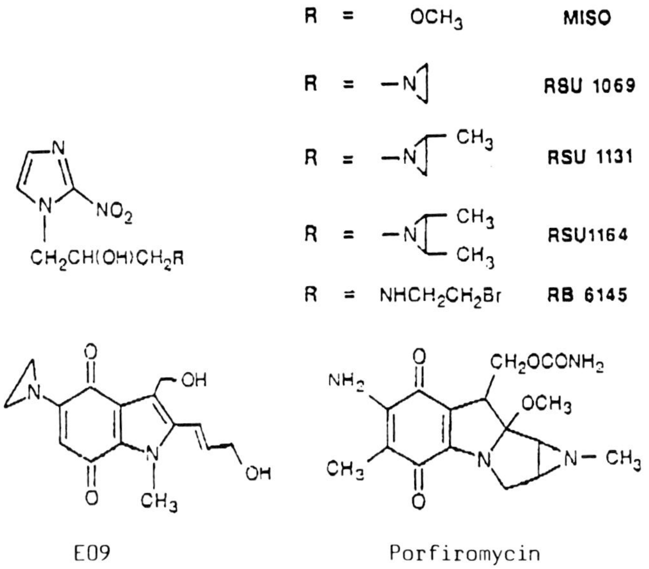

FIGURE 7. Hypoxia-selective cytotoxins.

Compounds of interest in this context are shown in Figure 7. All are chosen because of their increased hypoxia-selective cytotoxicity compared with the lead compounds. For example, EO9[56] and porfiromycin[57] show greater differential cytotoxicity against hypoxic cells than mitomycin C.

RB 6145 will shortly undergo phase I evaluation,[58] and its mode of action closely complements the capacity of microspheres for directed induction of tumor ischemia *in vivo*. Figure 7 shows that RB 6145 is designed as an inactive prodrug that on cyclization and halogen elimination yields the active aziridine ring containing compound RSU 1069. Thus, being a prodrug, high doses could be administered via the regional artery following angiotensin II infusion to achieve adequate tumor tissue concentrations; this would be immediately followed by embolization with microspheres. With regard to treatment of primary and secondary liver tumors, because selective tumor embolization can be achieved (Chapter 8) and unlike normal liver solid tumors in this organ do not possess a portal blood supply[44] (Chapter 7), tumor ischemia will be correspondingly greater than in surrounding normal liver.

B. RADIONUCLIDES FOR RADIOEMBOLIZATION

Radionuclides potentially valuable for therapy can be classified on the basis of their decay characteristics. Thus, β-emitters, such as ^{90}Y, ^{131}I, and ^{32}P, emit electrons over a continuous range of energies up to a maximum that is characteristic of the radionuclide. Penetration through tissue by β-particles is dependent on the energy of emission and ranges from 1 to 12 mm. They are of low linear energy transfer and accordingly have a low biological effectiveness, comparable to X-rays. α-

Emitters, such as ^{211}At and ^{212}Bi, emit particles (helium nuclei) that, relative to β-particles, are high linear energy transfer and correspondingly high relative biological effectiveness. However, their range of activity (<70μm) is shorter than for β-particles. Another type of radiological decay is associated with the release of Auger electrons. These produce extremely high localized doses over a range of 10 nm.[59]

Clearly the choice of radionuclide will depend on its anticipated location relative to the target (i.e., nucleus of tumor cell). If the radionuclide can be localized in the nucleus, the short range Auger effect is particularly cytotoxic as demonstrated *in vitro*.[59] α-Emitters when localized *in vitro* at or near the cell surface via monoclonal antibodies also produced marked cytotoxicity.[60] The α-emitter ^{211}At in the form of a radiocolloid has been examined *in vivo* in an ascites tumor model in mice, which permitted contact between tumor cells and radionuclide.[61] Here ^{211}At was effective, producing cures and toxicity at slightly higher doses. However, using mathematical modeling it is predicted that, due to the relatively short range of its α-particles, this radionuclide will only yield maximal cytotoxicity when a homogeneous distribution is achieved within a solid tumor.[62] Moreover, with regard to toxicity, it is axiomatic that ^{211}At must be localized within the tumor deposit with a high degree of specificity and that this must be achieved shortly after administration because of its short half-life (7.2 h). The conditions relating to efficacy and toxicity have still to be met by most carrier systems thus far developed.

Table 6 shows that the β-emitting radionuclide ^{90}Y has a number of desirable features for therapy of solid tumors. For example, it emits high energy β-particles with a maximal range in tissue of 12 mm compared with ^{131}I with a maximal range of 2.4 mm. Thus, it maintains activity over a range of >50 cell diameters. In addition, it does not emit γ-radiation, which could contribute to whole body dose without appreciably affecting viability of the tumor. A potential disadvantage of β-radiation is that, like X-rays, it is of low linear energy transfer and response is dependent on tissue oxygen tension, well-oxygenated cells showing greater radiation sensitivity than hypoxic cells.[59] This effect is illustrated in Figure 8 and shows fraction of cells surviving irradiation under both physiologically normal oxygen tension (air) and hypoxic conditions (nitrogen). As discussed, one consequence of microsphere embolization is tissue ischemia, and although this is a potentially valuable adjunct to the use of hypoxic cell cytotoxins, it may reduce efficacy of β-emitters incorporated within microspheres. Should this indeed be the case, Figure 8 also suggests how this may be at least partially overcome by the use of a class of compounds of high electron affinity known as oxygen-mimetic sensitizers.[63] These agents can be considered to mimic the effect of oxygen and sensitize hypoxic cells to the effects of radiation.[64]

IV. SUMMARY

Drugs within microsphere matrices are generally assumed to be incorporated in a native form by readily reversible interactions with the matrix, e.g., physical entrapment and ionic bonding (Chapter 1). This chapter indicates that for certain

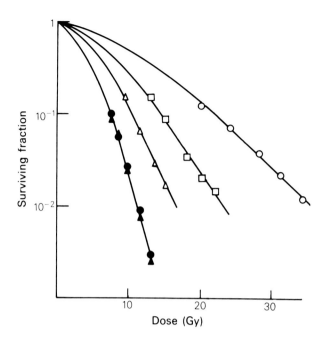

FIGURE 8. Survival curves for irradiated V79 cells. Sensitization by RSU 1069. Solid symbols (air): control (●); 0.15 mmol · dm⁻³ sensitizer (▲). Open symbols (nitrogen): control (○); 0.1 mmol · dm⁻³ sensitizer (□); 0.2 mmol · dm⁻³ sensitizer (△). (From Adams et al., *Br. J. Cancer*, 49, 571, 1984. With permission.)

drug molecules covalent attachment to matrices of appropriate chemical structure can overcome the "burst" effect of native drug release commonly seen with microspherical systems. For protein microspheres the data suggest that biodegradative processes are important for release of drug in a form covalently bound to matrix components. Although antitumor activity may not be markedly greater than drug in solution in simple model systems involving direct intratumoral injection, the tumor localization properties of microspheres observed clinically (see Chapter 8) may reveal the superiority of drug in microspherical form.

Also highlighted is the complementarity between the ischemia-inducing properties of microspheres and hypoxia-selective cytotoxins, a class of cytotoxic drug that is maximally active under conditions of reduced oxygen tension. Although theoretically attractive, it is recognized that formulation problems may be encountered when incorporating labile compounds within microspheres. With regard to the use of therapeutic radionuclides incorporated within microspheres, a comparison of radiological characteristics of available radionuclides with *in vivo* fate of carrier microspheres suggests that depth of penetration of emitted radiation will be important. Low linear energy transfer β-emitters with high emission energy, e.g., ⁹⁰Y and ³²P, appear most suitable for radioembolization of solid tumors. Again, rigorous preclinical formulation will be necessary to prevent premature radionuclide release and marrow toxicity. Another caveat is that low linear energy transfer β-emitters are less active against hypoxic cells compared with cells at normal oxygen tension. It remains to be seen whether microsphere-induced ischemia will prejudice the effect of incorporated radionuclides; if so, the use of oxygen-mimetic radiosensitizers may be required.

REFERENCES

1. **Anderson, J. H., Angerson, W. J., Willmott, N., Kerr, D. J., McArdle, C. S., and Cooke, T. G.,** Regional delivery of microspheres to liver metastases: effects of particle size and concentration on intrahepatic distribution, *Br. J. Cancer,* 64, 1031, 1991.
2. **Willmott, N., Goldberg, J., Anderson, J., Bessent, R., McKillop, J., and McArdle, C. S.,** Abnormal vasculature of solid tumors: significance for microsphere-based targeting strategies, *Int. J. Radiat. Biol.,* 60, 195, 1991.
3. **Tritton, T. R. and Yee, G.,** The anticancer agent adriamycin can be actively cytotoxic without entering cells, *Science,* 217, 248, 1982.
4. **Tritton, T. R. and Wingard, L. B., Jr.,** Targeting anticancer drugs to the cell surface by preparation of immobilised derivatives, in *Microspheres and Drug Therapy,* Davis, S. S., Illum, L., McVie, J. G., and Tomlinson, E., Eds., Elsevier, Amsterdam, 1985, 129.
5. **Gupta, P. K., Hung, C. T., and Perrier, D. G.,** Albumin microspheres. II. Effect of stabilisation temperature on the release of adriamycin, *Int. J. Pharm.,* 33, 147, 1986.
6. **Willmott, N., Chen, Y., and Florence, A. T.,** Haemoglobin, transferrin and albumin/polyaspartic acid microspheres as carriers for the cytotoxic drug adriamycin. II. *In vitro* drug release, *J. Controlled Release,* 8, 103, 1988.
7. **Natsume, H., Sugibayashi, K., and Morimoto, Y.,** *In vitro* release profile of mitomycin C from albumin microspheres: extrapolation from macrospheres to microspheres, *Pharm. Res.,* 8, 185, 1991.
8. **Juni, K., Ogata, J., Nakano, M., Ichihara, T., Mori, K., and Akagi, M.,** Preparation and evaluation *in vitro* and *in vivo* of polylactic acid microspheres containing doxorubicin, *Chem. Pharm. Bull.,* 33, 313, 1985.
9. **Kaneo, Y., Tanaka, T., and Iguchi, S.,** Preparation and properties of a mitomycin C-albumin conjugate, *Chem. Pharm. Bull.,* 38, 2614, 1990.
10. **Roos, C. F., Matsumoto, S., Takakura, Y., Hashida, M., and Sezaki, H.,** Physicochemical and antitumor characteristics of some polyamino acid prodrugs of mitomycin C, *Int. J. Pharmaceutics,* 22, 75, 1984.
11. **Wingard, L. B. and Narasimhan, K.,** Immobilisation of a primary amine-containing drug, adriamycin: coupling to a crosslinked polyvinyl alcohol and mechanistic comparison of hydrolytic stability, *Appl. Biochem. Biotechnol.,* 19, 117, 1988.
12. **Laakso, T., Stjarnkvist, P., and Sjoholm, I.,** Biodegradable microspheres. VI. Lysosomal release of covalently bound antiparasitic drugs from starch microspheres, *J. Pharm. Sci.,* 76, 134, 1987.
13. **Cummings, J., Willmott, N., Marley, E., and Smyth, J. F.,** Covalent coupling of doxorubicin in protein microspheres is a major determinant of tumor drug disposition, *Biochem. Pharmacol.,* 41, 1849, 1991.
14. **Tokes, Z. A., Rogers, K. E., and Rembaum, A.,** Synthesis of adriamycin-coupled polyglutaraldehyde microspheres and evaluation of their cytostatic activity, *Proc. Natl. Acad. Sci. USA,* 79, 2026, 1982.

15. **Zunino, Z., Savi, G., Guiliani, F., Gambetta, R., Supino, R., Tinelli, S., and Pezzoni, G.,** Comparison of anti-tumor effects of daunorubicin covalently linked to poly-L-amino acid carriers, *Eur. J. Cancer Clin. Oncol.,* 20, 121, 1981.

16. **Matsumoto, S., Yamamoto, A., Takakura, Y., Hashida, M., Tanigawa, N., and Sezaki, H.,** Cellular interaction and *in vitro* antitumor activity of mitomycin C-dextran conjugate, *Cancer Res.,* 46, 4463, 1986.

17. **Takakura, Y., Matsumoto, S., Hashida, M., and Sezaki, H.,** Physicochemical properties and antitumor activities of polymeric prodrugs of mitomycin C with different regeneration rates, *J. Controlled Release,* 10, 97, 1989.

18. **Tomasz, M., Chawla, A. K., and Lipman, R.,** Mechanism of monofunctional and bifunctional alkylation of DNA by mitomycin C, *Biochemistry,* 27, 3182, 1988.

19. **Yoshioka, T., Hashida, M., Muranishi, S., and Sezaki, H.,** Specific delivery of mitomycin C to the liver, spleen and lung: nano- and microspherical carriers of gelatin, *Int. J. Pharmaceutics,* 8, 131, 1981.

20. **Duncan, R., Hume, I. C., Kopeckova, P., Ulbrich, K., Stroholm, J., and Kopecek, J.,** Anticancer agents coupled to N-(2-hydroxypropyl) methacrylamide copolymers. III. Evaluation of adriamycin conjugates against mouse leukaemia L1210 *in vivo, J. Controlled Release,* 10, 51, 1989.

21. **Golightly, L., Brown, J. E., Mitchell, J. B., and Brown, J. R.,** Trypanocidal activity of free and carrier bound daunorubicin, *Cell. Biol. Int. Rep.,* 12, 77, 1988.

22. **Visscher, G. E., Pearson, J. E., Fong, J. W., Argentieri, G. J., Robison, R. L., and Maulding, H. V.,** Effect of particle size on the *in vitro* and *in vivo* degradation rates of poly(DL-lactide-co-glycolide) microcapsules, *J. Biomed. Mater. Res.,* 22, 733, 1988.

23. **Willmott, N., Chen, Y., Goldberg, J., McArdle, C. S., and Florence, A. T.,** Biodegradation rate of embolised protein microspheres in lung, liver and kidney of rats, *J. Pharm. Pharmacol.,* 41, 433, 1988.

24. **Trouet, A., Masquelier, M., Baurain, R., and Deprey-de-Campaneere, D.,** A covalent linkage between daunorubicin and protein that is stable in serum and reversible by lysosomal hydrolases, is required for a lysosomotropic drug carrier, *Proc. Natl. Acad. Sci., USA,* 79, 626, 1982.

25. **Duncan, R., Cable, H. C., Lloyd, J. B., Reymanova, P., and Kopecek, J.,** Polymers containing enymically degradable bonds. VII. Design of oligopeptide side chains in poly[N-(2-hydroxypropyl)methacrylamide] copolymers to promote efficient degradation by lysosomal enzymes, *Makromol. Chem.,* 184, 1997, 1983.

26. **Chen, Y., Willmott, N., Anderson, J., and Florence, A. T.,** Haemoglobin, transferrin and albumin/polyaspartic acid microspheres as carriers for the cytotoxic drug adriamycin. I. Ultrastructural appearance and drug content, *J. Controlled Release,* 8, 93, 1988.

27. **Kamel, M. H., Willmott, N., McNicol, A. M., and Toner, P. G.,** The use of electron microscopy and immunocytochemistry to characterise spontaneously arising, transplantable rat tumors, *Virchows Arch. B,* 57, 11, 1989.

28. **Willmott, N. and Cummings, J.,** Increased anti-tumor effect of adriamycin-loaded albumin microspheres is associated with anaerobic bioreduction of drug in tumor tissue, *Biochem. Pharmacol.,* 36, 521, 1987.

29. **Chen, Y., Willmott, N., Anderson, J., and Florence, A. T.,** Comparison of albumin and casein microspheres as carrier for doxorubicin, *J. Pharm. Pharmacol.,* 39, 978, 1988.

30. **Thomas, W. A.,** Peptide derivatives as prodrugs, *Biochem. Soc. Trans.,* 14, 383, 1986.

31. **Sharkey, R. M., Kaltovich, F. A., Shih, L. B., Fand, I., Govelitz, G., and Goldenberg, D. M.,** Radioimmunotherapy of human colonic cancer xenografts with ^{90}Y-labeled monoclonal antibodies to carcinoembryonic antigen, *Cancer Res.,* 48, 3270, 1988.

32. **Stewart, J. S. W., Hird, V., and Epenetos, A. A.,** Alternative to toxicity and dosimetry of Y-90 labeled antibody, *Int. J. Radiat. Oncol. Biol. Phys.,* 17, 241, 1989.

33. **Goldberg, J. A., Willmott, N., Anderson, J. H., McCurrach, G., Bessent, R. G., McKillop, J. H., and McArdle, C. S.,** The biodegradation of albumin microspheres used for regional chemotherapy in patients with colorectal liver metastases, *Nucl. Med. Commun.,* 12, 57, 1991.

34. **Ermias, A., Beau, P., Perdrisot, R., Le Jeune, J. J., Pouliquen, D., Leger, J., Lepape, A., and Jallet, P.**, Development of microencapsulated β-emitting radionuclides for selective tumor radioembolisation, *Eur. J. Nucl. Med.*, 15 (Abstr.), 401, 1989.

35. **Llaurado, J. G., Brewer, L. A., Elam, D. A., Ing, S. J., Raiszadeh, M., Slater, J. M., Hirst, A. E., and Zielinski, F. W.**, Radioisotopic pulmonary lobectomy: feasibility study in dogs, *J. Nucl. Med.*, 31, 594, 1990.

36. **Gray, B. N., Burton, M. A., Kelleher, D., Klemp, P., and Matz, L.**, Tolerance of the liver to the effects of yttrium-90 radiation, *Int. J. Radiat. Biol. Oncol. Phys.*, 18, 619, 1990.

37. **Ehrhardt, G. J. and Day, D. E.**, Therapeutic use of ^{90}Y-microspheres, *Nucl. Med. Biol.*, 14, 233, 1987.

38. **Jain, R. K.**, Transport of molecules across tumor vasculature, *Cancer Metastasis Rev.*, 6, 559, 1987.

39. **Dvorak, H. E., Nagy, J. A., Dvorak, J. T., and Dvorak, A. M.**, Identification and characterisation of the blood vessels of solid tumors that are leaky to circulating macromolecules, *Am. J. Pathol.*, 133, 95, 1988.

40. **Ohkouchi, K., Imoto, H., Takakura, Y., Hashida, M., and Sezaki, H.**, Disposition of anticancer drugs after bolus arterial administration in a tissue-isolated tumor perfusion system, *Cancer Res.*, 50, 1640, 1990.

41. **Kallinowski, F., Schlenger, K. H., Kloes, M., Stohrer, M., and Vaupel, P.**, Tumor blood flow: the principal modulator of oxidative and glycolic metabolism, and of the metabolic micromilieu of human tumor xenograft *in vivo*, *Int. J. Cancer*, 44, 266, 1989.

42. **Lindberg, B., Lote, K., and Teder, H.**, Biodegradable starch microspheres: a new medical tool, in *Microspheres and Drug Therapy*, Davis, S. S., Illum, L., McVie, J. G., and Tomlinson, E., Eds., Elsevier, Amsterdam, 1984, 153.

43. **Miyake, K., Tanonaka, K., Minematsu, R., Inove, K., and Takeo, S.**, Possible therapeutic effect of naftidrofuryl oxalate on brain energy metabolism after microsphere-induced cerebral embolism, *Br. J. Pharmacol.*, 98, 389, 1989.

44. **Sigurdson, E. R., Ridge, J. A., Kemeny, N., and Daly, J. M.**, Tumor and liver uptake following hepatic artery and portal vein infusion, *J. Clin. Oncol.*, 5, 1836, 1987.

45. **Stratford, I. J., Walling, J. M., and Silver, A. R. J.**, The differential cytotoxicity of RSU 1069: cell survival studies indicating interaction with DNA as a possible mode of action, *Br. J. Cancer*, 53, 339, 1986.

46. **Jenner, T. J., Sapora, O., O'Neill, P., and Fielden, E. M.**, Enhancement of DNA damage in mammalian cells upon bioreduction of the nitroimidazole-aziridines RSU-1069 and RSU-1131, *Biochem. Pharmacol.*, 37, 3837, 1988.

47. **Brown, J. M.**, Targeting bioreductive drugs to tumors: is it necessary to manipulate blood flow?, *Int. J. Radiat. Biol.*, 60, 231, 1991.

48. **Bremner, J. C. M., Stratford, I. J., Bowler, J., and Adams, G. E.**, Bioreductive drugs and the selective induction of tumor hypoxia, *Br. J. Cancer*, 61, 717, 1990.

49. **Willmott, N., Cummings, J., Marley, E., and Smyth, J. F.**, Relationship between reductive drug metabolism in tumor tissue of anthracyclines in microspherical form and anti-tumor activity, *Biochem. Pharmacol.*, 39, 1055, 1990.

50. **Beijnen, J. H., Lingeman, H., Van Munster, H. H., and Underbeg, W. J. H.**, Mitomycin antitumor agents: a review of their physico-chemical and analytical properties and stability, *J. Pharm. Biomed. Anal.*, 4, 275, 1986.

51. **Powis, G.**, Metabolism and reactions of quinoid anticancer agents, *Pharmacol. Ther.*, 35, 57, 1987.

52. **Keizer, H. G., DeLee, S. J., Van Vijn, J., Pinedo, H. M., and Joenje, H.**, Effect of artificial electron acceptors on the cytotoxicity of mitomycin C and doxorubicin in human lung tumor cells, *Eur. J. Cancer Clin. Oncol.*, 25, 1113, 1989.

53. **Gupta, V. and Costanzi, J. J.**, Role of hypoxia in anticancer drug-induced cytotoxicity for Ehrlich ascites cells, *Cancer Res.*, 47, 2407, 1987.

54. **Teicher, B. A., Holden, S. A., Al-Achi, A., and Herman, T. S.,** Classification of antineoplastic treatments by their differential toxicity toward putative oxygenated and hypoxic tumor subpopulations *in vivo* in the FSaIIc murine fibrosarcoma, *Cancer Res.,* 50, 3339, 1990.

55. **Ramakrishnan, K. and Fisher, J.,** 7-Deoxydaunomycinone quinone methide reactivity with thiol nucleophiles, *J. Med. Chem.,* 29, 1215, 1986.

56. **Lelieveld, P. and Hendriks, H. R.,** New EORTC compounds, *Cancer Treat. Rev.,* 17, 119, 1990.

57. **Sartorelli, A. C.,** Therapeutic attack on hypoxic cells of solid tumors, *Cancer Res.,* 48, 755, 1988.

58. **Showalter, H. D. H., Sercel, A. D., Winters, R. T., Leopold, W. R., Elliot, W. L., Fry, D. W., Arundel-Suto, C. M., and Sobolt-Leopold, J. S.,** A new class of bifunctional nitroimidazole radiosensitizers incorporating soft alkylating and acylating functionality, *Proc. Am. Assoc. Cancer Res.,* 32 (Abstr.), 389, 1991.

59. **Adelstein, S. J. and Kassis, A. I.,** Radiobiologic implications of the microscopic distribution of energy from radionuclides, *Nucl. Med. Biol.,* 14, 165, 1987.

60. **Kurtzman, S. H., Russo, A., Mitchell, J. B., De Graff, W., Sindelar, W., Brechbiel, M. W., Gansow, O. A., Friedman, A. M., Hines, J. J., Gamson, J., and Atcher, R. W.,** [212]Bismuth-linked to an antipancreatic carcinoma antibody: model for alpha-particle-emitter radiotherapy, *J. Natl. Cancer Inst.,* 80, 449, 1988.

61. **Bloomer, W. D., McLaughlin, W. H., Lambrecht, R. M., Atcher, R. W., Mirzadeh, S., Madara, J. L., Milius, R. A., Zalutsky, M. R., Adelstein, S. J., and Wolf, A. P.,** [211]At-radiocolloid therapy: further observations and comparison with radiocolloids of ^{32}P, [165]Dy and ^{90}Y, *Int. J. Radiat. Oncol. Biol. Phys.,* 10, 341, 1984.

62. **Humm, J. L.,** A microdosimetric model of astatine-211 labeled antibodies for radioimmunotherapy, *Int. J. Radiat. Oncol. Biol. Phys.,* 13, 1767, 1987.

63. **Coleman, C. N.,** Hypoxia in tumors: a paradigm for the approach to biochemical and physiologic heterogeneity, *J. Natl. Cancer Inst.,* 80, 310, 1988.

64. **Adams, G. E., Ahmed, I., Sheldon, P. W., and Stratford, I. J.,** Radiation sensitization and chemopotentiation: RSU 1069, a compound more efficient than misonidazole *in vitro* and *in vivo, Br. J. Cancer,* 49, 571, 1984.

Chapter 6

DRUG ANALYSIS OF PROTEIN MICROSPHERES: FROM PHARMACEUTICAL PREPARATION TO *IN VIVO* FATE

Jeffrey Cummings, David Watson, and John F. Smyth

TABLE OF CONTENTS

I. INTRODUCTION

The focus of this chapter will be on the analysis of anticancer drugs once incorporated in protein microspheres and will feature techniques relevant to studying chemical interactions between the drug and the microsphere matrix and between the drug and the biological matrix the microsphere finds itself in. It is therefore not intended as a general review or long list of all possible analytical techniques for cancer chemotherapeutic agents; the interested reader is referred to excellent reviews.[1,2] The importance of drug analysis to microspheres and regional cancer therapy can be stressed as follows: because the ultimate aim of a cancer drug delivery system is to target its payload selectively to the tumor, then a proper evaluation of its efficacy can only be achieved by rigorous drug analysis. The essential element in this drug analysis, as in any drug analysis, is that the method employed reflects accurately the real situation in the samples being studied, which is especially important with drug delivery systems that can potentially alter the chemical properties of the incorporated drug and its *in vivo* fate after administration.

To achieve our goal a proper understanding of the physicochemical properties of the compounds of interest and their *in vivo* pharmacology is a prerequisite and this has been included. As will be seen throughout this chapter and especially with doxorubicin, unexpected events can occur both during the pharmaceutical process and after administration, which only become evident when critical analysis is applied from more than one direction. Finally, a large part of this chapter will concentrate on the results of drug analyses to illustrate some of the points made herein.

II. ANTHRACYCLINES

The anthracyclines consist of a large group of naturally occurring and semi-synthetic antibiotic compounds based on a highly colored benzanthraquinone nucleus and carbohydrate side chain and are structurally and functionally divided into three classes. The class I compounds (Figure 1A), including doxorubicin and daunorubicin, the prototypes of the whole group, are all monosaccharides in which the sugar is the unusual daunosamine moiety, which contains a positively charged basic amino group on position 3' that is critical for anticancer activity. The class II compounds (Figure 1B), including aclacinomycin and marcellomycin, are poly-saccharides. They inhibit RNA synthesis at concentrations several hundredfold lower than required to inhibit DNA synthesis, which distinguishes them from class I. Included in this class is the nonsugar containing semisynthetic antibiotic menogaril. The third class has more recently emerged and is characterized by high activity (1000-fold greater cytotoxicity *in vitro* than doxorubicin). These compounds are based on class I but with substitution of morpholino and cyanomorpholino (MRA-CN) ring systems on the amino group of daunosamine but are distinguished from class I and II by a mechanism of action that probably involves covalent binding to DNA.

The unique structural backbone of the anthracyclines confers three general properties, which are the key to their *in vivo* pharmacology:

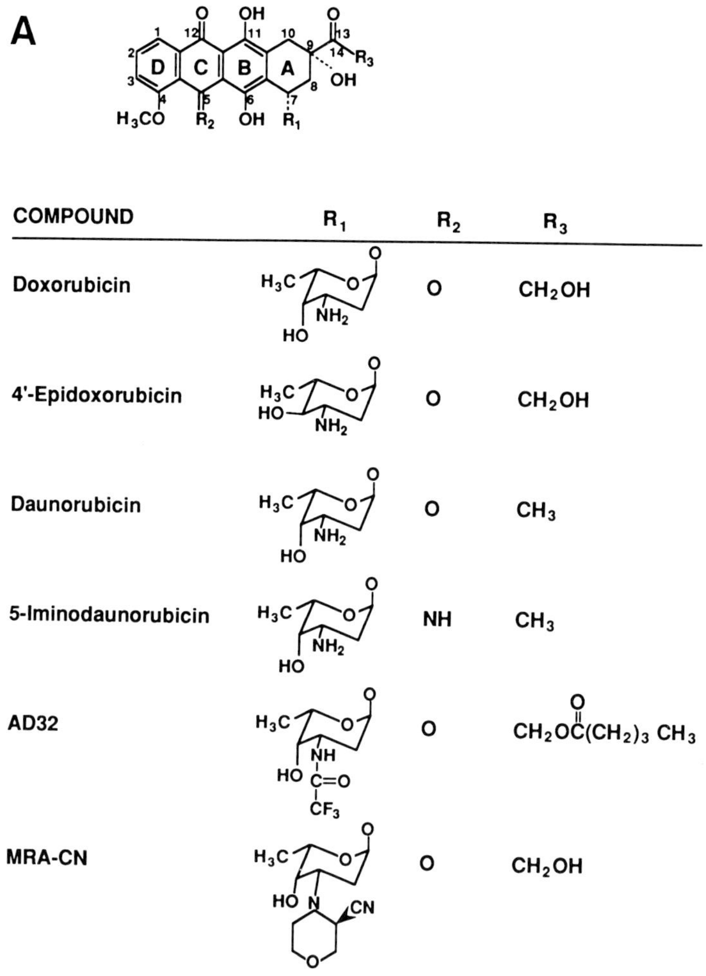

A

COMPOUND	R_1	R_2	R_3
Doxorubicin		O	CH_2OH
4'-Epidoxorubicin		O	CH_2OH
Daunorubicin		O	CH_3
5-Iminodaunorubicin		NH	CH_3
AD32		O	$CH_2OC(CH_2)_3 CH_3$
MRA-CN		O	CH_2OH

FIGURE 1. (A) Chemical structures of anthracyclines of class I and class III (cyanomorpholino compound MRA-CN). (B) Chemical structures of class II anthracyclines.

1. The planar ring system and charged side chains enable high affinity noncovalent binding to DNA by a process termed "intercalation" in which the drug binds in parallel to the base pairs of DNA.
2. The quinone moiety undergoes bioreduction to produce a semiquinone drug-free radical, which in turn can redox cycle with molecular oxygen to generate a cascade of reactive oxygen species.
3. The quinone (C ring) and hydroquinone (B ring) moiety can chelate iron III.

Comprehensive reviews of anthracycline pharmacokinetics and metabolism[3] and their interactions with DNA[4] have recently been published.

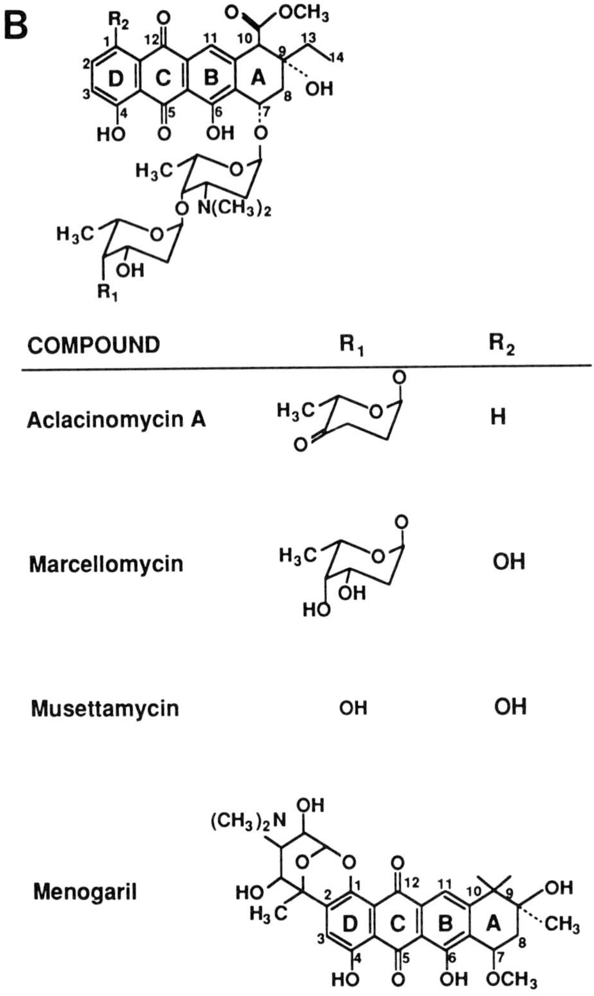

FIGURE 1B (Continued).

A. DOXORUBICIN AND DAUNORUBICIN

Daunorubicin (daunomycin, rubidomycin) was the first anthracycline antibiotic to be discovered (in 1963) followed by doxorubicin (adriamycin) (in 1969), and together these two remain the most useful clinically.[5] Both drugs are used extensively in combination chemotherapy, with doxorubicin having the wider spectrum of clinical activity. Both exhibit the classic toxicity profiles of cytotoxic drugs: nausea and vomiting, gastrointestinal tract toxicity, hair loss, and myelosuppression. In addition, they induce a unique toxicity to the heart, which is related to cumulative dose and peak plasma drug concentrations and is irreversible. Originally, this cardiotoxicity stimulated the drive for new compounds and analog development, but drug resistance, both in the form of the multidrug resistance phenotype[6,7] and the atypical (altered topoisomerase II) multidrug resistance phenotype,[8] is generally considered the major clinical problem to be overcome by the pharmacologist. Cardiotoxicity can be controlled by altering dose schedules without loss of anticancer activity.[9] Because doxorubicin is the more active drug and has been incorporated in microspheres, the following sections will deal exclusively with doxorubicin.

B. PHYSICOCHEMICAL PROPERTIES AND ANALYSIS

Doxorubicin is chemically reactive, chemically unstable, and particularly sensitive to light-induced degradation, as well as acid catalyzed hydrolysis of its glycosidic bond to a 7-hydroxyaglycone and undergoes rapid decomposition above pH 9 (the pka of the B ring hydroquinone). Of importance to the analyst, at all levels of doxorubicin determination, is the fact that the drug binds tightly, although noncovalently, to inert materials, such as glass vessels, tissue culture plastics, and cellulose membranes as well as forms tight complexes with proteins, nucleic acids, phospholipids (especially cardiolipin), amino acids, nucleotides, biogenic amines, and even self-associates at high drug concentrations.[10] This phenomenon is particularly problematic for the estimation of drug covalent binding to biomolecules because even a very low level of nonspecific binding will be sufficient to invalidate these analyses, which are normally measuring 1 drug adduct per 10^6 to 10^9 DNA nucleobases. A high performance liquid chromatography (HPLC) assay has been published recently, which can determine doxorubicin covalent binding to DNA down to 1 adduct per 10^6 bases without interference from noncovalently bound intercalated drug or nonspecifically bound drug.[11]

Doxorubicin stability studies have consistently produced different results despite using similar experimental conditions (35 min to 14 h for 5% decomposition at room temperature and lighting).[12] The reason for this large discrepancy is probably due to the fact that different methods of analysis are employed to measure the drug: most commonly HPLC with either ultraviolet detection or fluorescence detection, although electrochemical detection can be used, but this method has been shown to give rise to spurious peaks in biological specimens.[13] In early pharmacokinetic and metabolism studies of doxorubicin thin layer chromatography (TLC) was used extensively, but this technique is prone to producing metabolite artifacts due to both the acidic nature of the silica gel and the acidic solvent systems employed cleaving the glycosidic bond.[14,15] Gas chromatography and/or mass spectrometry have not been applied to doxorubicin analysis because of its poor volatility and stability.

Although doxorubicin can be detected with superb sensitivity by fluorescence, which has now been extended down to the low picogram level with the introduction of lasers, the drug degrades to nonfluorescent products and is biotransformed to nonfluorescent intermediates each with unique ultraviolet visible absorption spectra. As a consequence of this and the large number of metabolites of the drug that are formed *in vivo,* we believe the technique of choice for the analysis of doxorubicin is HPLC coupled to a diode array detector (DAD) and have reported the extensive use of this technique.[16]

C. PHARMACOLOGY

We have reviewed both the clinical and molecular pharmacology of doxorubicin in detail recently.[17,18] From an analytical standpoint the key question is what other forms the drug is converted into that have to be determined to properly evaluate the effects of microsphere entrapment on drug pharmacology.

1. Drug Metabolism

The major metabolite of doxorubicin is the C13 carbonyl-reduced alcohol referred to as doxorubicinol. This metabolite is formed by a ubiquitously distributed group of cytoplasmic aldo-ketoreductases. It is important to note that aldo-ketoreductase activity resides in blood elements and possibly plasma and that doxorubicinol can be produced *in situ*. Conjugates of doxorubicin (a 4-*0*-sulfate and 4-*0*-glucuronide) have been identified in patient urine by TLC,[15] but their presence in urine or plasma awaits confirmation using more sensitive HPLC methods. Removal of the daunosamine sugar group can occur at two points by different mechanisms to produce a series of aglycone metabolites. 7-Hydroxyaglycones, as mentioned, are formed by hydrolytic cleavage, which can occur *in vitro* at acid pH or, less probably, *in vivo* by microsomal hydrolases. 7-Deoxyaglycones are formed after doxorubicin quinone reduction by a process originally termed "reductive deglycosylation"[19] and are not *in vitro* degradation products but genuine drug metabolites. A full separation of doxorubicin, doxorubicinol, and their respective 7-hydroxyaglycones and 7-deoxyaglycones can be achieved by reversed phase HPLC with isocratic elution.[20]

2. Free Radical Chemistry

Possessing a quinone group doxorubicin can undergo bioreduction to a semiquinone free radical. Although not highly reactive, the radical is unstable and has a probable half-life of 10^{-7} s. Therefore, under normal circumstances detection of the radical is impossible in most biological matrices. It falls on the analyst, therefore, to measure the consequences of free radical formation rather than the event directly. There are three possible consequences of doxorubicin bioreduction (Figure 2):

1. Under aerobic conditions the semiquinone reacts preferentially with molecular oxygen, resulting in generation of reactive oxygen species, lipid peroxidation, and DNA damage induced most probably by the hydroxyl radical (OH·).
2. Under anaerobic conditions the semiquinone rearranges by eliminating daunosamine to give a C7 centered radical aglycone. Alternatively, either two electron reduction of doxorubicin (or disproportionation of the doxorubicin semiquinone free radical) to the hydroquinone followed by elimination of daunosamine yields a quinone methide (half-life several seconds). These reactive species are potentially capable of covalently binding to biological macromolecules.
3. Rather than binding covalently, the aglycone intermediates abstract a solvent proton to form the noncytotoxic stable 7-deoxyaglycone metabolite. Recent data suggest that *in vivo*, in tumor, tissue pathway 3 is preferred.[21]

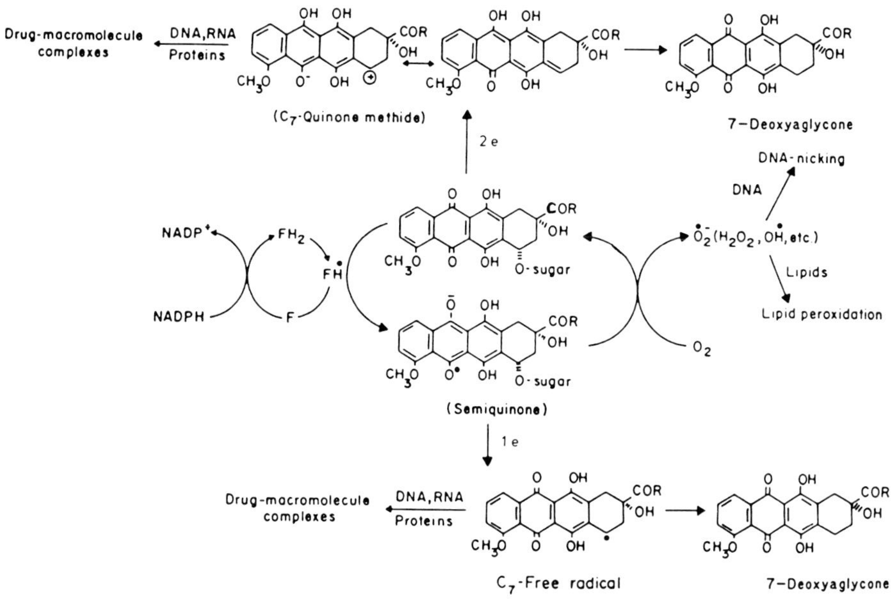

FIGURE 2. The three possible outcomes of doxorubicin quinone reduction.

3. Complexation of Iron

Chelation of iron (III) at C11 and C12 results in both quenching and a shift in the doxorubicin visible absorption spectrum, allowing the process to be monitored spectrophotometrically.[22] Also, complexation with iron can result in auto-oxidation of doxorubicin producing a series of metabolites, including the eventual end product a C9-COOH metabolite, which can be resolved from the parent drug by HPLC.[23] However, at physiological pH it is unlikely that *in vivo* a doxorubicin-iron preformed complex would remain intact or that doxorubicin would bind iron adventitiously. This is strengthened by the fact that pharmacokinetic studies of doxorubicin have never reported detection of iron complexes.

D. INCORPORATION IN MICROSPHERES

Protein microspheres are made under conditions that could impair the incorporated drug either through the use of chemically reactive cross-linkers, such as glutaraldehyde or by heat denaturation at temperatures in excess of 100°C. HPLC with DAD has been applied to assess whether or not the pharmaceutical process of making doxorubicin-albumin microspheres using glutaraldehyde affects the chemical structure of the drug both incorporated within and then released from the microparticles[24] and confirmed chromatographically pure doxorubicin in both cases. These studies have been extended to freeze-drying for production of a lyophilized, stable formulation, and the same results were obtained.[25] In the first of these two studies analysis involved extraction of tryptic digests of protein microspheres into 5 volumes of chloroform:propan-2-ol (2:1).[26,27] Subsequently, it came to light that if the total drug content was determined directly on the digest, without extraction, either by DAD or by use of ^{14}C-labeled drug, then there was always a discrepancy between the total amount of drug present in the digest and the value determined by HPLC in the extract. In this case significantly less was determined by HPLC, indicating a fraction of the drug remained with the digested microspheres and was not freely extractable into organic solvents. Eventually it was demonstrated that this fraction of drug was probably covalently bound to the matrix via a molecule of glutaraldehyde.[28] The covalently bound component was only identified by a combination of techniques using both ^{14}C-labeled drug and HPLC with DAD.

Not all protein microspheres studied contained a bound fraction of drug, which was shown to be dependent on the nature of the protein matrix and amount of glutaraldehyde used during preparation. Bound fraction could account for between 40 and 80% of total drug content (see also Chapter 5). Therefore, it appears that the pharmaceutical process can alter the structure of incorporated anthracyclines, and this has a profound effect on the biological properties of the microspheres (Section II.F.1.). A similar interaction has been confirmed with the other class I anthracycline, 4'-deoxydoxorubicin.

E. *IN VITRO* ACTIVITY

The *in vitro* activity of doxorubicin-loaded albumin microspheres has been studied in our laboratory against a panel of human ovarian carcinoma cell lines, including a multidrug-resistant variant. On a molar basis the microspheres were equipotent with free doxorubicin and did not circumvent drug resistance. These results are not unexpected because the real advantage of a drug delivery system is *in vivo*. Nevertheless, previous reports of doxorubicin covalently coupled to polyglutaraldehyde microspheres have shown potential to overcome drug resistance.[29]

F. *IN VIVO* FATE

It should now be clear that a proper evaluation of the fate of doxorubicin incorporated in microspheres *in vivo* ought to involve determination of native drug, its metabolites (especially the 7-deoxyaglycones), drug microsphere covalent complexes, drug covalent binding to DNA, and lipid peroxidation. The following two sections describe techniques that have been applied successfully to the analysis of doxorubicin microspheres *in vivo*.

1. Animal Models

To follow the fate of native doxorubicin and its metabolites plus the covalently bound fraction in the target organ *in vivo* after administration of microspheres, it is necessary to perform two separate drug determinations on each tissue or tumor sample. For both determinations tissues/tumor are treated as follows. After thawing from storage at $-20°C$, they are suspended in distilled water (20% w/v), then disaggregated mechanically, and finally homogenized using a Potter-type unit. Homogenates are then treated with 33% (w/v) silver nitrate (0.2 ml/ml homogenate) at 4°C for 10 min to free DNA intercalated drug and precipitate proteins.[30]

The free drug and 7-deoxyaglycone metabolites (determination 1) are extracted from the homogenate in 5 vol of chloroform:propan-2-ol (2:1 v/v) for 30 min, which is dried down at 50°C under vacuum and is then ready for isocratic HPLC with fluorescent detection.[20] Extracts can be stored for up to 1 week at −20°C without drug loss.

Total drug content in homogenates (determination 2) is measured by counting the activity of ^{14}C-doxorubicin (0.5 mCi/mmol) incorporated into microspheres as a radioactive tracer and the covalently bound fraction is calculated as the difference between the values (i.e., 2 − 1). For determination 2 soluene (2 ml) is added to 1 ml homogenate, which is then incubated at 37°C overnight. After incubation samples are thoroughly mixed with 15 ml of scintillation fluid and counted twice with a 24-h interval in between to control for spurious counts due to chemiluminescence and photoluminescence. Using these techniques several interesting observations have been made, which highlight that rather than being a passive instrument of drug transport, microspheres actively alter the metabolism of doxorubicin. Thus, albumin microspheres have been found to stimulate anaerobic quinone reduction of doxorubicin to 7-deoxyaglycones in the tumor itself by a factor of 155-fold from almost negligible levels of 0.02 μg/g up to 3.1 μg/g almost approaching the parent drug itself (3.9 μg/g) at 48 h after intratumoral treatment.[31] Although this was not totally unexpected because microspheres may induce hypoxia, the magnitude of the effect was surprising.

Covalent coupling to the protein matrix of microspheres has a dual effect on the fate of doxorubicin *in vivo:* (1) it actually reduces the degree of stimulation of anaerobic quinone reduction, which is probably beneficial because this has now been shown to be a pathway of drug inactivation,[21] and (2) it alters the pharmacokinetics of the parent drug producing elevated levels by reducing its rate of elimination from the tumor, thus acting as a sustained release depot, which may contribute to antitumor efficacy.[28] Complexation between doxorubicin and protein microsphere matrix is discussed in detail in Chapter 5.

2. Clinical Studies

Until recently no data were available on the analysis of clinical specimens after administration of doxorubicin incorporated in microspheres. Table 1 shows such data for 5 mg of doxorubicin incorporated in albumin microspheres, administered via the regional artery to a patient with breast cancer, compared with 25 mg of native doxorubicin in solution administered intravenously.[32] Native drug concentrations were measured after organic solvent extraction of silver nitrate-treated homogenates as described herein. Although these data are at present limited to one patient, it validates that drug-loaded microspheres, incorporating a fraction of the dose of drug administered in solution, can target higher drug levels to the tumor accompanied by lower systemic exposure. The data also show that microspheres localize high levels of doxorubicin in breast tissue adjacent to the tumor and caution that microspheres used in this context require further pharmacological manipulation to improve tumor selectivity (see Chapters 2 and 8).

TABLE 1

The *In Vivo* Fate of Doxorubicin Incorporated in Albumin Microspheres or Free in Solution in Cancer Patients 30 min to 1 h after Administration[a]

	Free solution 25 mg			Microspheres 5 mg		
	Plasma	Liver	Breast carcinoma	Plasma	Breast carcinoma	Adjacent normal breast tissue
Doxorubicin (μg/g or ml) (mean ± SD)	0.17 ± 0.13	5.6 ± 1.5	0.82 ± 0.48	0.07	1.68	14.7

[a] Microspheres were administered locally into an artery supplying the breast; free solution was administered systemically by the intravenous route.

Adapted from Cummings, J. and McArdle, C. S., *Br. J. Cancer*, 53, 835, 1986. With permission.

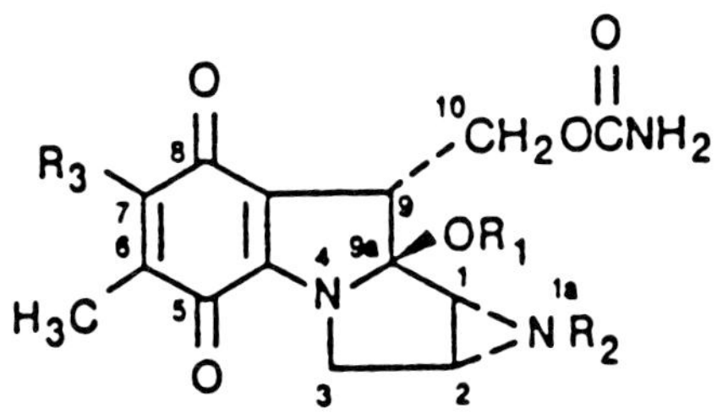

Compound	R_1	R_2	R_3
Mitomycin A	CH_3	H	OCH_3
Mitomycin B	H	CH_3	OCH_3
Mitomycin C	CH_3	H	NH_2
Porfiromycin	CH_3	CH_3	NH_2
KW 2083	CH_3	H	$HN-\langle\rangle-OH$
BMY-25282	CH_3	H	$N=CH-N\langle^{CH_3}_{CH_3}$
BMY-25067	CH_3	H	$NH-CH_2-S-S-\langle\rangle-NO_2$
RR-150	CH_3	H	$NH-CH_2-CH_2-SH$

FIGURE 3. Chemical structures of mitomycins.

III. MITOMYCINS

The original mitomycins were antibiotics isolated from *Streptomyces caespitosis,* and the first two compounds, discovered in 1956, were designated mitomycin A and B (Figure 3). Although they exhibited potent anticancer activity, toxicity was also evident in animals. Mitomycin C, subsequently isolated in 1958, proved to have superior antitumor activity and was less toxic and soon after was shown in Japan to have activity in humans.[33] Many promising semisynthetic compounds have been produced based mainly on substitution at C7 of the mitosane nucleus (Figure 3). The mitomycins contain three significant chemical features: a quinone moiety capable of free radical formation and redox cycling; a fused aziridine ring, which can promote DNA alkylation (covalent binding); and carbamate function, which is also implicated in DNA alkylation. Their anticancer activity is believed to be due to these unique chemical properties. Mitomycin C is the only clinically useful natural product anticancer drug believed to work by DNA alkylation. Structure activity studies indicate that a favorable quinone reduction potential, good water solubility, and low lipophilicity improve antitumor activity.[34]

A. MITOMYCIN C

The initial clinical trials with mitomycin C, despite revealing a broad spectrum of activity, showed that the drug was profoundly bone marrow myelotoxic, which discouraged further clinical trials in the U.S. for many years. Subsequently, it was ascertained that the use of intermittent high dose therapy with a 4 to 6-week interval reduced toxicity without affecting activity and established mitomycin C as a clinically useful cancer chemotherapeutic agent.[35] It is probably the drug of first choice for local intravesical administration in superficial bladder cancer, but it is more often found in combination chemotherapy regimens. As well as bone marrow toxicity, pulmonary toxicity has been reported that may be related to the high local concentration of oxygen and production of reactive oxygen species. There is a counterindication that mitomycin C may interact with doxorubicin to compound the cardiotoxicity of the latter.

Due to its low therapeutic index mitomycin C has been given both locally and in different forms, such as drug-dextran conjugates or absorbed onto activated carbon particles to reduce toxicity. Of particular interest, the drug has been incorporated into or admixed with a variety of microspherical drug delivery systems, such as ethylcellulose microparticles,[36] biodegradable starch microspheres,[37] albumin protein microspheres,[38] and polylactic acid microcapsules.[39] Despite having been microencapsulated for more than 10 years, little is known about the effect of the pharmaceutical process on the chemical and biological properties of the drug. This is more than likely due to the drug's complex chemistry, pharmacology, and mechanism of action, which have proved surprisingly difficult to analyze comprehensively *in vivo*.

B. PHYSICOCHEMICAL PROPERTIES

Despite containing two potentially reactive groups, carbamate function and fused aziridine ring, mitomycin C in aqueous solution at neutral pH is relatively stable (3 weeks at 5°C and 24 h at room temperature for 5% degradation).[12] In the solid state as the commercially available lyophilized powder, the drug is stable for up to 2 years and enhanced stability has been reported in tissue culture media (stable for several weeks at 37°C). Several different sets of conditions are known to activate the drug, and it has been long known that mitomycin C requires bioactivation before it is converted into DNA alkylating species. At basic pH the drug is unstable due to destruction of the quinone moiety. Under mild acid conditions the C9a *O*-methyl group leaves the mitosane nucleus as methanol (Figure 4), a C9, 9a double-bond forms producing the mitosene nucleus, and the aziridine ring opens to generate an electrophilic carbon center at C1. Water can act as a nucleophile to form the 1,2-*cis*- and 1,2-*trans*-1-hydroxy 2,7-diaminomitosene hydrolysis products.

The products of nucleophilic attack on C1 are highly dependent on stereochemical considerations, and this also has major ramifications for the type of DNA adducts formed. Acid hydrolysis results in a ratio of the *cis*- to *trans*-isomers of 3:1.[40] At lower pH the C1 center preferentially abstracts a solvent proton to form 2,7-diaminomitosene. In the presence of phosphate buffer ions 1,2-*cis*- and 1,2-*trans*-1-phosphate 2,7 diaminomitosene are formed, and in an acetic acid/acetate buffer acetylated mitosenes are observed.[41] At neutral pH reducing agents, such as sodium borohydride, sodium dithionite, or H_2/palladium, will catalyze similar chemistry due to conversion of the quinone ring from being electron-deficient into the electron-rich semiquinone or hydroquinone moieties, which then promote the *O*-methyl group to leave. Therefore, great caution has to be taken in the analysis of

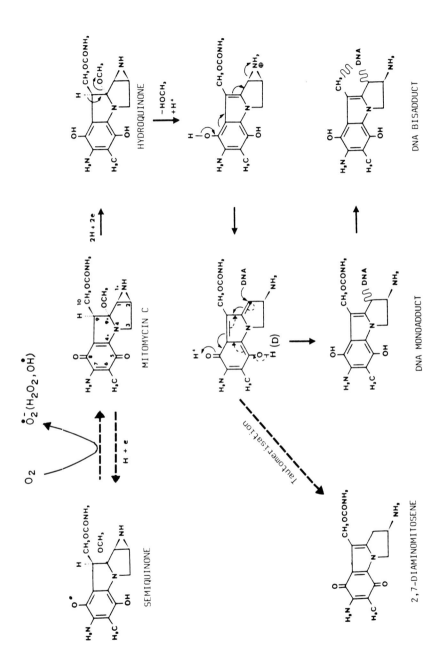

FIGURE 4. The three possible outcomes of mitomycin C quinone reduction. Note the analogy with Figure 2 with regard to possible metabolic pathways.

samples containing mitomycin C because although normally stable, it can be easily activated and degraded.

C. PHARMACOLOGY

After a typical therapeutic dose (10 mg/m²) mitomycin C is cleared rapidly from plasma in a biexponential manner with a terminal half-life of ≐60 min.[35] The kidney is the major organ of elimination with 10 to 15% of the administered dose appearing in the urine as the intact parent drug and possibly only 1 to 2% is excreted in the bile unchanged.[42] No relationship has been observed between mitomycin C pharmacokinetics and either patient response or toxicity;[43] however, inclusion in combination chemotherapy regimens appears to significantly increase total body clearance from 11 to 56 l/h/m².[44] Induction of drug metabolizing enzymes did not appear to alter terminal half-life.[42] Significantly, in all clinical pharmacokinetic studies known to the authors no metabolites have ever been detected; thus, more than 80% of the dose remains unaccounted for.

Using bioassay technology it has been demonstrated that no cytotoxic species are present in patient plasma other than mitomycin C itself.[45] It seems almost certain that native mitomycin C alone is the active form of the drug. In a group of female patients with cervical cancer the tumor-to-plasma ratio of drug concentration was determined to be 1.26, showing that equilibrium had occurred and suggesting a lack of a drug penetration problem in the tumor.[46] The ratio for ascites fluid to plasma was only 0.4. In rat tissues highest drug levels were seen in the lung (one of the main organs of toxicity), whereas only low levels were recorded in the liver, which is possibly due to a low hepatic extraction of 23%.[47]

D. MECHANISM OF ACTION

As long ago as 1964,[48,49] it was proposed that mitomycin C required biotransformation, preferentially under anaerobic conditions, before drug activation occurred resulting in cross-linking of DNA. To date, this mechanism, termed "anaerobic bioreductive alkylation", is still generally accepted as holding true, even though considerably more details are now available on the type of metabolism, the chemical intermediates involved, the types of adducts formed, and the sequence specificity of alkylation. The first stage in activation is quinone reduction (Figure 4), either through a 1-electron reduction pathway, which can be catalyzed by several enzymes, including cytochrome P-450 reductase, xanthine oxidase, or NADH dehydrogenase or through a 2-electron pathway catalyzed by DT-diaphorase (obligate 2-electron quinone reductase) or occurring by disproportionation of the semiquinone free radical to the hydroquinone form.

There is evidence in favor and supporters for both pathways.[4] In the presence of oxygen, the semiquinone will enter a futile redox cycle, which although potentially evolving reactive oxygen species is generally accepted as not being critical for antitumor activity but may be involved in the drug's toxic side effects. Two-electron reduction by DT-diaphorase should be unaffected by oxygen, and several reports with cancer cell lines, which express high and low levels of the enzyme, suggest that under aerobic conditions this enzyme does play an important role in drug activation.[50-52] Additionally, DT-diapharose may be involved in drug resistance to mitomycin C.[53,54] It is probable that the preferred pathway of drug activation *in vivo* will eventually depend on local conditions, such as the following: (1) the levels of endogenous reducing enzymes, (2) the levels of defense mechanisms to free radicals, and (3) the level of molecular oxygen. Either way quinone reduction results in methanol elimination, formation of a C9a, 9 double bond, aziridine ring opening, and production of a C1 reactive center, analogous to acid catalyzed activation.

Where acid catalyzed activation results only in monofunctional alkylation, bioreduction results in bifunctional alkylation now shown to occur at C10 after elimination of carbamate to produce another electrophilic center. Activation at C1 is believed always to proceed before activation at C10. Using a broad range of physicochemical techniques, primarily HPLC but also ultraviolet visible spectrophotometry, nuclear magnetic resonance, and mass spectrometry, a variety of major drug/DNA adducts have been reported. Hashimoto et al.[55] and Pan et al.[56] claimed the major adduct site is at O-6 guanine followed by N-6 adenine, and then N-2 guanine. Tomasz et al.[57,58] claimed that N-2 guanine is the preferred site of monoalkylation after bioreduction, chemical reduction, and acid catalyzed activation and identified the first bifunctional alkylation product as the N-2 guanine/N-2 guanine cross-linked adduct.

Computer graphic studies show that the mitomycin C/N-2 guanine mono-adduct has the ideal structure to interact with the minor groove of DNA, bringing the drug in close contact with the N-2 position of guanine with the correct stereochemistry for a *trans* bond to form. The data of Tomasz et al.[57,58] have been verified more recently by electrophoresis techniques and sequencing gels and confirm an absolute requirement for guanine and a sequence specificity for 5'-CG repeats as well as possibly 5'-GG repeats.[59,60]

E. ANALYSIS

Because of the complex physical and stereochemical properties of mitomycin C, a wide range of analytical techniques have been employed, and only recently (1983), its absolute stereochemical configuration was reassigned into C1 (S), C2 (S), C9a (R), and C9 (S) by heavy atom X-ray crystallography. Circular dichroism has been used in adduct identification and electrochemistry in the characterization of reactive intermediates.[61] For more routine analysis chromatographic methods have proved invaluable. Originally TLC was employed before the introduction of HPLC, and this technique is capable of effectively separating isomers, although it is limited in its sensitivity. Gel filtration chromatography has been extensively used in the identification of DNA adducts where larger molecules are involved. By far the most commonly used technique is HPLC with the majority of methods employing reversed phase stationary phases and a mobile phase consisting of an aqueous buffer in the pH range of 4 to 7 and an organic modifier of either methanol or acetonitrile. For the separation of stereoisomers gradient elution has been recommended but by careful use of pH, resolution of *cis*- and *trans*-1-hydroxy 2, 7-diaminomitosenes is achievable, by isocratic elution.

HPLC has proved useful for identifying conversion of mitomycin C into 2,7-diaminomitosene *in vitro* and likewise for the resolution of DNA adducts *in vitro*. Detection of chromatographic peaks is normally by ultraviolet visible spectrophotometry because mitomycin C has a strong absorption maximum at 360 nm (molar extinction coefficient 21,800 M^{-1} cm^{-1}), allowing for both good sensitivity and selectivity in biological matrices. It is important to stress that mitosene products exhibit a hypsochromic shift to 310 nm (molar extinction coefficient 6026 M^{-1} cm^{-1}) with considerable quenching, which is unusual considering the increase in conjugation. Effectively, this means that either dual wavelength detection or preferably DAD should be obligatory.

A combination of liquid-liquid and solid-liquid sample preparation methods has been described for plasma, which offers high efficiency.[61] Porfiromycin, which differs from mitomycin C only by an additional methyl group, is frequently used as an internal standard. Most common solvents are chloroform/propan-2-ol and chloroform/propan-2-ol/ethyl acetate and most common solid phases are C18 bonded silica, amberlite XAD-2, and Porapak-Q. Both solid phase and liquid extraction have been applied to tissues. Using the former, evidence has been presented that an unidentified tissue metabolite of mitomycin C is also extracted,[46] and using the latter evidence is presented that mitomycin C is relatively stable in tissue homogenates prior to extraction with only a 30% decline in concentration over 24 h.[62] Nevertheless, where possible, samples should be immediately frozen in either solid CO_2 or liquid nitrogen and after thawing analyzed as quickly as possible.

F. INCORPORATION IN MICROSPHERES

Only a limited number of studies are available on the effect of microsphere incorporation on the chemical nature of mitomycin C. Additionally, tracer studies with radioactively labeled mitomycin C have not been done due to a lack of general availability of labeled drug. In a detailed study, HPLC with DAD was applied to the analysis of mitomycin C incorporated into both albumin and polylactic acid microspheres.[63] The albumin microspheres were prepared by chemical cross-linking with 0.5 M biacetyl or by heat denaturation of the protein. In the case of heat denaturation 37% degradation occurred to a mixture of products, including 2,7-diaminomitosene and with biacetyl apparently complete degradation of the incorporated drug occurred. It was not possible to determine whether or not covalent coupling to the protein matrix was partly responsible for degradation. Once coupled it is unlikely that the drug would remain biologically active or capable of DNA alkylation.

Incorporation in polylactic acid microspheres, prepared by emulsification at 55°C, resulted in no apparent degradation. In a separate study, albumin microspheres (45 ± 8 μm diameter) prepared by heat denaturation at 120°C and/or cross-linked with glutaraldehyde were shown only to release 20% of their drug payload *in vitro* over a 3-day period, suggesting that considerable loss, either through degradation or covalent coupling, had occurred.[64] In this study, the drug was measured by bioassay, which is nonspecific for parent drug and derivatives; therefore, chemical degradation could have been even greater.

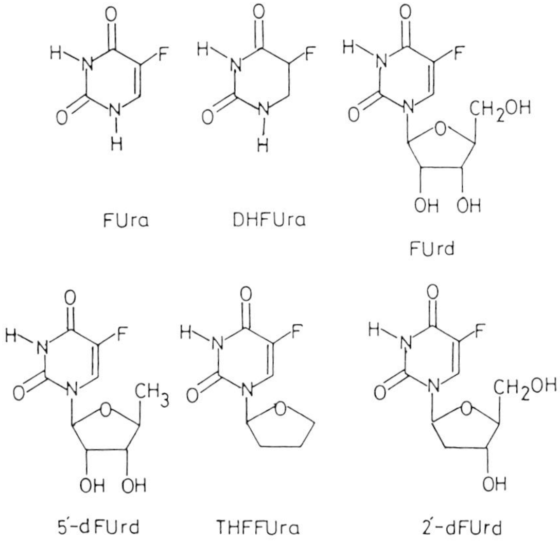

FIGURE 5. Chemical structures of 5-FU and some of its analogs and metabolites. See text for full nomenclature.

Studies with polylactic acid microspheres have shown that drug release is a function of drug loading; with 2.65% (w/w) loading only 20% is released over 10 days, but with 13.8% loading 100% is released over 10 days.[39] Because polylactic acid microspheres are prepared under more mild conditions, the data are probably unique to this system. Rapid release of apparently intact mitomycin C (80% of total loading in 30 min) has been reported with ethylcellulose microcapsules when the drug was determined by HPLC.[65]

IV. FLUOROPYRIMIDINES

The most important compound in this class is 5-fluorouracil (FUra), but its analogs 5'-deoxy-5-fluorouridine (5'-dFUrd), N[1]-tetrahydrofuran-2-yl 5-fluorouracil (THFFUra), 5-fluoro-2'-deoxyuridine (2'-dFUrd, floxuridine), and 5-fluorouridine (FUrd) have also been evaluated as therapeutic agents (Figure 5). 5-FUra was synthesized in 1957[66] and remains the most commonly used agent in its class: FUrd and 2'-dFUrd were synthesized shortly afterwards. FUrd was too toxic to be useful and 2'-dFUrd appeared to be a prodrug of 5-FUra. THFFUra was synthesized in 1967.[67] It yields FUra *in vivo* through hydrolysis by liver enzymes, although release is slow and may offer an advantage in terms of reduced systemic toxicity. 5'-dFUrd also probably acts via conversion to FUra, and the levels of phosphorylase enzymes causing this conversion may be higher in tumor cells conferring some selectivity.[68]

Recent work has produced other experimental prodrugs of FUra in attempts to control its release and reduce its systemic toxicity, e.g., myelosuppression. Chemical combinations of the drug with nitrosoureas resulted in a series of drugs with properties differing from the two agents used in combination with no chemical bond.[69] FUra has been chemically combined with polysaccharides, such as chitosan, and such conjugates were found to exhibit higher growth inhibitory effects and reduced toxicity compared with FUra[70,71] Similar conjugates have been prepared between FUra and dextrans.[72] Controlled release formulations of FUra have been prepared where the drug is incorporated into matrices, such as polycaprolactone[73] and polyphosphoester.[74] Alkyl and alkylcarbonate prodrugs have been prepared and found to improve oral bioavailability of FUra.[75]

A. 5-FLUOROURACIL

Because it is the most widely used fluoropyrimidine (both conventionally and with microspherical systems) and many analogs (Figure 5) are its prodrugs, a separate consideration of this compound may be informative.

1. Mechanism of Action

FUra belongs to the antimetabolite class of antitumor drugs, and although various mechanisms of action have been defined, it is still uncertain which is the most significant.[68] FUra has been shown to inhibit thymidylate synthetase after being first converted to 5-fluoro-2'-deoxyuridine monophosphate via a series of enzymic steps and then forming a ternary complex with N^5,N^{10}-methylene tetra-hydrofolate and thymidylate synthetase, thus inhibiting the conversion of uracil into thymine.[76,77] The incorporation of thymine into DNA forms an essential step in DNA synthesis. This effect may be modulated by intracellular pools of nucleosides. As well as inhibiting DNA synthesis, it is possible that an appropriate metabolite of FUra, such as 2'-dFUrd triphosphate, might become incorporated into DNA: the significance of this in terms of cytotoxicity is not known.[78,79] FUra is incorporated into all species of RNA with the greatest effects being on mRNA and rRNA, and in some cell lines there is a link between incorporation into RNA and cytotoxicity.[80-82]

The mechanism of action of FUra may be dependent on the concentration used and the duration of exposure.[83] Consistent with effects on both DNA and RNA synthesis, FUra kills cells both during the rapid growth phase and during the stationary phase of the cell cycle.[84] *In vitro* studies indicate that prolonged exposure to FUra greatly increases cell kill, but this is not necessarily borne out by *in vivo* work.[85,86] The half-life of FUra following bolus intravenous administration is about 15 min; protocols designed to give prolonged exposure to the drug have used continuous infusion into the hepatic artery or portal vein.[87-89]

2. Physicochemical Properties and Analysis

FUra is chemically stable and only has a tendency to degrade in solution above pH 9. It is weakly acidic with a pKa value of 8. Under strongly alkaline conditions it degrades by opening of the pyrimidine ring followed by decarboxylation and further degradation to yield urea, fluoride, and an aldehyde.[90] Chemically, it is not particularly reactive; the nitrogen atoms may be acylated or alkylated by suitable reagents, such as alkyl iodides, which form the basis of a number of analytical procedures.

The most commonly used analytical technique for the determination of FUra is HPLC. The chromophore of FUra is only of moderate strength; this is not a problem with regard to analysis of the drug in formulations. However, when applied to biological fluids many HPLC methods based on ultraviolet detection with chromatography on octadecyl silica gel have a relatively poor sensitivity of $\doteq 100$ ng/ml. Improved extraction techniques in combination with the use of styrene-divinylbenzene polymeric columns and ion-pairing reagents have yielded HPLC-ultraviolet procedures with limits of detection down to 10 ng/ml.[91-93] Extended "cleanup" procedures after extraction also improve sensitivity.[94] An advantage of HPLC methods is that they can detect fluoropyrimidines, such as 5′-dFUrd and FUrd, which are not ideal compounds for analysis by gas chromatography. The highest sensitivities afforded by HPLC involve alkylation of FUra with a fluorescent reagent,[95,96] and these procedures might be improved further by using column switching to remove excess derivatization reagent. A specialized technique with high sensitivity involves derivatization of FUra to enable chemiluminescence detection.[97]

Gas chromatography methods usually involve derivatization of FUra to improve chromatographic behavior and limits of detection for most methods lie in the range 25 to 100 ng/ml for FUra extracted from plasma.[98,99] The most sensitive and specific methods available are based on GC-MS and the most reliable of these use $^{15}N_2$-FUra as internal standard for accurate quantitation.[100] Chlorouracil has been used as an internal standard, but because GC-MS analysis often involves alkylation of FUra, problems may arise from different rates of alkylation of FUra and chlorouracil, which is less reactive. Other methods of analysis that may be relevant to the analysis of fluoropyrimidines in microspheres include the possibility of using Fourier transform IR to obtain data on the nature of the formulated drug because its characteristically strong carbonyl absorption will be affected by its form in the solid state. Similarly, solid state nuclear magnetic resonance of microsphere-encapsulated material might provide a means of quality control of the formulated product. Fluorine nuclear magnetic resonance has been used in metabolic studies; its use as an imaging technique has enabled dynamic monitoring of the metabolism of FUra in animal systems.[101,102] Such data demonstrate a negative correlation between tumor uptake of FUra and its degradation by the liver and also a lack of catabolism of FUra by hepatic tumor tissue.

3. Drug Metabolism

Unlike doxorubicin and mitomycin C, metabolism of FUra is probably not affected by incorporation into microspheres. Therefore, metabolites will only be described briefly. When administered in conventional form FUra is metabolized extensively by the liver and its concentration falls below the limit of detection within $\doteq 2$ h. As plasma levels of FUra decline those of 5,6-dihydro-5-fluorouracil (DHFUra), α-fluoro-β-ureido-propionic acid (FUPA) and α-fluoro-β-guanido-propionic acid (FABL) increase, reaching a peak at 90 min after injection.[103,104] These metabolites possess no strong chromophores, but an HPLC method using ultraviolet detection at 200 nm was developed for their analysis. N-glycosylation of FUra and subsequent phosphorylation to species that can be incorporated into DNA or inhibit enzymes involved in formation of DNA precursors were described by Valeriote and Santelli.[68]

B. MICROSPHERICAL SYSTEMS INCORPORATING FLUOROPYRIMIDINES

Although fluoropyrimidines have been used in simple admixture with either starch[105] or albumin[106] microspheres, this section describes systems in which drug is actually incorporated within the matrix. Such systems should be better able to take advantage of the targeting properties of microspheres (Chapter 8). Floxuridine (2'-dFUrd) has been incorporated into different matrix materials (monoglyceride, monodiglyceride, natural wax, cellulose polymer, and lactic acid) and the effectiveness of the different systems at promoting uptake of drug by the kidney assessed.[107] This compound has also been incorporated within ion-exchange microspheres and *in vitro* release rates studied.[108] When FUra was incorporated into albumin microspheres, it was reported that up to 30% of drug was released within the first few hours *in vitro,* but thereafter the rate of release was slow. Almost 100% of incorporated FUra was recovered when the microspheres were digested by pronase. The rate of drug release was dependent on the temperature at which the microspheres were formed.[109] In another study these authors selected a system in which FUra incorporated into albumin microspheres was released *in vitro* over 7 days. *In vivo* it was found that the drug formulated in this way exhibited antitumor activity.[110] FUra has been incorporated into ethylcellulose microspheres and *in vitro* release characteristics studied in 0.1 M HCl; 100% of the drug was recovered over 4 h and the most gradual release was from microspheres made with the highest molecular weight polymer of the three grades used. Release rate was even slower from FUra incorporated into a gel matrix.[111] Incorporation of FUra in polylactic acid (molecular weight 30 to 47 kDa) microspheres was about 40% w/w. The drug was released steadily from this system both *in vitro* and *in vivo* up to 48 h when release was 100%.[112] This form of FUra had a greater therapeutic effect than free drug in a model of carcinomatous peritonitis. Drug release was due to the permeability of the microsphere matrix rather than its degradation.

REFERENCES

1. **Eksborg, S. and Ehrsson, H.,** Drug level monitoring: cytostatics, *J. Chromatogr.,* 340, 31, 1985.
2. **Tjaden, U. R. and De Bruijn, E. A.,** Chromatography of anticancer drugs, *J. Chromatogr.,* 531, 235, 1991.
3. **Powis, G.,** Metabolism and reactions of quinoid anticancer agents, *Pharmacol. Ther.,* 35, 57, 1987.

4. **Fisher, J. F. and Aristoff, P. A.**, The chemistry of DNA modification by antitumor antibiotics, *Prog. Drug Res.*, 32, 411, 1988.
5. **Casazza, A. M.**, Preclinical selection of new anthracyclines, *Cancer Treat. Rep.*, 70, 43, 1986.
6. **Endicott, J. A. and Ling, V.**, The biochemistry of P-glycoprotein-mediated multidrug resistance, *Annu. Rev. Biochem.*, 58, 137, 1989.
7. **Ling, V.**, Does P-glycoprotein predict response to chemotherapy?, *J. Natl. Cancer Inst.*, 81, 84, 1989.
8. **Beck, W. T.**, The cell biology of multiple drug resistance, *Biochem. Pharmacol.*, 36, 2879, 1987.
9. **Smith, I. E.**, Optimal schedule for anthracyclines, *Eur. J. Cancer Clin. Oncol.*, 21, 159, 1985.
10. **Dalmark, M. and Johansen, P.**, Molecular associations between doxorubicin (adriamycin) and DNA derived bases, nucleosides, nucleotides, other aromatic compounds, and proteins in aqueous solution, *Mol. Pharmacol.*, 22, 158, 1982.
11. **Cummings, J., Bartoszek, A., and Smyth, J. F.**, Determination of covalent binding to intact DNA, RNA and oligonucleotides by intercalating anticancer drugs using high-performance liquid chromatography: studies with doxorubicin and NADPH cytochrome P-450 reductase, *Anal. Biochem.*, 194, 146, 1991.
12. **Bosanquet, A. G.**, Stability of solutions of antineoplastic agents during preparation and storage for *in vitro* assays. II. Assay methods for adriamycin and the other antitumor antibiotics, *Cancer Chemother. Pharmacol.*, 17, 1, 1986.
13. **Schwartz, H. S.**, Enhanced antitumor activity of adriamycin in combination with allopurinol, *Cancer Lett.*, 26, 69, 1983.
14. **Israel, M., Pegg, W. J., Wilkinson, P. M., and Garnick, B. M.**, Liquid chromatographic analysis of adriamycin and its metabolites in biological fluids, *J. Liquid Chromatogr.*, 1, 795, 1978.
15. **Takanashi, S. and Bachur, N. R.**, Adriamycin metabolism in man: evidence from urinary metabolites, *Drug Metab. Dispos.*, 4, 79, 1976.
16. **Cummings, J., Morrison, J. G., and Willmott, N.**, Determination of anthracycline purity in patient samples and identification of *in vitro* chemical reduction products by application of a multi-diode array high-speed spectrophotometric detector, *J. Chromatogr.*, 381, 373, 1986.
17. **Cummings, J. and Smyth, J. F.**, Pharmacology of adriamycin: the message to the clinician, *Eur. J. Cancer Clin. Oncol.*, 24, 579, 1988.
18. **Cummings, J., Anderson, L., Willmott, N., and Smyth, J. F.**, The molecular pharmacology of doxorubicin *in vivo*, *Eur. J. Cancer*, 27, 532, 1991.
19. **Asbell, M. A., Schwartzbach, E., Bullock, F. J., and Yesair, D. W.**, Daunomycin and adriamycin metabolism via reductive glycosidic cleavage, *J. Pharmacol. Exp. Ther.*, 182, 63, 1972.
20. **Cummings, J., Stuart, J. F. B., and Calman, K. C.**, Determination of adriamycin, adriamycinol and their 7-deoxyaglycones in human serum by high-performance liquid chromatography, *J. Chromatogr.*, 311, 125, 1984.
21. **Cummings, J., Willmott, N., Hoey, B., Butler, J., and Smyth, J. F.**, The role of quinone reduction in the mechanism of action of doxorubicin-loaded albumin microspheres, *Br. J. Cancer*, 63, 37, 1991.
22. **Gianni, L., Zweier, J. L., Levy, A., and Myers, C. E.**, Characterisation of the cycle of iron-mediated electron transfer from adriamycin to molecular oxygen, *J. Biol. Chem.*, 260, 6820, 1985.
23. **Gianni, L., Vigano, L., Lanzi, C., Niggeler, M., and Malatesta, V.**, Role of daunosamine and the hydroxyacetyl side chain in reaction with iron and lipid peroxidation by anthracyclines, *J. Natl. Cancer Inst.*, 80, 1104, 1988.
24. **Cummings, J. and Willmott, N.**, Adriamycin-loaded albumin microspheres: qualitative assessment of drug incorporation and *in vitro* release by high-performance liquid chromatography and high-speed multi-diode array spectrophotometric detection, *J. Chromatogr.*, 343, 208, 1985.
25. **Willmott, N. and Harrison, P. J.**, Characterisation of freeze-dried albumin microspheres containing the anti-cancer drug adriamycin, *Int. J. Pharmaceutics*, 43, 161, 1988.

26. **Willmott, N., Cummings, J., and Florence, A. T.**, *In vitro* release of adriamycin from drug-loaded albumin and haemoglobin microspheres, *J. Microencap.*, 2, 293, 1985.

27. **Chen, Y., Willmott, N., Anderson, J., and Florence, A. T.**, Haemoglobin, transferrin and albumin/polyaspartic acid microspheres as carriers for the cytotoxic drug adriamycin. I. Ultrastructural appearance and drug content, *J. Controlled Release*, 8, 93, 1988.

28. **Cummings, J., Willmott, N., Marley, E., and Smyth, J. F.**, Covalent coupling of doxorubicin in protein microspheres is a major determinant of tumor drug disposition, *Biochem. Pharmacol.*, 41, 1848, 1991.

29. **Tokes, Z. A., Rogers, K. E., and Rembaum, A.**, Synthesis of adriamycin-coupled polyglutaraldehyde microspheres and evaluation of their cytostatic activity, *Proc. Natl. Acad. Sci. USA*, 79, 2026, 1982.

30. **Cummings, J., Merry, S., and Willmott, N.**, Disposition kinetics of adriamycin, adriamycinol and their 7-deoxyaglycones in AKR mice bearing a sub-cutaneously growing ridgway osteogenic sarcoma (ROS), *Eur. J. Cancer Clin. Oncol.*, 22, 451, 1986.

31. **Willmott, N. and Cummings, J.**, Increased anti-tumor effect of adriamycin-loaded albumin microspheres is associated with anaerobic bioreduction of drug in tumor tissue, *Biochem. Pharmacol.*, 36, 521, 1987.

32. **Cummings, J. and McArdle, C. S.**, Studies on the *in vivo* disposition of adriamycin in human tumors which exhibit different responses to the drug, *Br. J. Cancer*, 53, 835, 1986.

33. **Frank, W. and Osterberg, A.**, Mitomycin C (NSC 26980): an evaluation of the Japanese reports, *Cancer Chemother. Rep.*, 9, 114, 1960.

34. **Remers, W. A. and Schepman, C. S.**, Structure activity relationships of the mitomycins and certain synthetic analogues, *J. Med. Chem.*, 17, 729, 1974.

35. **Dorr, R. T.**, New findings in the pharmacokinetic, metabolic and drug resistance aspects of mitomycin C, *Semin. Oncol.*, 15, 32, 1988.

36. **Kato, T., Nemoto, R., Mori, A., and Kumagai, I.**, Sustained-release properties of microencapsulated mitomycin C with ethylcellulose infused into the renal artery of the dog, *Cancer*, 46, 14, 1980.

37. **Ensminger, W. D., Gyves, J. W., Stetson, P., and Walker-Andrews, S.**, Phase I study of hepatic arterial degradable starch microspheres and mitomycin, *Cancer Res.*, 45, 4464, 1985.

38. **Fujimoto, S., Miyazaki, M., Endoh, F., Takahshi, O., Shrestha, R. D., Okui, K., Morimoto, Y., and Terao, K.**, Effects of intra-arterially infused biodegradable microspheres containing mitomycin C, *Cancer*, 55, 522, 1985.

39. **Tsai, D. C., Howard, S. A., Hogan, T. F., Malanga, C. J., Kandzari, S. J., and Ma, J. K. H.**, Preparation and *in vitro* evaluation of polylactic acid-mitomycin C microcapsules, *J. Microencap.*, 3, 181, 1986.

40. **Hoey, B. M., Butler, J., and Swallow, A. J.**, Reductive activation of mitomycin C, *Biochemistry*, 27, 2608, 1988.

41. **Tomasz, M. and Lipman, R.**, Reductive metabolism and alkylating activity of mitomycin C induced by rat liver microsomes, *Biochemistry*, 20, 5056, 1981.

42. **Kerpel-Fronius, S., Verway, J., Stuurman, M., Kanyar, B., Lelieveld, P., and Pinedo, H. M.**, Pharmacokinetics and toxicity of mitomycin C in rodents given alone, in combination, or after induction of microsomal drug metabolism, *Cancer Chemother. Pharmacol.*, 22, 104, 1988.

43. **Verweij, J., Den Hartigh, J., Stuurman, M., de Vries, J., and Pinedo, H. M.**, Relationship between clinical parameters and pharmacokinetics of mitomycin C, *J. Cancer Res. Clin. Oncol.*, 113, 91, 1987.

44. **Verweij, J., Stuurman, M., de Vries, J., and Pinedo, H. M.**, The difference in pharmacokinetics of mitomycin C given either as a single agent or as a part of combination chemotherapy, *J. Cancer Res. Clin. Oncol.*, 112, 283, 1986.

45. **Marshall, R. S., Erlichman, C., and Rauth, A. M.**, A bioassay to measure cytotoxicity of plasma from patients treated with mitomycin C, *Cancer Res.*, 45, 5939, 1985.

46. **Malviya, V. K., Young, J. D., Boike, G., Gove, N., and Deppe, G.,** Pharmacokinetics of mitomycin C in plasma and tumor tissue of cervical cancer patients and in selected tissues of female rats, *Gynecol. Oncol.,* 25, 160, 1986.

47. **Hu, E. and Howell, S. B.,** Pharmacokinetics of intra-arterial mitomycin C in humans, *Cancer Res.,* 43, 4474, 1981.

48. **Iyer, V. N. and Szybalski, W.,** Mitomycins and porfiromycin: chemical mechanism of action and cross linking of DNA, *Science,* 45, 55, 1964.

49. **Moore, H. W.,** Bioactivation as a model for drug design: bioreductive alkylation, *Science,* 197, 527, 1977.

50. **Rockwell, S., Keyes, S. R., and Sartorelli, A. C.,** Modulation of the cytotoxicity of mitomycin C to EMT6 mouse mammary tumor cells by dicoumarol *in vitro, Cancer Res.,* 48, 5471, 1988.

51. **Rockwell, S., Keyes, S. R., and Sartorelli, A. C.,** Modulation of the antineoplastic efficacy of mitomycin C by dicoumarol *in vivo, Cancer Chemother. Pharmacol.,* 24, 349, 1989.

52. **Siegel, D., Gibson, N. W., Preusch, P. C., and Ross, D.,** Metabolism of mitomycin C by DT-diaphorase: role in mitomycin C induced DNA damage and cytotoxicity in human colon carcinoma cells, *Cancer Res.,* 50, 7483, 1990.

53. **Dulhanty, A. M. and Whitmore, G. F.,** Chinese hamster ovary cell lines resistant to mitomycin C under aerobic but not hypoxic conditions are deficient in DT-diaphorase, *Cancer Res.,* 51, 1860, 1991.

54. **Marshall, R. S., Paterson, M. C., and Rauth, A. M.,** Studies on the mechanism of resistance of mitomycin C and porfiromycin in a human cell strain derived from a cancer-prone individual, *Biochem. Pharmacol.,* 41, 1351, 1991.

55. **Hashimoto, Y., Shudo, K., and Okamoto, T.,** Modification of deoxyribonucleic acid with reductively activated mitomycin C: structures of modified nucleotides, *Chem. Pharm. Bull.,* 31, 861, 1983.

56. **Pan, S.-S., Iracki, T., and Bachur, N. R.,** DNA alkylation by enzyme activated mitomycin C, *Mol. Pharmacol.,* 29, 622, 1986.

57. **Tomasz, M., Chowdary, D., Lipman, R., Shimotakahara, S., Veiro, D., Walker, V., and Verdine, G. L.,** Reaction of DNA with chemically or enzymatically activated mitomycin C: isolation and structure of the major covalent adduct, *Proc. Natl. Acad. Sci. USA,* 83, 6702, 1986.

58. **Tomasz, M., Lipman, R., Chowdary, D., Pawlak, J., Verdine, G. L., and Nakanishi, K.,** Isolation and structure of a covalent cross-link adduct between mitomycin C and DNA, *Science,* 235, 1204, 1987.

59. **Weidner, M. F., Sigurdsson, S. T., and Hopkins, P. B.,** Sequence preferences of DNA interstrand cross-linking agents at 5'CG by structurally simplified analogues of mitomycin C, *Biochemistry,* 29, 9225, 1990.

60. **Li, V.-S. and Kohn, H.,** Studies on the bonding specificity for mitomycin C-DNA monoalkylation process, *J. Am. Chem. Soc.,* 113, 275, 1991.

61. **Beijnen, J. H., Lingman, H., Van Munster, H. A., and Underberg, W. J. M.,** Mitomycin antitumor agents: a review of their physico-chemical and analytical properties and stability, *J. Pharm. Biomed. Anal.,* 4, 275, 1986.

62. **Wientjes, M. G., Dalton, J. T., Badalament, R. A., Dasani, B. M., Drago, J. R., and Au, J. L.-S.,** A method to study drug concentration-depth profiles in tissues: mitomycin C in dog bladder wall, *Pharm. Res.,* 8, 168, 1991.

63. **Mehta, R. C., Hogan, T. F., Mardmomen, S., and Ma, J. K. H.,** Chromatographic studies of mitomycin C degradation in albumin microspheres, *J. Chromatogr.,* 430, 341, 1988.

64. **Fujimoto, S., Miyazaki, M., Endoh, F., Takahashi, O., Okui, K., Sugibayashi, K., and Morimoto, Y.,** Mitomycin C carrying microspheres as a novel method of drug delivery, *Cancer Drug Delivery,* 2, 173, 1985.

65. **Goldberg, J. A., Kerr, D. J., Blackie, R., Whately, T. L., Pettit, L., Kato, T., and McArdle, C. S.,** Mitomycin C-loaded microcapsules in the treatment of colorectal liver metastases, *Cancer,* 67, 952, 1991.

66. **Duschinski, R., Pleven, E., and Heidelberger, C.,** Synthesis of 5-fluoropyrimidines, *J. Am. Chem. Soc.,* 79, 4559, 1957.

67. **Hiller, S. A., Zhuk, R. A., and Lidak, M. Y.,** Analogues of pyrimidine nucleosides. I. N'-(-tetrahydrofuryl) derivatives of natural pyrimidine bases and their antimetabolites, *Dokl. Akad. Nauk. SSSR,* 176, 332, 1967.

68. **Valeriote, F. and Santelli, G.,** 5-Fluorouracil (FUra), *Pharmacol. Ther.,* 24, 107, 1984.

69. **McElhinney, S., McCormick, J. E., Bibby, M. C., Double, J. A., Atassi, G., Dumont, P., Pratesi, G., and Radacic, M.,** Nucleoside analogues. VIII. Some isomers of B 3839 the original 5-fluorouracil/nitrosourea molecular combination and their effect on colon, breast and lung tumors in mice, *Anti-Cancer Drug Design.,* 4, 1, 1989.

70. **Ouchi, T., Banba, T., Huang, T. Z., and Ohya, Y.,** Design of polysaccharide-5-fluorouracil conjugates exhibiting anti-tumor activities, *Polym. Prepr.,* 31, 202, 1990.

71. **Ouchi, T.,** Design of biodegradable polymer-5-fluorouracil conjugates exhibiting antitumor activities, *Polym. Mater. Sci.,* 62, 412, 1990.

72. **Mora, M. and Pato, J.,** Synthesis and hydrolytic behavior of dextran bound anticancer agents, *Makromol. Chem.,* 191, 1051, 1990.

73. **Geblein, C. G., Chapman, M., and Mirza, T.,** The release of 5-fluorouracil from polycaprolactone matrices, *Polym. Sci. Technol.,* 38, 151, 1988.

74. **Tashev, E., Shi, F. Y., and Leong, K. W.,** Potential applications of poly(phosphoester-urethanes) in controlled drug delivery, *Polym. Mater. Sci. Eng.,* 63, 43, 1990.

75. **Buur, A., Yamamoto, A., and Lee, V. H. L.,** Penetration of 5-fluorouracil and prodrugs across the intestine of albino rabbit: evidence for shift in absorption site from upper to lower gastrointestinal tract by prodrugs, *J. Controlled Release,* 14, 43, 1990.

76. **Santi, D. V., McHenry, C. S., and Sommer, H.,** Mechanism of interaction of thymidylate synthetase with 5-fluorodeoxyuridylate, *Biochemistry,* 3, 471, 1974.

77. **Sommer, H. and Santi, D. V.,** Purification and amino acid analysis of an active site peptide from thymidylate synthetase containing covalently bound 5-fluoro-2'-deoxyuridylate and methylenetetrahydrofolate, *Biochem. Biophys. Res. Commun.,* 57, 689, 1974.

78. **Kufe, D. W., Major P. P., Egan, M., and Loh, E.,** 5-fluoro-2'-deoxyuridine incorporation into L1210 DNA, *J. Biol. Chem.,* 256, 8885, 1981.

79. **Ingraham, H. A., Tseng, B. Y., and Goulian, M.,** Mechanism for exclusion of 5-fluorouracil from DNA, *Cancer Res.,* 40, 998, 1980.

80. **Glazer, R. I. and Hartman, K. D.,** The effects of 5-fluorouracil on the synthesis and methylation of low molecular weight nuclear RNA in L1210 cells, *Mol. Pharmacol.,* 17, 245, 1980.

81. **Glazer, R. I. and Hartman, K. D.,** Analysis of the effect of 5-fluorouracil on the synthesis and translation of polysomal poly(A) RNA for Ehrlich ascites cells, *Mol. Pharmacol.,* 19, 117, 1981.

82. **Galzer, R. I. and Lloyd, L. S.,** Association of lethality of incorporation of 5-fluorouracil and 5-fluorouridine into nuclear RNA in human colon carcinoma cells in culture, *Mol. Pharmacol.,* 21, 468, 1982.

83. **Kanzawa, F., Hoshi, A., and Kuretani, K.,** Differences between 5-fluoro-2'-deoxycytidine and 5-fluorouridine in their cytotoxic effect on the growth of murine lymphoma L5178Y cells in *in vivo* and *in vitro* systems, *Eur. J. Cancer.,* 16, 1087, 1980.

84. **Drewinko, B., Yang, L. Y., Ho, D. H. W., Benuto, J., Loo, T. L., and Freirich, E. J.,** Treatment of cultured human colon carcinoma cells with fluorinated pyrimidines, *Cancer,* 45, 1144, 1980.

85. **Kovacsa, C. J. Kopkins, H. A., Simon, R. M., and Looney, W. B.,** Effect of 5-fluorouracil on the cell kinetic and growth parameters of heptoma 3924 A, *Br. J. Cancer,* 32, 42, 1975.

86. **Pallavacini, M. G., Cohen, A. M., Dethelefsen, L. A., and Gray, J. W.,** *In vivo* effects of 5-fluorouracil and ftorafur [1-(tetraydrofuran-2-yl)-5-fluorouracil] on murine mammary tumors and small intestine, *Cell Tissue Kinet.,* 12, 177, 1979.

87. **Daly, J. M., Kemeny, N., Sigurdson, E., Oderman P., and Thom, A.,** Regional infusion for colorectal hepatic metastases, *Arch. Surg.,* 122, 1273, 1987.

88. **Koks, C. H. W., Brouwers, J. R. B. J., and Sleijfer, D. Th.,** Regional infusion of fluoro-pyrimidines for hepatic metastases of colorectal cancer, *Pharm. Weekbl.,* 10, 69, 1988.

89. **Archer, S. G. and Gray, B. N.,** Comparison of portal vein chemotherapy with hepatic artery chemotherapy in the treatment of liver micrometastases, *Am. J. Surg.,* 159, 325, 1990.

90. **Bayomi, S. M. and Al-Badr, A. A.,** Analytical profile of 5-fluorouracil, in *Analytical Profiles of Drug Substances,* Vol. 18, Florey, K., Ed., Academic Press, New York, 1989, 599.

91. **Rustum, A. M. and Hoffman, N. E.,** Determination of 5-fluorouracil in plasma and whole blood by ion pair high performance liquid chromatography, *J. Chromatogr.,* 426, 121, 1986.

92. **Peters, G. J., Kraal, I., Laurensse, E., Leyra A., and Pinedo, H. M.,** Separation of 5-fluorouracil and uracil by ion pair reverse phase HPLC on a column with porous polymeric packing, *J. Chromatogr.,* 307, 464, 1984.

93. **Tjaden, U. R., Reewijk, H. J. E. M., de Bruuijn, E. A., Keize, H. J., and van der Greef, J.,** Bioanalysis of 5-fluorouracil applying liquid chromatography and valve switching, *Chromatographia,* 25, 806, 1988.

94. **La Creata, F. L. and Williams, W. M.,** High performance liquid chromatographic analysis of fluoropyrimidine nucleosides and 5-fluorouracil in plasma, *J. Chromatogr.,* 414, 197, 1987.

95. **Iwamoto, M., Yoshida, S., and Hirose, S.,** Fluorescence determination of 5-fluorouracil and 1-(tetrahydro-2-furanyl) 5-fluorouracil in blood serum by high performance liquid chromatography, *J. Chromatogr.,* 310, 151, 1984.

96. **Yoshida, S., Adachi, T., and Hirose, S.,** 4-Bromomethyl-6,7-dimethoxy coumarin as a fluorescence reagent for precolumn derivatisation of 5-fluorouracil compounds in high performance liquid chromatography, *J. Chromatogr.,* 430, 156, 1988.

97. **Yoshida, S., Urakami, K., Kito, M., Takeshima, S., and Hirose, S.,** High performance liquid chromatography with chemiluminescence detection of serum levels of precolumn derivatised fluoropyrimidine compounds, *J. Chromatogr.,* 530, 57, 1990.

98. **De Bruijn, E. A., Driessen, O., van den Bosch, N., van Stijen, E., Slee, P. H. Th. J., van Oosterom, A. T., and Tjaden, U. R. A.,** A gas chromatographic assay for the determination of 5,6-dihydrouracil and 5-fluorouracil in human plasma, *J. Chromatogr.,* 278, 283, 1983.

99. **Williams, W. M., Barbour, W. S., and Fu-hsiung, L.,** Gas liquid chromatographic analysis of fluoropyrimidine nucleosides and fluorouracil in plasma and urine, *Anal. Biochem.,* 147, 478, 1985.

100. **Bates, C. D., Watson, D. G., Willmott, N., Logan, H., and Goldberg, J.,** The analysis of 5-fluorouracil in human plasma by gas chromatography-negative ion chemical ionisation mass spectrometry (GC-NICIMS) with stable isotope dilution, *J. Pharm. Biomed. Anal.,* 9, 19, 1991.

101. **Sijens, P. E., Huang, Y., Baldwin, N. J., and Ng, T. C.,** ^{19}F magnetic resonance spectroscopy studies of the metabolism of 5-fluorouracil in murine RIF-1 tumors and liver, *Cancer Res.,* 51, 1384, 1991.

102. **de Brauw, L. M., Marinelli, A., van de Velde, C. J. H., Hermans, J., Tjaden, U. R., Erkelens, C., and de Bruijn, E. A.,** Pharmacological evaluation of experimental isolated liver perfusion and hepatic artery infusion with 5-fluorouracil, *Cancer Res.,* 51, 1694, 1991.

103. **Heggie, G. D., Sommadossi, J.-P., Cross, D. S., Huster, W. J., and Diasio, R. B.,** Clinical pharmacokinetics of 5-fluorouracil and its metabolites in plasma, urine and bile, *Cancer Res.,* 47, 2203, 1987.

104. **Sommadosi, J.-P., Gerwirtz, D. A., Diasio, R. B., Aubert, C., Cano, J.-P., and Goldman, I. D.,** Rapid catabolism of 5-fluorouracil in freshly isolated rat hepatocytes as analysed by high performance liquid chromatography, *J. Biol. Chem.,* 257, 8171, 1982.

105. **Thom, A. K., Sigurdson, E. R., Bitar, M., and Daly, J. M.,** Regional hepatic arterial infusion of degradable starch microspheres increases fluorodeoxyuridine (FUdR) tumor uptake, *Surgery,* 105, 383, 1989.

106. **Goldberg, J. A., Kerr, D. J., Willmott, N., McKillop, J. H., and McArdle, C. S.,** Pharmacokinetics and pharmacodynamics of locoregional 5-fluorouracil (5FU) in advanced colorectal liver metastases, *Br. J. Cancer,* 57, 186, 1988.

107. **Bechtel, W., Wright, K. C., Wallace, S., Mosier, B., Mosier, D., Mir, S., and Kudo, S.,** An experimental evaluation of microcapsules for arterial chemoembolization, *Radiology,* 161, 601, 1986.

108. **Jones, C., Burton, M. A., Gray, B. N., and Hodgkin, J.,** *In vitro* release of cytotoxic agents from ion exchange resins, *J. Controlled Release,* 8, 251, 1989.
109. **Sugibayashi, K., Akimoto, M., Morimoto, Y., Nadai, T., and Kato, Y.,** Drug-carrier property of albumin microspheres in chemotherapy: III, effect of microsphere entrapped 5-fluorouracil on Ehrlich ascites carcinoma in mice, *J. Pharm. Dyn.,* 2, 350, 1979.
110. **Morimoto, Y., Akimoto, M., Sugibayashi, K., Nadai, T., and Kato, Y.,** Drug carrier property of albumin microspheres in chemotherapy: IV, antitumor effect of single-shot or multiple-shot administration of microsphere-entrapped 5-fluorouracil on Ehrlich ascites or solid tumor in mice, *Chem. Pharm. Bull.,* 28, 3087, 1980.
111. **Ghorab, M. M., Zia, H., and Luzzi, L. A.,** Preparation of controlled release anticancer agents: I, 5-fluorouracil ethyl cellulose microspheres, *J. Microencap.,* 7, 447, 1990.
112. **Yamada, T., Sakatoku, M., Onhira, M., Watanabe, Y., and Iwa, T.,** A new anticancer drug delivery system for the management of carcinomatous peritonitis, *Surgery,* 109, 706, 1991.

Chapter 7

REGION THERAPY OF LIVER METASTASES: A SURGEON'S VIEW

H. J. Gallagher and John M. Daly

TABLE OF CONTENTS

I. INTRODUCTION

A. THE CURRENT SITUATION

Although finding curative therapies for cancer remains the ultimate medical goal, palliation and prolongation of life, in particular a good quality of life, is a priority for most patients with malignant disease. Colorectal cancer is the second most common cancer in women and third most common cancer in men exceeded only by prostate and lung carcinomas.[1] The following statistics apply to the U.S. only: in 1991 there were 157,500 new cases of large bowel cancer.[1] Approximately 50% of these patients will develop progressive disease after resection of the primary tumor and die within 5 years. The liver is the most common site of metastases with 10 to 25% of patients having synchronous metastases at the time of diagnosis and up to 71% of patients having liver secondaries at death.

Although initial surgical resection will cure approximately 53% of patients,[1] the outlook for patients with liver metastases is extremely poor with virtually no survivors at 5 years and only a 20% 3-year survival rate in those who present with a single metastasis.[2] Hepatic resection offers the only realistic curative therapeutic option, with 25 to 30% of carefully selected patients surviving more than 5 years.[3,4] Unfortunately, only a small minority of patients are suitable for hepatic surgery. Of 78,000 patients per year with recurrent cancer, 60% will have liver disease of which only 20%, or 9400, will have the disease restricted to the liver.[5-7] Only 25% of those (2300) will be suitable for surgical resection.[8] Thus, approximately 45,000 patients annually are candidates for nonsurgical therapy for colorectal liver metastases. In the majority the aim will be palliation; however, in those patients whose disease is confined to the liver but are not candidates for hepatic resection, cure may be contemplated.

B. THE GOALS OF PALLIATIVE THERAPY

The goal of palliation is to improve survival with minimal morbidity and an acceptable quality of life. The efficacy of palliative therapy can only be judged against the natural progression of the disease process. Studies show that the duration of survival is directly related to the extent of liver metastases and the patient's functional index. Whereas asymptomatic patients with less than three metastases at diagnosis had a median survival of 24 months,[9] patients with a large tumor bulk had a median survival of 3 to 6 months.[10,11] Bengmark[12] suggested that, as a guideline, any therapy that does not quadruple life expectancy from the aforementioned total should not be used outside controlled studies. Although this might appear extreme, the side effects of palliative therapy are tolerated best by healthier patients who benefit the most. Markedly symptomatic patients, with a life expectancy of weeks, have little to gain from aggressive intervention.

C. TREATMENT OPTIONS

Major liver resection should be reserved for carefully selected patients with liver metastases for whom major surgery offers a reasonable opportunity for cure.

Patients with extensive bilobar, multiple (>4) metastases or concurrent health problems, which preclude major surgery, should be considered for adjunctive therapy provided benefits outweigh the side effects and quality of life remains adequate or is improved.

Options for adjunctive therapy include the following: radiation therapy (targeted or external); chemotherapy (systemic, portal, or intra-arterial); and ischemic therapy involving whole liver devascularization (long-term or intermittent) or localized ischemia targeted against metastatic deposits using embolization strategies involving injected foreign particles, particularly microspheres. Several regimens involve a combination of therapies, for example, chemoembolization in which chemotherapy is delivered along with the embolic particles. This chapter will focus on chemotherapy of liver metastases and, in particular, chemoembolization using degradable starch microspheres (DSM) in combination with chemotherapeutic agents. It discusses the benefits and side effects of such therapies as well as the various delivery methods available to the surgeon or oncologist and the rationale on which they are used.

D. RATIONALE FOR THERAPY

The susceptibility of cancer cells to chemotherapy often varies in a dose-dependent fashion. Higher drug levels often translate into higher tumor response rates. Unfortunately, high doses of chemotherapy are toxic to normal cells as well as cancer cells. Thus, systemically administered drug concentrations should remain within a narrow therapeutic window, maintaining a careful balance between therapeutic efficacy and host toxicity. The latter may preclude attaining systemic drug concentrations effective for tumor cytotoxicity. This problem can be addressed in a number of ways. Selectively increasing drug delivery to tumor cells can be performed by targeting, in which the agent is delivered directly to the liver as opposed to systemic administration. Drug delivery may be further enhanced by manipulating regional blood flow. Tumor cell drug uptake, metabolism, and release can also be altered.

II. DETECTION AND ASSESSMENT OF METASTATIC DISEASE

Early detection of metastases is a prerequisite to improving the beneficial effect of therapy. The smaller the tumor load, the more effective any therapy aimed at metastatic disease will be. It is also important for the surgeon contemplating curative hepatic resection for metastatic disease to preoperatively estimate the extent of disease. However, not uncommonly, at the time of surgery patients are found to be unresectable due to previously undetected metastases or, perhaps of greater concern, patients are resected and further liver metastases or extrahepatic metastases are detected within a few weeks of surgery.

A number of advances in early diagnosis and recurrence detection have been made in the last few years. The most promising methods are discussed below.

A. INTRAOPERATIVE ULTRASONOGRAPHY

Intraoperative ultrasonography (IOUS) has become the investigation of choice in detecting liver metastases and determining the feasibility of resection at the time of surgery. It may be performed at the initial surgical procedure in which the primary tumor is resected and synchronous metastases detected, or it may be used at second-look surgery to assess metachronous lesions, which appear amenable to curative hepatic resection by determining the lesion's relationship to vascular and biliary structures. Perhaps more importantly, it can also detect small metastases that would otherwise go unnoticed; thus, an unnecessary procedure could be abandoned and intra-arterial chemotherapy commenced instead.

A number of studies have compared IOUS with more conventional diagnostic techniques. Machi et al.[13] evaluated the accuracy of the procedure at 18 months or more postoperatively in 188 patients with large bowel cancer. IOUS had a significantly increased sensitivity of 82.3% compared with preoperative ultrasonography (38.1%), conventional computed tomography (CT) (42.8%), and surgical exploration (60.2%). Specificity was uniformly high with all procedures (Table 1). They noted that of 104 liver metastases detected at operation, 22 were detected by IOUS alone. This involved 18 patients (9.5%) and the tumor sizes ranged from 4×4 to 15×18 mm, a size below the limit of detection for preoperative ultrasonography and CT. Moreover, being deep-seated, they were invisible to the surgeon. It should be noted that of the 22 tumors detected only by IOUS, 8 were present in 7 patients with no other involvement.

Although apparently ruled out by conventional preoperative diagnostic techniques and surgical exploration, liver metastatic recurrence is known to occur in 10 to 20% of patients after resection of the primary colorectal tumor.[13] In comparison, the recurrence rate of 6.9% (i.e., 13 of 188 patients who were apparently free of liver metastasis when assessed by IOUS) appears markedly lower and can presumably be attributed to the improved sensitivity of IOUS. Overall IOUS identified metastases in 18 of the 31 patients in whom liver metastases were otherwise unrecognized at the time of surgery.

Similar data from Norway were produced by Olsen[14] in a study of 213 patients with colorectal cancer. Using IOUS 19 patients with known metastatic disease were found to have additional previously undetected lesions. In 21 patients preoperative and intraoperative exploration failed to identify small lesions. Following IOUS 59 lesions ranging in size from 0.3 to 3.5 cm were identified in these patients. IOUS sensitivity was calculated to be 98% compared with 66% for preoperative ultrasonography, clinical visual inspection, and palpation during operation.

Several other studies reported similar results. Stadler et al.[15] reported that the use of IOUS altered patient management and the choice of operation in 15% of the cases evaluated. Other Japanese,[16] Italian,[17] British,[18] and Dutch[19] studies all confirmed IOUS as the investigation of choice in detecting hepatic metastases at the time of initial surgery or at the time of second-look surgery for hepatic resection or a rising circulating plasma carcinoembryonic antigen (CEA) level.

Although detecting liver metastases is of major concern, it is important to search diligently for extrahepatic recurrences in the lungs and the abdominal cavity/pelvis.

TABLE 1
Results and Accuracy of Diagnostic Procedures Evaluated at >18 Months Follow-Up

	Preoperative ultrasonography	Preoperative computed tomography	Surgical exploration	Intraoperative ultrasonography	p value
True-positive	43	48	68	93	
True-negative	141	136	129	134	
False-positive	5	10	17	12	
False-negative	70	65	45	20	
Sensitivity (%)	38.1	42.8	60.2	82.3	<0.0005[a]
Specificity (%)	96.6	93.2	88.4	91.8	NS[b]
Predictive value of positive test (%)	89.6	82.8	80.0	88.6	NS
Predictive value of negative test (%)	66.8	67.7	74.1	87.0	<0.005[a]

[a] Intraoperative ultrasonography versus each of the other three procedures.
[b] No significant differences.

Adapted from Machi, J., Isomoto, H., Kurohiji, T., Yamashita, Y., Shirouzu, K., Kakegawa, T., Sigel, B., Zaren, H., and Sariego, J., *World J. Surg.*, 15, 551, 1991. With permission.

A rising plasma CEA level is indicative of recurrent disease and warrants further investigation. Standard investigations, such as colonoscopy, CT, blood tests, chest roentgenogram, and ultrasonography frequently fail to reveal the site of recurrence in the otherwise healthy, asymptomatic patient. A second-look operation is often performed in these situations to remove residual tumor if possible. Such procedures offer the only curative approach. Alternatively, these procedures allow the implantation of an intra-arterial catheter for chemotherapy if hepatic metastases are detected and cannot or should not be removed.

B. ANTIBODY-BASED TECHNIQUES

In cases in which conventional investigations fail to detect tumor recurrence, promising results have been obtained with radioimmunological external scanning and radioimmunologically guided surgery (RIGS®). Monoclonal antibodies against CEA or other tumor antigens are radiolabeled with [111]Indium or [131]Iodine and administered to the patient. Antibody should be taken up by the residual tumor and detected by planar and single photon emission computed tomography (SPECT) scanning, showing as a "hot" spot or spots.

A number of antibodies have been used with varying degrees of success. Griffin et al.[20] used an ^{111}In-labeled antibody to CEA, designated clone 110, in 21 patients with previous surgery and a histological diagnosis of colorectal carcinoma. All demonstrated a rising plasma CEA level or had clinical evidence of recurrent disease. Abnormal areas of localization were seen in 20 of 21 patients. This was confirmed histologically in 19 patients either by operation or fine needle aspiration biopsy. One patient with a negative scan had a negative laparotomy despite a suspicious CT scan.

In another study by Patt et al.[21] ^{111}In-labeled anti-CEA antibody (ZCE-025) was used in 20 patients with rising plasma CEA levels despite previous complete resectional surgery. A thorough conventional investigative workup, including colonoscopy and CT scanning, had failed to localize any recurrent disease. The patients were scanned 72 and 144 h after administration of the antibody. Scans were positive in 19 of 20 patients, 13 of whom underwent exploratory surgery (recurrent tumor was found in 10) and 2 of whom had a diagnostic biopsy (positive in both cases). The 3 patients with a negative laparotomy and all 4 patients who did not have surgery were subsequently monitored using conventional radiological techniques. In all 7 patients recurrent tumor was eventually identified at the sites suggested by their ZCE-025 scan. The authors pointed out that all patients with a positive ZCE-025 scan eventually developed tumor and that 5 patients actually benefited from the scan, 4 having all their recurrent disease resected and 1 patient receiving definitive pelvic radiation therapy.

Gasparini et al.[22] also used an anti-CEA antibody (FO23C5) labeled with ^{111}In or ^{131}I in 51 patients with primary or secondary colorectal carcinoma; 77% (37 of 48) of immunoscintigraphs were positive in areas known to contain primary tumor or local recurrence; however, the ability to detect liver metastases was much lower (only 4 of 16 being accurately diagnosed), probably due to the high uptake of antibody within normal hepatic parenchyma.

RIGS uses a hand-held gamma detector (Neoprobe® 1000) to detect gamma emissions from, for example, ^{125}I-labeled monoclonal antibody localized in tissue. The murine monoclonal antibody B72.3 is an IgG_1 that reacts with a high molecular weight (220,000 to 500,000) tumor-associated glycoprotein complex (TAG-72) found on several human cancers of epithelial origin, including colonic adenocarcinoma.[23] With this reagent, Nieroda et al.[24] used the following protocol in 30 patients with primary colorectal cancer. First, patients were prepared on an oral regimen of supersaturated potassium iodide to saturate the thyroid gland and prevent uptake of ^{125}I-labeled antibody. The patients were also tested for immediate-type hypersensitivity using an intradermal forearm injection of the unlabeled antibody and observing for a reaction after 15 min; no patient had such a reaction. Each patient then received radiolabeled antibody intravenously. The timing of each operation was determined by measuring gamma counts over the heart to assess blood clearance of radiolabel. A mean of 22 days (8 to 34 days) elapsed between injection of the antibody and operation.

On the day of operation the patient had preoperative external count rate measured over the liver, perineum, and heart, noting areas of high activity. At laparotomy the abdomen was explored using the probe and areas containing high activity were noted. The primary tumor was then removed and the abdomen scanned again to detect other areas of radioactivity. Regions of high counts were biopsied and sent for frozen section. B72.3 localized in 23 of the 30 patients (77%). Unsuspected metastases were identified in 7 of the 23 patients (30%): 2 with occult liver metastases, 3 with lymph node metastases, and 3 with invasion of adjacent structures. Tumor margins were clearly identified in 20 of the 23 patients. The results altered patient management in 7 of 23 patients and changed adjuvant therapy in an additional 4 patients. The probe also allowed the distinction between a number of benign liver lesions and one benign ovarian cyst. These results demonstrate the usefulness of a procedure that may, after further development, become a standard part of colorectal cancer surgery.

Nieroda et al.[25] used RIGS in 191 patients undergoing surgery for recurrent colorectal cancer. A similar protocol to that described herein was followed. The antibody localized histologically documented tumor in 140 patients (73%), failing in 35 (18%). As shown in Table 2, RIGS redefined the margins of resection in 60 patients (43%) to include occult tumor in tissue considered normal by palpation and visual examination, detected occult lymph node disease in 27 patients (19%), and was responsible for probe-directed positive biopsies in another 15 patients (11%). Adjuvant therapy was instituted in 8 patients (6%).

Further studies confirmed the usefulness of the B72.3 antibody. Martin and Carey[26] reported that 53 of 86 patients (62%) with recurrent cancer were assessed as resectable by surgical inspection at second-look operations; however, use of RIGS reduced that to 40 patients (47%). Survival of the group defined by RIGS as resectable was 83% at 3 years and 60% at 5 years. For the RIGS-nonresectable group survival was 30% at 3 years, but there were no survivors at 5 years. Thus, use of RIGS proved useful in identifying patients who appeared resectable by clinical assessment but had more extensive disease than was initially appreciated. Sickle-

TABLE 2
Effects of Radioimmunologically Guided
Surgery (RIGS) on Patient Management
(N = 140)[a]

	No.	%
No added information	58	41
Margins redefined	60	43
Occult nodes delineated	27	19
Probe-directed biopsy	15	11
Adjuvant therapy		
Radiation therapy	4	3
Chemotherapy	4	3

[a] Number of patients considered positive for tumor by
   RIGS probe.

From Nieroda, C. A., Mojzisik, C., Hinkle, G., Thurston,
M. O., and Martin, E. W., *Cancer Detec. Prev.*, 15, 225,
1991. With permission.

Santanello et al.[27] also reported the usefulness of RIGS in patients with recurrent disease. Other, newer antibodies also show promise. Dawson et al.[28] reported a 98% localization of primary tumors and 89% of secondary tumors using a mouse monoclonal antibody to CEA (A5B7).

Numerous investigators have documented the inaccuracy of the surgeon in identifying metastases, for example, in lymph nodes. Herrera-Ornelas et al.[29] showed that 64% of lymph node metastases were in nodes less than 5 mm in diameter. Although these may be palpable, they may also be overlooked despite a careful and diligently performed laparotomy. Rosemurgy and Block[30] reported a sensitivity of 71% and an accuracy of only 66% for the ability of the surgeon to identify the true extent of nodal involvement. Thus, a major advantage of RIGS may lie in the sensitivity of the probe, which under certain circumstances can identify tumor foci consisting of as few as 3.9×10^4 cells.[31] However, it should be noted that this remarkable sensitivity is obtained not under conditions resembling a surgical exploration but in a model system where radiolabeled antibody-coated cells are injected into the serosa of segments of biopsied human colon. Another advantage of RIGS is that the small size of the transducer allows it to be used intrarectally or intravaginally to detect local tumor deposits and to direct needle biopsies.

There are several drawbacks to this modality. First, a portion of tumors do not localize the antibody, especially in the case of B72.3. Second, the long interval following administration while waiting for the background radioactivity of the antibody to subside (usually 3 to 4 weeks) is distressing to patients who are aware of their condition and awaiting operation. It also precludes use in patients requiring more urgent surgery for acute or subacute obstruction or severe symptoms. Because this modality appears most useful in patients with recurrent disease, this is perhaps less of a drawback because many patients are identified on the basis of a rising serum CEA level, are asymptomatic, and are usually scheduled for several investigative procedures that can be performed in the intervening time. Third, false-positives (which reduce specificity) occur especially in patients with inflammatory lesions, such as duodenal ulcers, inflammatory bowel disease, ischemic bowel disease, and adenomatous polyps. The presence of inflammation and cellular atypia may contribute to cross-reactivity with the diagnostic antibody or alternatively cause increased capillary permeability to macromolecules. Antibody concentrations may be falsely elevated due to delayed excretion in patients with bowel obstruction.

Eventually, the diagnostic techniques described may reduce the number of patients with tumor recurrences due to surgical failure to remove all tumor at the time of the original operation. Moreover, determining the extent of recurrent disease and its resectability is necessary to determine which patients are incurable by current surgical strategies and which are candidates for regional infusional (e.g., implantable pump) or embolic (e.g., microsphere) therapy.

III. DRUG DELIVERY ROUTES

A. BLOOD SUPPLY TO METASTASES

Regional blood flow to the liver and hepatic metastases are important factors in drug delivery. Whereas micrometastases are seeded to the liver by portal blood flow, the growing metastasis derives its nutrient supply from branches of the hepatic artery. Breedis and Young[32] and others[33-35] using injection casting techniques in post-mortem specimens and other methods were among the first to observe that this was the case: corroborating studies have used methods, such as the uptake of radiolabeled microspheres[37] (see also Chapter 8), macroaggregated albumin radiolabeled with ^{99m}Tc (^{99m}Tc-MAA),[37] and arteriography[38] to confirm these results.

The cited studies all involved relatively large tumors with a well-established blood supply and did not investigate the role of portal injection blood flow in the earliest stages of metastatic implantation. Injection studies in cadaver specimens demonstrate a combined portal and arterial blood supply in metastases <1 cm in size with dominance of the arterial flow.[32,35] Other studies using implanted hepatic tumors in rats show that these artificial lesions derive at least some blood flow from portal vessels in or surrounding the tumors;[39,40] similarly, chemically induced hepatocellular cancers in rats appear to be sustained at least in part by portal blood flow up to a size of approximately 2 mm.[41]

The question of the importance of portal blood supply in micrometastases was addressed by Archer and Gray.[42] Using a rat model of liver metastases, induced by intraportal injection of cultured tumor spheroids, they quantified the relative contribution of the portal vein and hepatic artery to the internal circulation of small liver tumors. Using simultaneous injections of two differing radiolabeled microspheres into the left ventricle (^{57}Co) and the portal vein (^{113}Sn or ^{131}I), they recorded the relative tumor/normal tissue ratio (T/N) from hepatic arterial flow and portal venous flow. The mean hepatic artery T/N ratio was significantly greater than that of the portal vein for all tumor sizes studied. In tumors as small as 0.5 mm, the mean hepatic artery T/N ratio ± SEM was 1.50 ± 0.12 compared with a portal vein T/N ratio of 0.13 ± 0.04. Tumors ≥2 mm in size had T/N ratios of 1.26 ± 0.11 versus 0.06 ± 0.01 for hepatic arterial and portal blood, respectively. The study showed that tiny metastases, 0.5 mm in size, have already established a well-defined arterial blood supply with only a minor portal contribution. These studies imply that for locoregional chemotherapy of established tumors higher tumor drug concentrations will be achieved by intra-arterial rather than intraportal administration.

In another study designed to identify those patients with hepatic metastases who would respond to intra-arterial chemotherapy, Kaplan et al.[43] used radionuclide angiography to predict response. Nineteen patients underwent hepatic artery catheterization; then patterns of perfusion were assessed using ^{99m}Tc-MAA infused at high and low flow rates. Responses to chemotherapy could be predicted: 10 of 11 patients with good flow to tumor areas responded to therapy; none of 8 patients with absent or poor flow responded. The study also examined the relationship between infusion rate of ^{99m}Tc-MAA and tumor perfusion. Two patients showed improved perfusion of tumor lesions when the infusion rate of ^{99m}Tc-MAA was increased.

Another study by Daly et al.[44] examined the role of the ^{99m}Tc-MAA scan in greater detail in patients with colorectal liver metastases. They noted that the radionuclide scan had greatest predictive value in previously untreated patients. This held true for response rates with treatment either by systemic or intra-arterial chemotherapy. Of 47 patients with an evaluable scan treated with intra-arterial therapy, 31 individuals had a positive scan in that ^{99m}Tc-MAA uptake was greater in tumor tissue than in normal liver. Sixteen of these patients responded to therapy (true-positive) and 15 did not (false-positive). Of 16 patients with a negative scan, 15 did not respond (true-negative), whereas only 1 of 16 patients did respond (false-negative). Overall, the radionuclide scan had a sensitivity of 94% and a specificity of 50%: in previously untreated patients the values were 91 and 77%, respectively.

Liver biopsies of two patients shortly after ^{99m}Tc-MAA administration, one with a positive and another with a negative scan, showed increased uptake in tumor tissue relative to liver in the patient with the positive scan and a reduced uptake in the tumor of the patient with the negative scan. This suggests that the ^{99m}Tc-MAA scan can be used to predict, in a relative fashion, tumor perfusion and hence exposure of metastases to chemotherapeutic agents. These results were confirmed by Kemeny et al.[45] in a study that examined 112 patients for prognostic variables of tumor response. Only the ^{99m}Tc-MAA scan predicted tumor response to chemotherapy.

B. A COMPARISON OF DRUG DELIVERY ROUTES

To correlate tumor drug uptake with route of delivery a number of studies have been performed in both animals and humans. Ridge et al.[46] compared the use of systemic, portal, and hepatic arterial delivery routes on the uptake of ^{14}C-labeled doxorubicin in rabbits with hepatic implants of VX2 carcinoma. Hepatic arterial infusion produced the highest tumor doxorubicin concentration (34.3 nmol/g tumor) compared with systemic (11.5 nmol/g tumor) or portal (6.3 nmol/g tumor) routes of administration. Normal liver tissue drug levels also varied with the route of delivery, being highest with portal administration (54.4 nmol/g liver). Uptake from the hepatic arterial route was 48.4 nmol/g liver and 32.4 nmol/g liver via the systemic route. Interestingly, cardiac levels of the drug were highest with systemic administration and lowest with the portal route. These data suggest that tumor uptake is significantly greater when chemotherapeutic agents are administered by the hepatic arterial route; thus, equivalent tumor levels might be achieved using lower doses. The reduced cardiac levels suggests that this route might also reduce systemic toxicity.

Archer and Gray[47] compared portal vein chemotherapy with hepatic artery chemotherapy in a rat model of liver metastases and investigated the importance of timing in the administration of the drug. Portal vein chemotherapy was effective only when administered concurrently with tumor inoculation via the portal vein, reducing final tumor burden in the liver by 91%. Administration by the same route at day 6 post-tumor inoculation demonstrated no difference in tumor incidence or growth relative to untreated controls. Commencement of chemotherapy via the hepatic artery at 0, 2, 4, and 6 days after tumor inoculation reduced the burden of hepatic metastases by approximately 66% relative to untreated controls.

Didolkar et al.[48] studied the pharmacokinetics of the delivery of 5-fluorouracil (5-FU) (Chapter 6) to the normal canine liver after continuous infusion. They measured inferior vena cava and hepatic venous drug concentrations after administration via one of four routes: systemic vein, portal vein, hepatic artery, or hepatic artery combined with hepatic ligation. The results showed that administration of the drug distal to the ligated artery resulted in the highest hepatic vein drug concentrations with the smallest systemic/hepatic vein ratio. Hepatic arterial administration was the next most advantageous with the systemic venous and portal venous routes a poor third. When compared with data from a bolus injection using the same dose of 5-FU, the results were similar. The rate of metabolism of 5-FU was significantly reduced in dearterialized animals, thus prolonging tumor exposure to the drug and potentially increasing tumor cell kill.

A number of human studies have been performed in which metastatic tumors have been biopsied after infusion of chemotherapeutic agents and the distribution of parent drug and/or their metabolic products recorded. Sigurdson et al.[49] examined fluorodeoxyuridine (FUdR, floxuridine) (Chapter 6) uptake by colorectal hepatic metastases after intrahepatic arterial infusion. Patients entered in this study underwent laparotomy for placement of a continuous infusion pump into the gastroduodenal artery. After ascertaining that the catheter was correctly placed, a mixture of ^{99m}Tc-MAA and ^{3}H-fluorodeoxyuridine was injected. Two to 5 minutes later both tumor and liver tissue were biopsied from the same lobe and the ^{99m}Tc- and ^{3}H- radioactivity counted. Results showed that there was a linear correlation between the tumor/liver ratios of fluorodeoxyuridine and ^{99m}Tc-MAA.

On the basis of the ^{99m}Tc-MAA scan patients were classified as having a ''hot'' or ''cold'' scan according to the localization of ^{99m}Tc-MAA in tumor regions. Ten of 15 patients evaluated had ''cold'' scans with 5 having a ''hot'' scan. Mean ^{3}H-fluorodeoxyuridine levels in tumor were 6.9 ± 2.2 in the ''cold'' group and 14.8

± 11.1 in the "hot" group. This difference fell just short of statistical significance ($p = 0.07$). Two months later the group was evaluated for tumor response. There were four partial responses to therapy, but this did not correlate with tumor fluorodeoxyuridine concentrations. The finding was explained as being due to small biopsy size and tumor tissue heterogeneity, which could lead to a tenfold variation in uptake of fluorodeoxyuridine within the same metastasis. The latter point was examined after infusion of ^{99m}Tc-MAA and ^{3}H-fluorodeoxyuridine[50] in four patients undergoing lobectomy or wedge resection where the whole tumor was available for analysis. In each case between 40 and 100 specimens of tumor and liver were assayed to map drug and MAA distribution. The study demonstrated a linear relationship between drug uptake (^{3}H localization) and tissue perfusion (^{99m}Tc localization) for both tumor and liver tissue.

Although investigations of the type described herein demonstrate a relationship between drug uptake and tumor perfusion, it is generally observed that tumor tissue has a much lower extraction and/or rate of drug metabolism than liver. Thus, methods that increase tumor blood flow with respect to the liver should increase tumor drug uptake and response. Alternatively, extraction may be increased by slowing blood flow through the liver, thus allowing increased time for tumor tissue extraction of the drug. Respectively, these can be achieved by pharmacological manipulation using vasoactive drugs or the infusion of microspheres causing microemboli, which obstruct and slow hepatic blood flow temporarily.

The results of studies described in this section combine to suggest that intra-arterial chemotherapy should be of greatest benefit to the patient with hepatic metastases (especially when the tumor load is small and the patient has a good Karnofsky performance score and a "hot" tumor ^{99m}Tc-MAA scan). Because intra-arterial therapy requires a laparotomy and is much more invasive, it remains to be seen whether such aggressive intervention is warranted in terms of survival benefit, tumor response, and palliation.

Kemeny et al.[51] randomized carefully matched patients without extrahepatic disease to receive either systemic intravenous or intrahepatic arterial fluorodeoxyuridine via an implanted pump. Patients received a continuous 14-day infusion each month after pump implantation. Of the initial 162 patients entered in the study, 63 were excluded after operation (25 had hepatic resections, 33 had extrahepatic disease, 4 had no detectable disease, and 1 had an infection). The remaining 99 patients were randomly assigned to intra-arterial (n = 48) or systemic (n = 51) fluorodeoxyuridine at 0.3 mg/kg/day or 0.15 mg/kg/day, respectively, these being equitoxic regimens. Results showed that intra-arterial therapy produced significantly higher complete/partial response rates, 50% versus 20%, when compared with systemic intravenous therapy. Plasma CEA was reduced by more than 50% in 60% of patients receiving intra-arterial therapy compared with 25% in those patients who received systemic therapy.

Thirty-one (60%) patients crossed over from the systemic intravenous group following progression of liver metastases: 25% achieved a partial response and 33% a minor response or stabilization of disease on intra-arterial therapy. Plasma CEA levels decreased by >50% in 10 of the 31 patients. The median survival was 17 months following regional fluorodeoxyuridine compared with 12 months for the systemic treatment. Because of the crossover nature of this study and the relatively small numbers, duration of survival could not be evaluated statistically. However, trends suggested a survival advantage for regional treatment and therapy was better tolerated compared with the group receiving systemic fluorodeoxyuridine.

In a similar study Daly et al.[52] compared intra-arterial and portal administration of fluorodeoxyuridine in 25 matched patients randomized preoperatively. Continuous infusion of the drug was given alternating in a 2-week cycle with saline. All patients entered into the study had previously failed systemic chemotherapy. Of the 25 randomized patients, 5 were excluded at operation on the basis of extrahepatic disease and 1 had the pump removed because of persistent pump pocket infection. Of the remaining 19 patients, 8 received intra-arterial and 11 received portal fluorodeoxyuridine. Tumor response occurred in 50% (4 of 8) of the intra-arterial group with no responders in the portal group. The responders in the intra-arterial group also showed a >50% reduction in their plasma CEA levels, whereas only 1 in the portal group showed such a reduction. Nine patients crossed over from the portal to the intra-arterial group and 3 of those showed a partial tumor response to therapy. The mean duration of response was 8 months. These results show that despite failing systemic chemotherapy 7 of 17 patients (41%) responded to intra-arterial chemotherapy.

In a study designed to examine survival benefit, Chang et al.[53] randomized patients to intra-arterial or systemic chemotherapy with fluorodeoxyuridine. They recorded better response rates in the intra-arterial group with 13 of 21 patients (62%) responding compared with 5 of 29 patients (17%) in the intravenous group. At 2 years the survival rates were 22 and 15%, respectively.

Cumulative evidence shows that, for lesions restricted to the liver, intensification of chemotherapy via intra-arterial administration offers the most effective regimen for inducing tumor regression with acceptable morbidity. The absence of a corresponding survival benefit may be due to systemic disease for which a systemic approach to therapy is mandatory. Regional was better tolerated than systemic therapy:[51] in the systemic group the major side effect was diarrhea with occasional colitis requiring hospitalization for supportive care and rehydration. Mucositis also occurred in 10% of patients. Side effects were less severe in the intra-arterial group and mainly related to gastrointestinal ulceration and hepatic enzyme elevation. Biliary sclerosis, the most serious complication (8% of patients), can be avoided by monitoring of liver function tests and adjusting the drug dose as necessary.

C. SURGICAL CONSIDERATIONS

The first attempts at hepatic arterial cannulation for chemotherapy were performed as long ago as 1962 by Clarkson et al.[54] Catheters were placed either surgically or by the Seldinger technique. In this study, 35% of patients had their therapy interrupted by complications, such as catheter occlusion, sepsis, arterial thrombosis, and catheter displacement. Other studies documented similar problems and included gastrointestinal tract hemorrhage.[55,56] Nevertheless, Reed et al.[57] reported a 73% tumor response rate (median duration 12 months) in 88 patients with liver metastases. Complications were common with an operative mortality of 12% and catheter-related morbidity of 24%.

Complications have been reduced with the development of a totally implantable delivery device, the Infusaid® infusion pump[58,59] (Infusaid Corporation, Norwood, MA). It is a lightweight Freon driven pump with a 50-ml capacity chamber that requires filling at 1- to 2-week intervals and a side port to allow direct access to the hepatic artery for flushing and to perform cognate studies. Initial evaluation described tumor response rates varying from 28 to 83% with minimal catheter-related complications.[60-65] A vital requirement of any regional approach to therapy, whether infusional via a pump or embolic using microspheres, is accurate surgical placement of the arterial catheter.

Daly et al.,[66] examined anatomical considerations, operative techniques, and treatment morbidity associated with the use of an implantable device. An initial retrospective review of 200 celiac and superior mesenteric angiograms was performed to clarify the anatomical variations of the blood supply to the liver with particular reference to the origin of the gastroduodenal artery. The anomalies were classified according to a modification of Michels scheme[67] (Figure 1 shows the major divisions of this classification). They noted that in 70% of cases the gastroduodenal artery arose proximal to the bifurcation of the common hepatic artery (type IA). This permitted complete hepatic perfusion by a catheter with its tip at the junction of the common hepatic and gastroduodenal arteries. Alternatively, to achieve liver perfusion via both left and right hepatic arteries in patients with type IB, II, or IV vascular anatomy, retrograde cannulation of the splenic artery could be performed so the catheter tip lies in the celiac artery. In patients with type III vascular anatomy the major blood supply to the right hepatic lobe arose from the superior mesenteric artery, whereas the left hepatic artery arose from the celiac artery. This required either placement of two catheters separately or anastomosis of the right to the left hepatic artery.

Preoperative patient assessment should include routine medical history, physical examination, and estimation of Karnofsky performance status. Investigations should include recent chest roentgenogram, complete blood cell count, blood chemistry analysis, CEA, prothrombin and partial thromboplastin times, electrocardiogram, abdominal and chest CT scan, and celiac and superior mesenteric arteriograms. Patients who are to have concurrent primary colon resection should also undergo investigations relevant to that procedure (especially colonoscopy or double-contrast barium enema).

Although surgery may be technically feasible in many patients, it is advisable to exclude patients if they have evidence of liver failure (serum bilirubin >4 mg/dl) or a poor performance status (<60). Other medical problems precluding anesthesia would also preclude surgery. Extrahepatic metastatic disease is also a relative contraindication to surgery.

Operative placement of the system starts with an exploratory laparotomy to assess the degree and extent of parietal and visceral disease. The diagnosis of metastatic disease can be confirmed histologically by frozen section if this has not

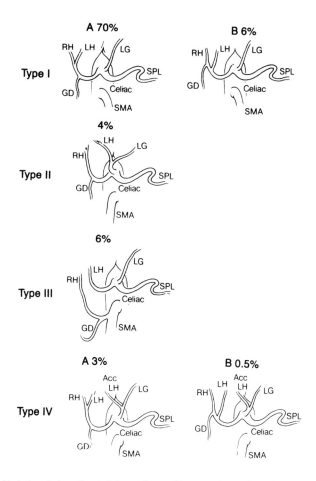

FIGURE 1. Variations in hepatic arterial vasculature. Retrospective review of 200 angiograms allowed calculation of percent of patients with arterial configurations as demonstrated. Celiac, celiac axis; SMA, superior mesenteric artery; LG, left gastric artery; SPL, splenic artery; LH, left hepatic artery; RH, right hepatic artery; GD, gastroduodenal artery; Acc LH, accessory left hepatic artery. (Adapted from Daly, J. M., Kemeny, N., Oderman, P., and Botet, J., *Arch. Surg.*, 119, 936, 1984. With permission.)

been previously established. The degree of hepatic replacement can be estimated manually and visually.

Preoperative arteriograms are assessed and compared with the operative assessment of the hepatic blood supply. With regard to patients with type IA vascular anatomy, the right gastric artery is ligated, and after duodenal mobilization small branches to the duodenal bulb are also divided. The common hepatic artery is dissected thoroughly to expose the gastroduodenal artery. It is essential to ligate all branches of the gastroduodenal artery, especially the supraduodenal branch, which arises within 2 cm of its hepatic artery origin. These ligations are performed to prevent infusion of the drug to the stomach and duodenum. The gastroduodenal artery is then ligated distally and the proximal end temporarily occluded. A transverse arteriotomy is made and a beaded Silastic catheter tip advanced retrogradely into the artery so that its tip lies at the junction of the common hepatic and gastroduodenal arteries. The catheter is then secured in place with nonabsorbable sutures.

Should splenic artery cannulation be required, the operation proceeds as before with ligation of the gastroduodenal artery and right gastric arteries but also includes ligation of the left gastric artery distal to the origin of the left hepatic artery. The splenic artery is then temporarily occluded and a transverse arteriotomy is performed. The vessel is then catheterized so that the tip lies within the celiac artery.

Position of the catheter is confirmed by the injection of fluorescein solution via the pump's side port. The abdomen is examined under a Wood's ultraviolet lamp to confirm uniform hepatic distribution with no other visceral fluorescence, especially of the stomach and duodenum. The pump is then placed in a subcutaneous pouch fashioned in the left or right lower quadrant below the belt line for patient comfort.

Prophylactic broad-spectrum antibiotics are given preoperatively and continued for 72 h postoperatively. Other methods used to reduce pocket infection include shaving the abdomen immediately prior to operation. Prophylactic cholecystectomy is recommended to avoid the risk of chemical cholecystitis. On the fifth postoperative day a ^{99m}Tc-MAA scan is performed to confirm uniform hepatic perfusion.

Arterial infusion is started 7 days after surgery. Fluorodeoxyuridine is the most commonly used agent and is started at a dose of 0.3 mg/kg/day for a 14-day cycle followed by a 14-day saline infusion. Heparin 10,000 IU is placed in the pump at each refill to prevent catheter occlusion. If this regimen is unsuccessful in preventing disease progression, mitomycin C can be given as a single 2-h infusion via the side port every 6 weeks at a dose of 15 mg/m.[2] It is advisable to prescribe some form of peptic ulcer prophylaxis, such as cimetidine 300 mg 4 times a day or sucralfate 1 g 4 times a day.

Patients are followed up with serial visits every 2 weeks when their pump is filled and they are asked about symptoms or side effects of therapy, such as weakness and abdominal pain. Liver function tests and complete blood counts are performed at each visit and plasma CEA levels are taken at alternate visits. An abdominal CT scan is performed at 2 months and thereafter as necessary. Esophagogastroduodenoscopy is performed for patients who describe epigastric pain, fullness, or vomiting.

Commonly, side effects associated with intra-arterial therapy involve the distal stomach and duodenum: the most commonly seen lesions on esophagogastroduodenoscopy are antral gastritis, gastric ulcer, duodenitis, and duodenal ulcer. To examine whether this was due to fluorodeoxyuridine still perfusing these organs, despite ligation of the right gastric and gastroduodenal arteries, Hohn et al.[68] additionally ligated all vessels supplying the superior border of the distal stomach and the proximal duodenum and in 35 patients had no cases of gastritis or ulceration related to therapy. It was also suggested that the placement of the tip of the catheter may be critical in that it should lie within the lumen of the common hepatic artery and not just in the gastroduodenal artery.

Hepatic toxicity is noted by elevation of the serum bilirubin above 3 mg/dl and elevation of serum SGOT above baseline levels. The bilirubin elevation occurs in approximately 27% of patients and is reversible on cessation of therapy in 55% of those. Serum SGOT levels were elevated in 22 of 34 (65%) patients, 19 of whom had levels greater than 3 times baseline. In all patients, serum SGOT levels returned to normal after cessation of therapy.[66] A more serious manifestation of toxicity is biliary sclerosis. In the series described by Daly et al.,[66] 2 of 34 patients developed extrahepatic biliary duct strictures that required external drainage and decompression.

IV. THE ROLE OF MICROSPHERES

A. THEORETICAL AND EXPERIMENTAL BACKGROUND

To gain a survival benefit newer approaches to delivery of antineoplastic agents must be considered to increase exposure of tumor to drug and improve response. The interaction of four factors determines tumor drug exposure (pharmacokinetics) and therefore response (pharmacodynamics): tumor blood flow, local plasma drug concentration, cellular drug uptake, and drug metabolism. Manipulation of hepatic blood flow, in particular tumor blood flow, can alter exposure of the neoplastic cell to the drug, permitting increased drug uptake and efficacy. Approaches to manipulation of tumor blood flow using vasoactive agents (see Chapters 2 and 8) and microspheres offer theoretical advantages. Various microspherical systems are described in other chapters of this volume: the remainder of this chapter will review the experience of our group and others with DSM.

DSM of 25 to 45 μm diameter, which initially lodge in precapillary arterioles but move into capillary beds as they break down and become smaller due to enzymatic degradation, can reduce blood flow by temporarily occluding vessels and preventing coinjected drug from being removed into the venous washout. This approach should be distinguished from that involving incorporation of active agents within microsphere matrix (see Chapters 1, 3, 4, 5, and 6).

DSM were originally developed to induce a temporary state of intestinal ischemia, thus protecting the bowel from radiation damage.[69,70] However, it was their ability to alter drug distribution that led to their use in drug targeting.[71] DSM are made from polysaccharides produced from potato starch hydrosylate and cross-linked by the process of emulsion polymerization. They are degraded by amylase and *in vitro* have been shown to have a half-life of 20 to 30 min depending on their diameter. *In vivo*, however, the half-life relates more closely to the product of the weight or number of microspheres and diameter.[72] Polysaccharide cross-linking, via epichlorohydrin bridges, is greatest in the outer shell of the microspheres; thus, at low amylase concentration the spherical microsphere structure is maintained for a reasonable length of time. At higher concentrations of amylase there is a gradual decrease in microsphere number and size.[73] Both these mechanisms probably work *in vivo* as the initial cessation of blood flow results in a low amylase state, which gradually increases with the restoration of blood flow.[74]

Regional infusion of DSM is followed by a temporary reduction in hepatic blood flow and is believed to increase local tissue drug concentrations by two mechanisms. First, it causes decreased drug elution, thus allowing greater cellular drug uptake. Prior injection of the drug followed by the microspheres delivers the drug to the tumor tissue before the microcirculation is occluded. It is postulated that this leads to a proportionally greater decrease in the drug elution from tumor tissue than normal hepatic parenchymal cells. In an experimental model involving the pig, Starkhammar et al.[75] demonstrated that portal blood flow was a major factor in clearance of a labeled marker in the normal liver. DSM-induced arterial occlusion after repeated doses reduced the passage of this marker significantly, but much of it still passed into the systemic circulation. Portal vein occlusion further reduced the clearance of the marker, suggesting that portal elution was an important factor in drug clearance. It may be less important in liver metastases because of the minimal role played by the portal system in supplying these lesions. Second, blood is diverted from normal liver tissue to tumor deposits. Liver metastases are hypovascular and receive a proportionally lower dose of microspheres than normal liver: the resulting occlusion of the normal hepatic microcirculation results in re-direction of blood flow to the microsphere-deficient capillary bed of the metastasis, thus increasing tumor perfusion and drug delivery.

Evidence supporting this hypothesis comes from a study by Civalleri et al.,[76] who studied changes in intrahepatic arterial blood flow in four patients receiving intra-arterial DSM and chemotherapy for hepatic metastases. They imaged the liver using contrast-enhanced CT scanning. An initial scan was performed prior to therapy following injection of a nonionic contrast medium and the integrated density (ID) calculated for both normal hepatic parenchyma and for areas of metastatic tumor. Immediately after injection of DSM the scan was repeated and the ID calculated for the same areas. Before DSM the ID for the colorectal metastases was lower than that of normal hepatic parenchyma in 9 of 10 samples. After DSM the paren-chymal tissue and single hyperdense metastasis all showed marked reduction in their ID, whereas the 9 hypodense lesions showed an average increase in their densities, albeit with great variability.

Civalleri later addressed the same issue using the ^{99m}Tc-MAA scan.[77] In 4 of 6 cases of hypovascular metastases the administration of DSM completely or par-tially reversed blood flow as imaged by the ^{99m}Tc-MAA scan and the lesions became "hot". Together, these studies suggest that DSM embolization might improve the efficacy of treatment by increasing drug extraction by the tumor or redistributing blood flow to hypovascular metastases.

With regard to the coadministration of active agents (or model drugs) with DSM, work in animal models has shown consistently that arterial blood flow can be interrupted temporarily without evidence of tissue ischemia or damage even after repeated doses. Complete cessation of arterial flow can be achieved for short periods if a large enough dose is used. In humans this dose can vary widely and needs to be calculated on an individual basis.[78]

In experimental models involving solid tumors of the liver, intrahepatic arterial injections of cytotoxic drugs in admixture with DSM have resulted in increased tumor tissue concentrations, reduction in peak plasma concentrations, and increased antitumor activity compared with drug alone. These results are summarized in Table 3.

Human studies have been performed to evaluate the effect of DSM on drug concentrations in liver metastases in patients receiving chemotherapy. Fourteen patients with liver metastases from colorectal cancer underwent hepatic arterial infusion of ^{14}C-fluorodeoxyuridine during surgery, followed within 2 to 5 min by another infusion of ^{3}H-fluorodeoxyuridine with or without DSM.[84] Seven patients had contemporaneous hepatic resections and four patients underwent open biopsy of normal liver and tumor 5 min after infusion. Results demonstrated that coadministration of fluorodeoxyuridine and DSM increased tumor drug levels almost threefold (5.9 ± 4.4 to 17.1 ± 9.4 nmol/g) without altering hepatic drug levels (35.7 ± 10.9 to 30.2 ± 30.2 nmol/g). The tumor/liver drug ratio of tritiated fluoropyrimidines was also altered in favor of the tumor from 0.16 ± 0.09 to 0.63 ± 0.13.

Similar findings were reported by Civalleri et al.[85] in four patients with colorectal metastases who received intrahepatic arterial cisplatin with or without DSM at the placement of an arterial catheter. Tissue biopsies were taken 15 min after drug administration and plasma platinum concentrations were also measured. Tumor platinum concentrations were significantly elevated after the coadministration of the drug with DSM (3.03 ± 1.6 μg/g) compared with cisplatin alone (0.67 ± 0.49 μg/g). Tumor/liver ratio of platinum concentration was also raised, although not significantly. Peak plasma drug concentrations occurred later and were significantly lower with DSM.

Other studies measured drug pharmacokinetics using mitomycin[86] or BCNU.[87] In the mitomycin study 16 patients received mitomycin alone followed later by the drug plus DSM. Systemic exposure to the drug was calculated from peripheral blood samples and the area under the curve calculated for each individual. Administration of DSM reduced the systemic exposure by between 17 to 70%. This decreased exposure was still evident 60 min after the drug was given with a mean reduction of approximately 40%. A similar study with BCNU[87] was performed which showed a reduction in systemic exposure to nitrosourea of 34 to 92%.

Both these studies showed marked variability in the degree of systemic exposure. This probably results from individual variability in the amount of arteriovenous shunting. Gyves et al.[86] examined this potential problem in the patient population discussed herein and calculated a percent shunt index for 6 of them. The values ranged from 8 to 29% and appeared to be related to the dose of DSM. Starkhammar et al.,[88] also recorded high levels of shunting. A study by Ziessman et al.[89] recorded baseline and DSM-induced shunting after sequential injections of microspheres (5 × 180 mg) at 2-min intervals. They found baseline shunting, expressed as percent shunt index, ranging from 5.8 to 26% (mean 12.6%). After 5 injections of DSM, tolerated only by half of the patients, the shunt index rose to 12.5 to 37% (mean 26.8%) (total 900 mg of DSM). The study showed an incremental increase in the degree of shunting in most patients, particularly after the later injections, although interpatient variation was considerable. They suggested that high levels of baseline

TABLE 3
Effect of Degradable Starch Microspheres (DSM)[a] in Models of Liver Metastases

Dose of DSM (mg/kg)	Drug used in admixture	Experimental model[b]	Effect of DSM on drug concentration/activity			Ref.
			Blood	Tumor	Liver	
Not stated	Doxorubicin (3 mg/kg)	VX-2 tumor (rabbit)	Peak concentration decreased by 60% (41 versus 17 nmol/ml)	Increased (17 versus 60 nmol/g)	No difference (55 versus 51 nmol/g)	79
60	Doxorubicin (4 mg/kg)	Carcinoma (rat)	WBC[c] increased (9.6 versus 13.9 × 10^9/ml)	Growth inhibition	Necrosis	80
60	5-Fluorouracil (0.8 mg/kg)	Carcinoma (rat)	NT[d]	No significant difference (7.6 versus 11.4 pmol/μg DNA)	No significant difference (22.4 versus 19.2 pmol/μg DNA)	81
100	5-Fluorouracil (150 mg/kg)	No tumor (rat)	Peak concentration reduced (1.9 versus 1.3% injectate)	—	Initial concentration increased (7.5 versus 10.9% injectate)	82
50	5-Fluorouracil (100 mg/kg)	Sarcoma (rat)	NT	Increased (0.2 versus 0.5 mg/g)	NT	83

a Effect of DSM and drug relative to drug alone.
b In all models tumor was transplanted in liver and treatment was by intrahepatic arterial injection.
c White blood cell count.
d Not tested.

shunting might serve as a relative contraindication to therapy with DSM as regional specificity is reduced.

The aforementioned studies all used ^{99m}Tc-MAA, a reagent that may overestimate the degree of shunting to the lung unless appropriate care is taken (see Chapter 8). Chapter 8 also shows that, at least for a single dose of a customized reagent (^{131}I-microspheres of 20 to 40 μm diameter), arteriovenous shunting is a minor factor in the consideration of microsphere-based strategies in regional treatment of liver metastases.

B. TUMOR VASCULAR MORPHOLOGY: IMPLICATIONS FOR MICROSPHERE-BASED DRUG DELIVERY STRATEGIES

Vascular morphology has important consequences for strategies to enhance tumor drug delivery and efficacy. Chapter 2 reviews the use of vasomodulators and Chapter 8 describes the application of the vasoconstrictor angiotensin II in delivery of microspheres to liver metastases. The following includes an account of the salient differences between tumor and normal tissue vasculature and our view of the mechanism of differential responsiveness to vasomodulators that may be of therapeutic advantage in regional therapy of liver metastases.

Tumor vasculature has been the source of many studies since Goldmann first described the vascular system of human and experimental tumors in 1907.[90] He noted a disruption of the normal vascular architecture in invasive tumors and described a zone of proliferation in which new vessels were being produced. A tumor cannot rely on diffusion of nutrients from normal tissues to survive and proliferate but must develop a blood supply of its own or incorporate normal vasculature. The success of this process varies from tumor to tumor, as can be seen in rapidly growing tumors that frequently outstrip their blood supply and undergo central necrosis and liquefaction.

In a review of tumor vascular morphology Warren[91] concluded that although solid tumors might differ with regard to vascular morphology, morphological pattern was not unique for a particular tumor. In another study on the subject, Day[92] suggested that the contradictory information in the literature could be rationalized by considering tumor vascularity as having two origins: one assimilated from normal tissue blood supply and the other produced by the tumor itself from a fibrovascular stromal reaction.

The vascular morphology of xenotransplanted human tumors has been described in some detail in a series of studies by Konerding et al.,[93-95] in which the tumor vasculature was examined by corrosion casting and both transmission and scanning electron microscopy. They found disorganized heterogeneous structures, immature endothelial cells with abnormal cell contacts, and even tumor cells incorporated into the vessel wall. Most studies agree that the heterogeneous nature of the tumor vascularity does not correlate with histology,[96,97] that is, tumors with similar histology often do not have a comparable vascular pattern.

The contractility and innervation of newly formed vessels of the tumor vasculature are believed to be deficient; however, incorporated normal vessels in the tumor may retain their contractility and function and thus the overall tumor response to vasoactive stimuli will depend on the ratio of incorporated normal vessels to newly developed vessels. Studies using histochemical techniques failed to identify adrenergic nerve endings in the vascular beds of human malignancies and a transplanted rat tumor.[98-100] In most rapidly growing tumors the neovasculature lacks a normal structure and retains a capillary-type circulation with varying intercapillary distances, arteriovenous malformations, and venous sinusoids frequently lacking endothelial cells. Tumor capillaries have also been demonstrated to consist of a mixture of endothelial and neoplastic cells. This disordered vasculature lacks contractility, thus suggesting that most tumor blood flow varies passively in response to factors altering regional blood flow and that intrinsic modulation of flow is lacking except in incorporated normal vessels.

Hemingway et al.,[101] using a rat model of hypovascular hepatic metastases, obtained similar results using two vasoconstrictors (angiotensin II and phenylephrine). They also noted that the vasoconstrictor effect in the liver lasted at least 90 min far exceeding any systemic hemodynamic effect. Thus, vasoconstriction is mediated by the liver arterioles and because tumor vasculature is immature and lacks innervation and smooth muscle, it does not respond to the vasoconstrictor activity of angiotensin. Therefore, blood is diverted to the relatively "dilated" tumor vasculature. This effect is complemented by an increase in blood pressure, which enhances tumor perfusion.

Modulation of hepatic blood flow with vasoactive agents in patients with liver metastases from colorectal cancer has been investigated in recent studies. Andrews et al.[102] performed infusions of epinephrine in 18 patients with hepatic arterial catheters. Using a coinfusion of ^{99m}Tc-MAA they estimated the tumor/liver ratio with varying doses of epinephrine using SPECT. The study reported an increased tumor/liver ratio after epinephrine infusion with a mean increase over baseline of 3.01 times.

Sasaki et al.[103] examined the effects of the potent hepatic arterial constrictor angiotensin II[104,105] following intrahepatic arterial administration in nine patients with liver cancer or metastases using the extremely short-lived radioisotope ^{81m}Kr (half-life 13 s). They found that after the start of the infusion radioactivity increased in the tumor region in comparison with normal liver, which decreased. Relative blood flow to the tumor region continued to increase to a maximal tumor/liver ratio of 3.30. The effect was maximal at 100 sec with a slow return to normal, a duration of action that is suited to bolus administration of microspheres rather than long-term infusion therapy.

More recently Goldberg et al. investigated the ability of angiotensin II to target radiolabeled microspheres to metastases in two studies that are described in detail in Chapter 8. Again, the increase in T/N ratio for microsphere embolization was twofold to threefold. Complications of angiotensin II therapy are few. No study reported excessive hypertension or rebound hypotension or an increase in extrahepatic shunting. Hepatic tachyphylaxis has been reported with intraportal infusion of angiotensin II;[106] however, it appears that this can be avoided by administering the agent intra-arterially.

C. CLINICAL TOXICITY AND EFFICACY STUDIES WITH DEGRADABLE STARCH MICROSPHERES (DSM)

In a phase I study 34 patients with hepatic cancer (mainly of colorectal origin) were treated with various doses of DSM admixed with mitomycin C (Chapter 6) at a dose of 10 mg/m^2 via the hepatic artery to establish a dose of microspheres that gave acceptable toxicity with maximal hepatic drug exposure.[107] This latter parameter was estimated indirectly by measuring the reduction in mitomycin C area under the plasma concentration time curve due to coinjection with DSM. Dose-limiting acute toxicities were nausea/vomiting and right upper quadrant hepatic pain. At a dose of 36 × 10^6 (360 mg) particle toxicity was manageable, but at a dose of 90 × 10^6 (900 mg) incidences of nausea and vomiting and upper quadrant pain were 50% and 40%, respectively. Although the higher dose of DSM gave the greatest decrease (60% of control) in systemic drug exposure (and by inference the greatest increase in hepatic exposure), the lower dose was not significantly inferior in this respect (70% of control): consequently, it was selected for phase II efficacy studies.

This study was carried out in 24 patients with solid tumors of the liver, mainly of colorectal origin, that had previously failed hepatic arterial chemotherapy with fluoropyrimidines.[108] Treatment consisted of mitomycin C (15 mg/m^2) in admixture with DSM (36 × 10^6) administered as a bolus via the hepatic artery every 6 to 8 weeks: the median number of courses per patient was 3 and all patients were evaluated for response and toxicity.

As evaluated by ^{99m}Tc-sulfur colloid liver/spleen scan or CT, there were no complete responses and 6 (25%) partial responses, defined as >50% decrease in size of lesion. Hematological toxicity was mild and consisted of thrombocytopenia in 3 patients (13%). In 5 patients alterations in liver perfusion were noted by hepatic arterial perfusion scintigraphy, which on further investigation were due to areas of luminal narrowing and irregularity consistent with chemical vasculitis.

In the only phase III prospective randomized trial published to date,[109] 61 patients were randomized to one of three groups: 20 control patients received no treatment, 22 patients received hepatic artery embolization with lyophilized dura mater, and 19 patients received hepatic artery infusions of 5-FU (Chapter 6) and DSM. Treatment in this latter group consisted of four daily, consecutive injections initially containing 500 mg 5-FU mixed with 900 mg DSM every 28 days. In each subsequent session the patient received two injections every 28 days. In these sessions the dose of DSM varied from 300 to 900 mg according to an amount determined for each individual patient. Hepatic artery embolization showed no survival benefit when compared with controls; however, there did appear to be some survival benefit with the third group receiving 5-FU and DSM, although this did not reach statistical significance. When the patient population was broken down into subgroups, the longest median survival was seen in a subgroup with smallest tumor burden (<50% hepatic replacement at presentation), a situation in which extrahepatic metastases should not be the sole determinant of survival: controls, 10 months; hepatic artery embolization, 10.2 months; and 5-FU + DSM, 23.6 months.

Morbidity related to the insertion of the arterial cannula was restricted to one wound infection and one deep venous thrombosis. All patients developed nausea during treatment sessions immediately after the administration of DSM. This was short-lived, lasting only 30 to 60 min. Occasional pain or discomfort was also experienced, but this was also of similar duration. Importantly, there were no systemic side effects, such as alopecia or hematological toxicities.

V. CONCLUSION

Although continuous regional infusion of cytotoxic agents has improved response rates, there is a clear and continuing need for improved regional treatment of liver metastases from colorectal cancer. Theoretical considerations and experimental data from animal models (Table 3) suggest a possible role for DSM in conjunction with cytotoxic agents. Clinical evaluation of this modality has demonstrated only relatively modest antitumor activity. However, it should be recalled that the use of DSM in admixture with cytotoxic drugs alters drug disposition to a comparatively small extent. For example, in the phase II study described herein,[108] the reduction in systemic exposure to mitomycin C attributable to DSM was approximately 30%, therefore, the increase in liver exposure would be expected to be no more than this. In the phase III study with 5-FU the change in drug disposition at a DSM dose of 5 to 15 mg/kg was not measured. However, it is unlikely to be substantial because in a rat model it was found that as much as 100 mg/kg of DSM was required for only a 50% increase in liver exposure to 5-FU that lasted for 10 min[82] (see also Table 3).

The large doses of DSM required to induce modest changes in disposition of admixed drug, and therefore response, are in contrast to the preliminary clinical data described in Chapter 3 involving the use of microspheres in which active agents are incorporated within the matrix. Consequently, these latter systems appear worthy of further clinical evaluation.

REFERENCES

1. **American Cancer Society,** *Cancer Facts and Figures — 1991,* American Cancer Society, Atlanta, 1991, 1.
2. **Wagner, J. S., Adson, M. A., Van Heerden, J. A., Adson, M. H., and Ilstrup, D. M.,** The natural history of hepatic metastases from colorectal cancer, *Ann. Surg.,* 199, 502, 1984.
3. Registry of Hepatic Metastases, Resection of the liver for colorectal carcinoma metastases: a multi-institutional study of patterns of recurrence, *Surgery,* 100, 278, 1986.
4. **Doci, R., Gennari, L., Bignami, P., Montalto, F., Morabito, A., and Bozzetti, F.,** One hundred patients with hepatic metastases from colorectal cancer treated by resection: analysis of prognostic determinants, *Br. J. Surg.,* 78, 797, 1991.

5. **Welch, J. P. and Donaldson, G. A.,** Detection and treatment of recurrent cancer of the colon and rectum, *Am. J. Surg.,* 135, 505, 1978.

6. **Olsen, R. M., Perencevich, N. P., Malcolm, A. W., Chaffey, J. T., and Wilson, R. E.,** Patterns of recurrence following curative resection of adenocarcinoma of the colon and rectum, *Cancer,* 45, 2969, 1980.

7. **Willet, C. G., Tepper, J. E., Cohen, A. M., Orlow, E., and Welch, C. E.,** Failure patterns following curative resection of colonic carcinoma, *Ann. Surg.,* 200, 685, 1984.

8. **Adson, M. A.,** Diagnosis and surgical treatment of primary and secondary solid hepatic tumors in the adult, *Surg. Clin. North Am.,* 61, 181, 1981.

9. **Steele, G. Jr. and Ravikumar, T. S.,** Resection of hepatic metastases from colorectal cancer, *Ann. Surg.,* 210, 127, 1989.

10. **Saenz, N. C., Cady, B., McDermott W. V. Jr., and Steele G. D. Jr.,** Liver surgery: experience with colorectal cancer metastatic to the liver, *Surg. Clin. North Am.,* 69, 361, 1989.

11. **Lahr, C. J., Soong, S., Cloud, G., Smith, J. W., Urist, M. M., and Balch, C. M.,** A multifactorial analysis of prognostic factors in patients with liver metastases from colorectal carcinoma, *J. Clin. Oncol.,* 1, 720, 1983.

12. **Bengmark, S.,** Palliative treatment of hepatic tumors, *Br. J. Surg.,* 76, 771, 1989.

13. **Machi, J., Isomoto, H., Kurohiji, T., Yamashita, Y., Shirouzu, K., Kakegawa, T., Sigel, B., Zaren, H., and Sariego, J.,** Accuracy of intraoperative ultrasonography in diagnosing liver metastasis from colorectal cancer: evaluation with postoperative follow up results, *World J. Surg.,* 15, 551 1991.

14. **Olsen, A. K.,** Intraoperative ultrasonography and the detection of liver metastases in patients with colorectal cancer, *Br. J. Surg.,* 77, 998, 1990.

15. **Stadler, J., Holscher, A. H., and Adolf, J.,** Intraoperative ultrasonographic detection of occult liver metastases in colorectal cancer, *Surg. Endosc.,* 5, 33, 1991.

16. **Yoshida, T., Matsue, H., Suzuki, M., Okazaki, N., Yoshino, M., Moriya, Y., and Hojo, K.,** Preoperative ultrasonography screening for liver metastases of patients with colorectal cancer, *Jpn. J. Clin. Oncol.,* 19, 112, 1989.

17. **Russo, A., Sparicino, G., Plaja, S., Cajozzo, M., La Rosa, C., Demma, A., and Bazan, P.,** Role of intraoperative ultrasound in the screening of liver metastases from colorectal carcinoma: initial experience, *J. Surg. Oncol.,* 42, 249, 1989.

18. **Thomas, W. M., Morris, D. L., and Hardcastle, J. D.,** Contact ultrasonography in the detection of liver metastases from colorectal cancer: an *in vitro* study, *Br. J. Surg.,* 74, 955, 1987.

19. **Boutkan, H., Meijer, S., Cuesta, M. A., Prevoo, W., Luth, W. J., and Van Heuzen, E. P.,** Intra-operative ultrasonography of the liver: a prerequisite for surgery of colorectal cancer, *Neth. J. Surg.,* 43, 89, 1991.

20. **Griffin, T. W., Brill, A. B., Stevens, S., Collins, J. A., Bokhari, F., Bushe, H., Stochl, M. C., Gionet, M., Rusckowski, M., Stroupe, S. D., Kiefer, H. C., Sumerdon, G. A., Johnson, D. K., and Hnatowich, D. J.,** Initial clinical study of Indium-111-labelled clone 110 anticarcinoembryonic antigen antibody in patients with colorectal cancer, *J. Clin. Oncol.,* 9, 631, 1991.

21. **Patt, Y. Z., Lamki, L. M., Shanken, J., Jessop, J. M., Charnsangavej, C., Ajani, J. A., Levin, B., Merchant, B., Halverson, C., and Muray, J. L.,** Imaging with Indium[111]-labelled anticarcinoembryonic antigen monoclonal antibody ZCE-025 of recurrent colorectal or carcinoembryonic antigen-producing cancer in patients with rising serum carcinoembryonic antigen levels and occult metastases, *J. Clin. Oncol.,* 8, 1246, 1990.

22. **Gasparini, M., Ripamonti, M., Seregni, E., Regalia, E., and Buraggi, G. L.,** Tumor imaging of colorectal carcinoma with an anti-CEA monoclonal antibody, *Int. J. Cancer Suppl.,* 2, 81, 1988.

23. **Colcher, D., Zalutsky, M., Kaplan, W., Kufe, D., Austin, F., and Schlom, J.,** Radiolocalization of human mammary tumors in athymic mice by a monoclonal antibody, *Cancer Res.,* 43, 736, 1983.

24. **Nieroda, C. A., Mojzisik, C., Sardi, A., Ferrara, P. J., Hinkle, G., Thurston, M. O., and Martin, E. W.,** Radioimmunoguided surgery in primary colon cancer, *Cancer Detect. Prev.,* 14, 651, 1990.

25. **Nieroda, C. A., Mojzisik, C., Hinkle, G., Thurston, M. O., and Martin, E. W.,** Radioimmunoguided surgery (RIGS) in recurrent colorectal cancer, *Cancer Detect. Prev.,* 15, 225, 1991.

26. **Martin, E. W. Jr. and Carey, L. C.,** Second look surgery for colorectal cancer: the second time around, *Ann. Surg.,* 214, 321, 1991.

27. **Sickle-Santanello, B. J., O'Dwyer, P. J., Mojzisik, C., Tuttle, S. E., Hinkle, G. H., Rousseau, M., Schlom, J., Colcher, D., Thurston, M. O., Nieroda, C., Sardi, A., Farrar, W. B., Minton, J. P., and Martin, E. W.,** Radioimmunoguided surgery using the monoclonal antibody B72.3 in colorectal tumors, *Dis. Colon Rectum,* 30, 761, 1987.

28. **Dawson, P. M., Blair, S. D., Begent, R. H. J., Kelly, A. M. B., Boxer, G. M., and Theodorou, N. A.,** The value of radioimmunological surgery in first and second look laparotomy for colorectal cancer, *Dis. Colon Rectum,* 34, 217, 1991.

29. **Herrera-Ornelas, L., Justiniano, J., Castillo, N., Petrelli, N. J., Stulc, J. P., and Mittelman, A.,** Metastases in small lymph nodes in cancer, *Arch. Surg.,* 122, 1253, 1987.

30. **Rosemurgy, A. S. and Block, G. E.,** Surgical treatment of carcinoma of the abdominal colon, *Surg. Gynecol. Obstet.,* 167, 399, 1988.

31. **Oredipe, O. A., Barth, R. F., Tuttle, S. E., Adams, D. M., Sautins, I., Bucci, D. M., Mojzisik, C. M., Hinkle, G. M., Jewell, S., and Steplewski, Z.,** Limits of sensitivity for the radioimmunodetection of colon cancer by means of a hand-held gamma probe, *Nucl. Med. Biol.,* 15, 595, 1988.

32. **Breedis, C. and Young, G.,** The blood supply of neoplasms in the liver, *Am. J. Pathol.,* 30, 369, 1954.

33. **Healy, J. E.,** Vascular patterns in human metastatic liver tumors, *Surg. Gynecol. Obstet.,* 120, 1187, 1965.

34. **Lien, W. M. and Ackerman, N. B.,** The blood supply of experimental liver metastases: II, a microcirculatory study of the normal and tumor vessels of the liver with the use of perfused silicone rubber, *Surgery,* 68, 334, 1970.

35. **Lin, B., Lunderquist, A., Hagerstrand, L., and Boijsen, E.,** Postmortem examination of the blood supply and vascular pattern of small liver metastases in man, *Surgery,* 96, 517, 1984.

36. **Blanchard, R. J. W., Grotenhuis, I., LaFave, J. W., and Perry, J. F.,** Blood supply to hepatic VX2 carcinoma implants as measured by radioactive microspheres, *Proc. Soc. Exp. Biol. Med.,* 118, 465, 1965.

37. **Ackerman, N. B., Lien, W. M., Kondi, E. B., and Silverman, N. A.,** The blood supply of experimental liver metastases: I, the distribution of hepatic artery and portal vein blood to "small" and "large" tumors, *Surgery,* 66, 1067, 1969.

38. **Suzuki, T., Sarumaru, S., Kawabe, K., and Honjo, I.,** Study of vascularity of tumors of the liver, *Surg. Gynecol. Obstet.,* 134, 27, 1972.

39. **Ackerman, N. B.,** Experimental studies on the role of the portal circulation in hepatic tumor vascularity, *Cancer,* 58, 1653, 1984.

40. **Ackerman, N. B.,** The blood supply of experimental liver metastases: IV, changes in vascularity with increasing tumor growth, *Surgery,* 75, 589, 1974.

41. **Conway, J. G., Popp, J. A., Sungchul, J., and Thurman, R. G.,** Effect of size on portal circulation of hepatic nodules from carcinogen-treated rats, *Cancer Res.,* 44, 3374, 1983.

42. **Archer, S. G. and Gray, S. N.,** Vascularization of small liver metastases, *B. J. Surg.,* 76, 545, 1989.

43. **Kaplan, W. D., Ensminger, W. D., Come, S. E., Smith, E. H., D'Orsi, C. J., Levin, D. C., Takvorian, R. W., and Steele, G. D. Jr.,** Radionuclide angiography to predict patient response to hepatic artery chemotherapy, *Cancer Treat. Rep.,* 64, 1217, 1980.

44. **Daly, J. M., Butler, J., Kemeny, N., Yeh, S. D. J., Ridge, J. A., Botet, J., Bading, J. R., DeCosse, J. J., and Benua, R. S.,** Predicting tumor response in patients with colorectal hepatic metastases, *Ann. Surg.,* 200, 384, 1985.

45. **Kemeny, N., Niedzwiecki, D., Shurgot, B., and Oderman, P.,** Prognostic variables in patients with hepatic metastases from colorectal cancer, *Cancer,* 63, 742, 1989.

46. **Ridge, J. A., Collin, C., Bading, J. R., Hancock, C., Conti, P. S., Daly, J. M., and Raaf, J. H.,** Increased adriamycin levels in hepatic implants of rabbit VX-2 carcinoma from regional infusion, *Cancer Res.,* 48, 4584, 1988.

47. **Archer, S. G. and Gray, B. N.,** Comparison of portal vein chemotherapy with hepatic artery chemotherapy in the treatment of liver micrometastases, *Am. J. Surg.,* 159, 325, 1990.

48. **Didolkar, M. S., Jackson, A. J., Covell, D. G., Walker, A. P., and Eddington, N. D.,** Influence of the routes of continuous intrahepatic infusion of 5-fluorouracil on its pharmacokinetics, *J. Surg. Oncol.,* 41, 187, 1989.

49. **Sigurdson, E. R., Ridge, J. A., and Daly, J. M.,** Fluorodeoxyuridine uptake by human colorectal metastases after hepatic artery infusion, *Surgery,* 100, 285, 1986.

50. **Ridge, J. A., Sigurdson, E. R., and Daly, J. M.,** Distribution of fluorodeoxyuridine uptake in the liver and colorectal hepatic metastases of human beings after arterial infusion, *Surg. Gynecol. Obstet.,* 164, 319, 1987.

51. **Kemeny, N., Daly, J. M., Reichman, B., Geller, N., Botet, J., and Oderman, P.,** Intrahepatic or systemic infusion of fluorodeoxyuridine in patients with liver metastases from colorectal carcinoma: a randomized trial, *Ann. Intern. Med.,* 107, 459, 1987.

52. **Daly, J. M., Kemeny, N., Sigurdson, E., Oderman, P., and Thom, A.,** Regional infusion for colorectal metastases: a randomized trial comparing the hepatic artery with the portal vein, *Arch. Surg.,* 122, 1273, 1987.

53. **Chang, A. E., Schneider, P. D., Sugarbaker, P. H., Simpson, C., Culnane, M., and Steinberg, S. M.,** A prospective randomized trial of regional versus systemic continuous 5-fluorodeoxyuridine chemotherapy in the treatment of colorectal metastases, *Ann. Surg.,* 206, 685, 1987.

54. **Clarkson, B., Young, C., Dierick, W., Kuehn, P., Kim, M., Berrett, A., Clapp, P., and Lawrence, W. Jr.,** Effects of continual hepatic artery infusion of antimetabolites on primary and metastatic cancer of the liver, *Cancer,* 15, 472, 1962.

55. **Narsete, T., Ansfield, F., Wirtanen, G., Ramirez, G., Walberg, W., and Jarret, F.,** Gastric ulceration in patients receiving intrahepatic infusion of 5-fluorouracil, *Ann. Surg.,* 186, 734, 1977.

56. **Patt, Y. Z., Mavligit, G. M., Chuang, V. P., Wallace, S., Johnston, S., Benjamin, R. S., Valdivieso, M., and Hersh, E. M.,** Percutaneous hepatic arterial infusion (HAI) of mitomycin C and floxuridine (FUDR): an effective treatment for metastatic colorectal carcinoma in the liver, *Cancer,* 46, 261, 1980.

57. **Reed, M. J., Vaitkevicius, V. K., Al-Sarraf, M., Vaughn, C. B., Singhakowinta, A., Sexon-Porte, M., Izbicki, R., Baker, L., and Straatsma, G. W.,** The practicality of chronic hepatic artery infusion therapy of primary and metastatic hepatic malignancies: ten year results of 124 patients in a prospective protocol, *Cancer,* 47, 402, 1981.

58. **Blackshear, P. J.,** Implantable drug delivery systems, *Sci. Am.,* 241, 66, 1979.

59. **Blackshear, P. J., Dorman, F. D., and Blackshear, P. J. Jr.,** The design and initial testing of an implantable infusion pump, *Surg. Gynecol. Obstet.,* 134, 51, 1972.

60. **Buchwald, H., Grage, T. B., Vassilopoulos, P. P., Röhde, T. D., Varco, R. L., and Blackshear, P. J.,** Intra-arterial infusion chemotherapy for hepatic carcinoma using a totally implantable infusion pump, *Cancer,* 45, 866, 1980.

61. **Balch, C. M., Urist, M. M., and McGregor, M. L.,** Continuous regional chemotherapy for metastatic colorectal cancer using a totally implantable infusion pump, *Am. J. Surg.,* 145, 285, 1983.

62. **Barone, R. M., Byfield, J. E., Goldfarb, P. B., Frankel, S., Ginn, C., and Greer, S.,** Intra-arterial chemotherapy using an implantable infusion pump and liver irradiation for treatment of hepatic metastases, *Cancer,* 50, 850, 1982.

63. **Cohen, A. M., Kaufman, S. D., Wood, W. C., and Greenfield, A. J.,** Regional hepatic chemotherapy using an implantable drug infusion pump, *Am. J. Surg.,* 145, 529, 1983.

64. **Ensminger, W., Niederhuber, J., Dakhil, S., Thrall, J., and Wheeler, R.,** Totally implanted drug delivery system for hepatic arterial chemotherapy, *Cancer Treat. Rep.,* 5, 394, 1981.

65. **Ensminger, W., Niederhuber, J., Gyves, J., Thrall, J., Cozzi, E., and Doan, K.,** Effective control of liver metastases from colon cancer with an implantable system for hepatic arterial chemotherapy, *Proc. Am. Soc. Clin. Oncol.,* 1, 94, 1982.
66. **Daly, J. M., Kemeny, N., Oderman, P., and Botet, J.,** Long-term hepatic arterial infusion chemotherapy, *Arch. Surg.,* 119, 936, 1984.
67. **Michels, N. A.,** *Blood Supply and Anatomy of Upper Abdominal Organs with Descriptive Atlas,* JB Lippincott, Philadelphia, 1955.
68. **Hohn, D. C., Stagg, R. J., Price, D. C., and Lewis, R. J.,** Avoidance of gastroduodenal toxicity in patients receiving hepatic arterial 5-fluoro-2′-deoxyuridine, *J. Clin. Oncol.,* 3, 1257, 1984.
69. **Arfors, K. E., Forsberg, J. O., Larssen, B., Lewis, D. H., Rosengren, B., and Odman, S.,** Temporary intestinal ischaemia induced by degradable microspheres, *Nature,* 262, 500, 1976.
70. **Lote, K.,** Hypoxic radioprotection by temporary intestinal ischaemia: degradable starch embolization in the cat, *Am. J. Roentgenol.,* 137, 909, 1981.
71. **Lindell, B., Aronsen, K., Nosslin, B., and Rothman, U.,** Studies in pharmacokinetics and tolerance of substances temporarily retained in the liver by microsphere embolization, *Ann. Surg.,* 187, 95, 1978.
72. **Lindberg, B., Lote, K., and Teder, H.,** Biodegradable starch microspheres: a new medical tool, in *Microspheres and Drug Therapy,* Davis, S. S., Illlum, L., McVie, J. G., and Tomlinson, E., Eds., Elsiever, Amsterdam, 1984, 153.
73. **Ball, A. B. S.,** Regional chemotherapy for colorectal hepatic metastases using degradable starch microspheres: a review, *Acta Oncol.,* 30, 309, 1991.
74. **Dakhil, S., Ensminger, W. D., Cho, K., Niederhuber, J., Doan, K., and Wheeler, R.,** Improved regional selectivity of hepatic arterial BCNU with degradable microspheres, *Cancer,* 50, 631, 1982.
75. **Starkhammar, H., Håkansson, L., Sjödahl, R., Svedberg, J., and Ekberg, S.,** Effect of portal blood flow and intra-arterially injected starch microspheres on the passage of a labeled tracer through the liver: an experimental study in pigs, *Acta Oncol.,* 26, 217, 1987.
76. **Civalleri, D., Rollandi, G., Simoni, G., Mallarini, G., Repotto, M., and Bonalumi, U.,** Redistribution of arterial blood flow in metastases-bearing livers after infusion of degradable starch microspheres, *Acta Chir. Scand.,* 151, 613, 1985.
77. **Civalleri, D., Scopinaro, G., Balletto, N., Claudiani, F., DeCian, F., Camerini, G., DePaoli, M., and Bonalumi, U.,** Changes in vascularity in liver tumors after hepatic arterial embolization with degradable starch microspheres, *Br. J. Surg.,* 76, 699, 1989.
78. **Starkhammar, H., Håkansson, L., Morales, O., and Svedberg, J.,** Intra-arterial mitomycin C treatment of unresectable tumors: preliminary results on the effect of degradable starch microspheres, *Acta Oncol.,* 26, 295, 1987.
79. **Sigurdson, E. R., Ridge, J. A., and Daly, J. M.,** Intra-arterial infusion of doxorubicin with degradable starch microspheres, *Arch. Surg.,* 121, 1277, 1986.
80. **El Hag, I. A., Teder, H., Roos, G., Christensson, P. I., and Stenram, U.,** Enhanced effect of adriamycin on a rat liver adenocarcinoma after hepatic artery injection with degradable starch microspheres, *Sel. Cancer Ther.,* 6, 23, 1990.
81. **Teder, H., Erichsen, C., Christensson, P. I., Jonsson, P.-E., and Stenram, U.,** 5-Fluorouracil incorporation into RNA of a rat liver adenocarcinoma after hepatic artery injection together with degradable starch microspheres, *Cancer Drug Delivery,* 4, 169, 1987.
82. **Teder, H., Aronsen, H. F., Björkman, S., Lindell, B., and Ljungsberg, J.,** The influence of degradable starch microspheres on liver uptake of 5-fluorouracil after hepatic artery injection in the rat, *J. Pharm. Pharmacol.,* 38, 939, 1986.
83. **Flowerdew, A. D. S., Richards, H. K., and Taylor, I.,** Temporary blood stasis with degradable starch microspheres (DSM) for liver metastases in a rat model, *Gut,* 28, 1201, 1987.
84. **Thom, A. K., Sigurdson, E. R., Bitar, M., and Daly, J. M.,** Regional hepatic arterial infusion of degradable starch microspheres increases fluorodeoxyuridine (FUdR) tumor uptake, *Surgery,* 105, 383, 1989.

85. **Civalleri, D., Esposito, M., Fulco, R. A., Vannozzi, M., Balletto, N., DeCian, F., Percivale, P. L., and Merlo, F.,** Liver and tumor uptake and plasma pharmacokinetics of arterial cisplatin administered with or without starch microspheres in patients with liver metastases, *Cancer,* 68, 988, 1991.

86. **Gyves, J. W., Ensminger, W. D., Van Harken, D., Niederhuber, J., Stetson, P., and Walker, S.,** Improved regional selectivity of hepatic arterial mitomycin by starch microspheres, *Clin. Pharmacol. Ther.,* 34, 259, 1983.

87. **Dakhil, S., Ensminger, W., Cho, K., Niederhuber, J., Doan, K., and Wheeler, R.,** Improved regional selectivity of hepatic arterial BCNU with degradable microspheres, *Cancer,* 50, 631, 1982.

88. **Starkhammar, H., Hakansson, L., Morales, O., and Svedberg, J.,** Effect of microspheres in intra-arterial chemotherapy: a study of arterio-venous shunting and passage of a labeled marker, *Med. Oncol. Tumor Pharmacother.,* 4, 87, 1987.

89. **Ziessman, H. A., Thrall, J. H., Ensminger, W. D., Niederhuber, J. E., Tuscan, M., and Walker, S.,** Quantitative hepatic arterial perfusion scintigraphy and starch microspheres in cancer chemotherapy, *J. Nucl. Med.,* 24, 871, 1983.

90. **Goldmann, E.,** Growth of malignant disease in man and the lower animals with special reference to vascular system, *Lancet,* 2, 1236, 1907.

91. **Warren, B. A.,** The vascular morphology of tumors, in *Tumor Blood Circulation,* Peterson, H.-I., Ed., CRC Press, Boca Raton, FL, 1979, 1.

92. **Day, E. D.,** Vascular relationships of tumor and host, *Prog. Exp. Tumor Res.,* 4, 57, 1964.

93. **Konerding, M. A., Steinberg, F., and Streffer, G.,** The vasculature of xenotransplanted human melanomas and sarcomas in nude mice: I, vascular corrosion casting studies, *Acta Anat.,* 136, 21, 1989.

94. **Konerding, M. A., Steinberg, F., and Streffer, G.,** The vasculature of xenotransplanted human melanomas and sarcomas in nude mice. II. Scanning and transmission electron microscopic studies, *Acta Anat.,* 136, 27, 1989.

95. **Konerding, M. A., Steinberg, F., and Budach, V.,** The vascular system of xenotransplanted tumors: scanning electron and light microscopic studies, *Scanning Electron Microsc.,* 3, 327, 1989.

96. **Solesvik, O. V., Rofstad, E. K., and Brustad, T.,** Vascular structure of five human melanomas grown in athymic nude mice, *Br. J. Cancer,* 46, 556, 1982.

97. **Vaupel, P. and Gabbert, H.,** Evidence for and against a tumor type-specific vascularity, *Strahlentherapie Onkol.,* 162, 633, 1986.

98. **Mattsson, J., Appelgren, L., Hamberger, B., and Peterson, H.-I.,** Adrenergic innervation of tumor blood vessels, *Cancer Lett.,* 3, 347, 1977.

99. **Mattsson, J., Appelgren, L., Hamberger, B., and Peterson, H.-I.,** Tumor vessel innervation and the influence of vasoactive drugs on tumor blood flow, in *Tumor Blood Circulation,* Peterson, H.-I., Ed., CRC Press, Boca Raton, FL, 1979, 129.

100. **Hafström, L., Nobin, A., Persson, B., and Sundqvist, K.,** Effects of catecholamines on cardiovascular response and blood flow distribution to normal tissue and liver tumors in rats, *Cancer Res.,* 40, 481, 1980.

101. **Hemingway, D. M., Cooke, T. G., Chang, D., Grime, S. J., and Jenkins, S. A.,** The effects of intra-arterial vasoconstrictors on the distribution of a radiolabeled low molecular weight marker in an experimental model of liver tumor, *Br. J. Cancer,* 63, 495, 1991.

102. **Andrews, J. C., Walker-Andrews, S. C., Juni, J. E., Warber, S., and Ensminger, W. D.,** Modulation of liver tumor blood flow with hepatic arterial epinephrine: a SPECT study, *Radiology,* 173, 645, 1989.

103. **Sasaki, Y., Imaoka, S., Hasegawa, Y., Nakano, S., Ishikawa, O., Ohigashi, H., Taniguchi, K., Koyama, H., Iwanaga, T., and Terasawa, T.,** Changes in distribution of hepatic blood flow induced by intra-arterial infusion of angiotensin II in human hepatic cancer, *Cancer,* 55, 311, 1985.

104. **Udhoji, V. N. and Weil, M. H.,** Circulatory effects of angiotensin, levarterenol, and metariminol in the treatment of shock, *N. Engl. J. Med.,* 270, 501, 1964.

105. **Richardson, P. D. and Withrington, P. G.,** Liver blood flow. I. Intrinsic and nervous control of liver blood flow, *Gastroenterology,* 81, 158, 1981.
106. **Richardson, P. D. I. and Withrington, P. D.,** The effects of intraportal injections of nor-adrenaline, adrenaline and angiotensin on the hepatic portal vascular bed of the dog: marked tachyphylaxis to angiotensin, *Br. J. Pharmacol.,* 59, 293, 1977.
107. **Ensminger, W. D., Gyves, J. W., Stetson, P., and Walker-Andrews, S.,** Phase I study of hepatic arterial degradable starch microspheres and mitomycin, *Cancer Res.,* 45, 4464, 1985.
108. **Wollner, I. S., Walker-Andrews, S. C., Smith, J. E., and Ensminger, W. D.,** Phase II study of hepatic arterial degradable starch microspheres and mitomycin, *Cancer Drug Delivery,* 3, 279, 1986.
109. **Hunt, T. M., Flowerdew, A. D. S., Birch, S. J., Williams, J. D., Mullee, M. A., and Taylor, I.,** Prospective randomized trial of hepatic arterial embolization of infusion chemotherapy with 5-fluorouracil and degradable starch microspheres for colorectal liver metastases, *Br. J. Surg.,* 77, 779, 1990.

Chapter 8

EVALUATION OF THE POTENTIAL OF MICROSPHERICAL SYSTEMS FOR REGIONAL THERAPY IN THE TUMOR-BEARING LIVER AND KIDNEY USING TECHNIQUES IN NUCLEAR MEDICINE

Jacqueline A. Goldberg, James H. McKillop, and Colin S. McArdle

TABLE OF CONTENTS

I. PRINCIPLES OF NUCLEAR MEDICINE

Nuclear medicine techniques use either radioisotopes of elements or radioisotopically labeled substances (radiopharmaceuticals). In diagnostic nuclear medicine both the level of radioactivity and the amount of radiopharmaceutical utilized are at such a low level that they do not have any discernible physiological or pharmacological effect. Nuclear medicine studies are based upon the tracer principle, which states that a radioactive substance or isotope behaves physiologically in an identical manner to a nonradioactive version of the same substance or element.[1]

In marked contrast to other imaging tests, nuclear medicine investigations evaluate function of the area studied rather than anatomy. When a radiopharmaceutical is injected, it will localize in a target organ as a result of some functional aspect of the organ. Thus, radioactive iodine is trapped by the thyroid using the physiological iodide trap. Technetium-99m (^{99m}Tc) can substitute for iodide in this trap and will thus be retained by the thyroid, although it will not be incorporated into the thyroid hormone synthetic pathway. Thallium-201 will substitute for potassium in the ATP-ase dependent sodium-potassium pump, which enables it to be used as a myocardial imaging agent. The ^{99m}Tc-iminodiacetic acid compounds are excreted by the liver by the same mechanism as bilirubin, which allows them to be used as biliary imaging agents.

Radiolabeled microspheres have long been used as markers for regional blood flow. This use depends on the injection of the microspheres into the feeding vessel of the area concerned in such a way that the microspheres are fully mixed with the blood flow. To ensure adequate mixing it is important that the injection avoids streaming and that there is adequate turbulence of blood flow.[2] The downstream distribution of the microspheres will then be proportional to relative regional blood flow. The size of the microspheres is such that they will physically impact in the first network of small blood vessels they encounter, and their distribution within the network will reflect relative regional blood flow.

The distribution of radiopharmaceuticals can be measured by obtaining tissue biopsies, which are then counted *in vitro*. This, however, is not usually a realistic proposition for clinical studies and some form of radiation detector is more often used to demonstrate distribution of activity in the patient. Early studies used non-imaging probes.[3] These were positioned over the organ of interest and the count rate from the organ was measured. By measuring counts on a number of occasions the turnover of the radiopharmaceutical could be measured. Studies of this nature are still occasionally performed in clinical practice, for example, in measuring thyroid radioiodine uptake or in probe renography.

Initial methods of radionuclide imaging utilized a probe that was moved over the organ of interest, with count rates being measured at a number of points.[4] In this way a map of distribution of the radiopharmaceutical was obtained. The probe was then connected to a motorized system, which moved it over the area being studied; this arrangement formed the basis of the rectilinear scanner.[1]

Rectilinear scanners have now been almost entirely replaced by the gamma camera. The gamma camera consists of a large radiation detector, in the form of

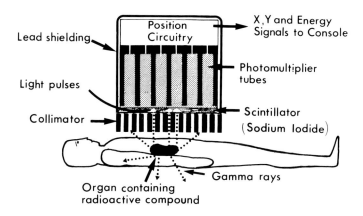

FIGURE 1. Schematic diagram of a gamma camera. Gamma rays are emitted from the organ containing the radiopharmaceutical. Only radiation traveling in the direction of the collimator passes through and reaches the scintillator. Radiation that reaches the scintillator gives rise to light pulses that are detected by the photomultiplier tubes and converted to an electrical signal. Because only rays traveling in a particular direction are allowed to reach the scintillator, the X and Y position signals generated by the position circuitry are a good indication of source of the gamma radiation. Thus, a map of the distribution of the radioactivity within the patient, i.e., a gamma camera image, may be constructed, (*Computer Techniques in Clinical Medicine*, Macfarlane, P. W., Ed., Heinemann-Butterworth, 1986. With permission.)

a sodium iodide scintillation crystal.[5] The scintillation crystal converts gamma rays emitted by the radiopharmaceutical into a light photon. The light photons are detected by photomultiplier tubes, which produce an electrical current. The electronic circuitry of the gamma camera then calculates the position of the incident gamma ray on the scintillation crystal. The distribution of the incident rays and their frequency are what constitutes the gamma camera image[1] This image reflects the distribution of tracer in the field of view and thus provides information on the organ function under study (Figure 1).

The radiopharmaceutical in the organ will emit radioactive photons randomly in all directions. If all these photons were allowed to strike the scintillation crystal, then it would not be possible to build up a map of distribution of the tracer because the origin of any photon striking the crystal could not be calculated. For this reason, the crystal has a collimator placed in front of it.[1] This consists of a lead sheet with many holes bored in it. Typically, these holes are parallel to one another, although other arrangements are also used in special circumstances. Only photons traveling in the direction of the holes will reach the crystal. Thus, in the case of parallel hole collimators oblique photons will be blocked and only those traveling at right angles to the crystal will be detected. This means that a reliable map of distribution of tracer in the patient can be constructed from events occurring in the scintillation crystal.

The maps of tracer distribution can be converted into images by photographing the camera oscilloscope, but increasingly the camera output is fed into a computer for later manipulation. Computer storage of the data is essential if quantitation of the data or image processing is to be undertaken. Even for routine studies that will

TABLE 1
Suitable Radionuclides for Use in Human
Radiolabeled Microsphere Studies

Radionuclide	Symbol	Principal gamma energies (keV)	Physical half-life
Technetium-99m	^{99m}Tc	140	6.0 h
Indium-111	^{111}In	173, 247	67.3 h
Indium 113m	^{113m}In	393	1.7 h
Iodine-123	^{123}I	159	13.2 h
Iodine-125	^{125}I	27.5, 35	60 days
Iodine-131	^{131}I	364	8.1 days

be analyzed visually, it is now generally accepted that a computer should be utilized to optimize image display.

II. RADIOLABELS FOR BIODEGRADABLE MICROSPHERES

For the purposes of diagnostic or research studies using microspheres a number of radiolabels are available. The most important of these radionuclides are listed in Table 1.

^{99m}Tc is widely used in nuclear medicine.[1,6] It has many advantages, including availability from a generator when required, gamma ray photons with a near-ideal energy for gamma camera detection, chemical properties that allow combination to many different substances (thus enabling it to be used for radiopharmaceuticals targeted on many different organs), and a relatively short half-life, which reduces radiation dose to the patient. ^{99m}Tc-labeled microspheres are ideal for studying the distribution of blood flow by gamma camera imaging. Because of their relatively short half-life they are not suitable for evaluating the long-term (i.e., more than 12 to 24 h) stability of microspheres *in vivo*.

Indium-111 (^{111}In) has complex metallic chemistry.[1,6] It emits gamma rays, which are somewhat above the ideal energy for gamma camera imaging, although reasonable images can still be obtained. It is not available from a generator and thus must be ordered specifically when required. The longer physical half-life results in an increased radiation dose to the patient for the same administered activity compared with ^{99m}Tc. The higher energy photons make ^{111}In suitable for use with ^{99m}Tc in dual-tracer studies, e.g., before and after an intervention, because the gamma camera or *in vitro* counter can be set up to discriminate between the different photon energies. The longer half-life makes ^{111}In a possible tracer for studying microsphere stability. Indium-113m (^{113m}In) has identical chemical properties to ^{111}In but a much shorter physical half-life. It is available from a generator and has photon energies sufficiently different from ^{99m}Tc to allow dual-tracer experiments.

Radioisotopes of iodine are widely used for radiolabeling of proteins.[1,6] None are available from a generator. Iodine-123 has near-ideal gamma rays for gamma camera detection and a relatively short half-life, thus reducing patient radiation dose. It is suitable for imaging microsphere distribution, but because of the similarity in photon energies it cannot be used with ^{99m}Tc in dual-tracer studies. The major disadvantage of ^{123}I relates to its lack of ready availability in many centers, the need to specifically order a tracer with a short half-life (and thus short shelf-life), and high cost. Iodine-125 (^{125}I) is widely used for *in vitro* studies, including radioimmunoassay. The low energy photons make ^{125}I completely unsuitable for gamma camera imaging or probe studies. It can be used, however, for studies involving tissue (or blood) sampling and *in vitro* counting. Because of radiation dosimetry, the activity administered to patients must be strictly controlled.

Iodine-131 (^{131}I) was the original radionuclide used clinically (for thyroid imaging). The high energy photons result in suboptimal gamma camera images. The long half-life and presence of β-emissions result in a substantial radiation dose, which limits the activity that can be administered. As a result ^{131}I is not now widely used for diagnostic nuclear medicine, although it does have an important therapeutic role, notably in thyroid disorders. ^{131}I is a suitable tracer to consider for dual-isotope studies with ^{99m}Tc and is valuable when studying longer-term stability of microspheres.

For all of the iodine tracers, it is important to remember that radionuclide which becomes detached from the microsphere, either because of leaching of the label or breakup of the microsphere, will concentrate in the thyroid. To protect the thyroid from an excessive radiation dose it is necessary to block uptake using either oral potassium iodide or potassium iodate. The duration of the blocking therapy will vary according to the particular radioisotope of iodine being used, the rate of breakup of the radiolabeled protein, and the administered activity.[7] For ^{99m}Tc, ^{111}In, and ^{113m}In, blockade is unnecessary.

A number of other tracers have been used for labeling microspheres,[1] but their use is much less common and beyond the scope of this chapter.

III. SINGLE PHOTON EMISSION COMPUTED TOMOGRAPHY

In planar gamma camera studies an image is obtained in a particular projection by placing the camera in the appropriate position in relation to the patient and maintaining that position throughout data acquisition. Thus, the image obtained will be a two-dimensional representation of the three-dimensional distribution of the tracer activity. The precise depth location of areas of activity cannot be measured precisely, although this can be overcome to some extent by obtaining more than one planar projection. In each projection, however, the activity of the area of interest will also be influenced by activity in adjacent areas or structures in front of or behind the target area. This can cause difficulties in visual analysis of images but is of particular importance when quantitation is being undertaken.

Nuclear medicine tomography offers a possible solution to these difficulties. In tomography the aim is to produce an image that contains information from a clearly identified (and usually thin) section or slice of the patient. Within the tomographic slice there is still two-dimensional representation of three-dimensional activity, but this is within a well-defined slice thickness and by analyzing sequential tomographic slices an approach to three-dimensional information is achieved.

Two nuclear medicine approaches to tomography are currently used in clinical practice. Positron emission tomography (PET) requires special facilities, notably a custom-built detection system and, preferably, an on site cyclotron. These requirements are expensive, both in terms of equipment and staffing, and PET facilities are therefore only available in a limited number of centers at present. The technique, however, is an exciting one because it allows the use of radiopharmaceuticals of biologically "relevant" elements, such as carbon, nitrogen, and oxygen, and enables accurate quantitation of tracer uptake. Because many of the tracers are short-lived, dynamic studies (e.g., before and after interventions) are possible. Further discussion of PET is beyond the scope of this book, but recent reviews are available.[8]

Single photon emission computed tomography (SPECT), by contrast, utilizes standard radiopharmaceuticals and equipment that are generally available. To produce tomographic information from a SPECT study images are acquired from a large number of projections over a wide range of angles. The information from these multiple projections is then integrated by computer programs to produce tomographic images. The process, which is analogous to that employed in CT scanning, is explained in more detail next.

SPECT studies are usually performed using a rotating gamma camera (Figure 2), although other forms of instrumentation can be utilized.[9-11] A single-headed rotating gamma camera is most often employed and such instruments are now available in most nuclear medicine imaging departments. This is rotated around the patient, usually over 360°, with stops at regular intervals for data acquisition. Typically, the stops occur at 3 to 6° intervals. The duration of acquisition per stop varies depending on the type of study but is usually of the order of 30 to 60 s. The statistical reliability of the study is increased by more prolonged data acquisition, but this has to be offset against the increased risk of patient movement with resultant image degradation. Recently, various multiple-headed gamma cameras have become available. Because they have the ability to acquire several projections simultaneously, it is possible to either increase the number of counts acquired or to cut the period of acquisition, or both.[12] The period of acquisition can also be reduced by acquiring data over less than 360° (e.g., 180°). Acquisition over 180° is advocated for Thallium-201 myocardial perfusion imaging by some workers but has significant shortcomings, especially when quantitation is envisaged.[13] For this reason 360° acquisition is generally recommended.

Another requirement for successful SPECT acquisition is that the distribution of the radiopharmaceutical should not change significantly during the acquisition time. In microsphere studies this has implications for the stability of the radiolabeling and of the microsphere integrity. In the reconstruction of SPECT images, two main approaches have been employed, namely, filtered back projection and iterative reconstruction.[11,13-16]

Filtered back projection is the more widely used. Back projection consists of reconstitution of the acquired data onto the reconstruction image plane, with an

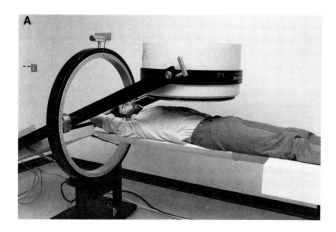

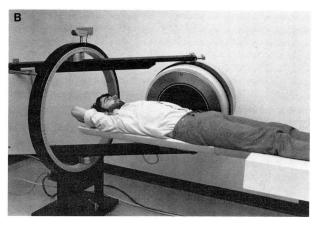

FIGURE 2 (A and B). Collection of data for a SPECT study. The gamma camera rotates around the patient, stopping at predetermined intervals to acquire an image. Data are usually obtained over a 180° or 360° arc. Some recently introduced gamma cameras speed up the acquisition of data by having multiple heads (usually 2 or 3), which acquire information simultaneously.

initial assumption that the original data were uniformly distributed throughout the object. When this is repeated for all angles, data are superimposed. The image, however, is blurred because each radioactive point in the section is reconstructed as a star-like structure with rays, which correspond to the back projection angles, although true activities will be accentuated by superimposition of data. The second step, filtering, is a mathematical process whereby the blurring of the data mentioned above and inconsistencies in the data are compensated. There are many filters available. Which is optimum depends upon the particular study being undertaken.[17]

Iterative reconstruction methods utilize repetitive back projections, starting with an initial estimate of the unknown activity distribution. Following each back projection the current estimate of the distribution of activities is compared with the measured projection data. The process is repeated until the differences between the calculated and observed data are reduced to a preselected level. Iterative techniques require much more powerful computing than filtered back projection and are often more time-consuming. The iterative methods are especially helpful when the data are incomplete or statistically noisy.

The quality of the reconstructed SPECT image is dependent on many factors, including the activity level within the organ of interest, the energy of the photons emitted, the resolution of the imaging system, the collimator used, and the reconstruction procedures employed. A detailed consideration of these factors is inappropriate in this chapter and the reader is referred to recent in-depth studies.[11,12,15,18-21]

Continued attention to quality control is essential for successful SPECT imaging[12,22,23] and should encompass the radiopharmaceuticals, the imaging equipment, and the computer hardware and software.

IV. TECHNIQUES FOR RADIOLABELING BIODEGRADABLE MICROSPHERE MATRIX COMPONENTS

Biodegradable microspheres have been used as both investigative and therapeutic agents in patients. Radiolabeled protein particles can be used to monitor arteriovenous shunting and tumor targeting. Starch[24,25] and albumin[26] microspheres have been used to improve the potential of regional chemotherapy. In this context, they can be admixed with cytotoxic drugs (Chapter 7) or used as vehicles for anticancer agents (Chapters 1, 4, and 5). Radiolabeling has been used to investigate the behavior of therapeutic microspheres *in vivo*. The rate of breakdown of particles in tumor and normal tissue and the effect of large doses of microspheres on arteriovenous shunting have been of particular interest with the advent of regional cytotoxic therapy.

A number of different techniques have been described for radiolabeling microspheres. Protein microspheres can be labeled after manufacture, such as with the commercially available kits for obtaining ^{99m}Tc-labeled albumin microspheres (TDK-5, Sorin Biomedica SpA, Vercelli, Italy). The Chloramine-T method described by Hunter and Greenwood[27] has been used to postlabel previously manufactured albumin microspheres with ^{131}I for use in tumor targeting studies.[28]

Both of the aforedescribed methods use postlabeling of preformed protein microspheres; consequently, radiolabel may be distributed primarily on the outer surface. To study biodegradation rate of microspheres *in vivo,* it is important for the radiolabel to be evenly distributed throughout the particle, rather than forming an outer shell. In this way, activity changes with time, detected by sequential gamma camera imaging of a target organ reflect the rate of degradation of the particles rather than loss of only the outer radiolabeled shell. Microspheres of this type are made by using radiolabeled protein in their synthesis.

^{111}In and ^{131}I have been compared for this purpose. ^{111}In was chelated to albumin using the technique of Paik et al.[29] or Hnatowich et al.[30] Both methods involve the use of the anhydride of the chelating agent cDTPA (cDTPAA), but the latter requires the use of chloroform as a solvent for cDTPAA, which is then evaporated prior to coupling cDPTAA to protein. In the former technique dimethyl sulfoxide is used without an evaporation step. In our hands, the former method was more straightforward and less likely to result in reduced labeling efficiency.[31]

Microspheres are then manufactured by stabilization with glutaraldehyde of a water-in-oil emulsion containing either [111]In- or ^{131}I-albumin using techniques developed by our group.[32] It was found that ^{111}In-labeled albumin microspheres were inadequate for biodegradation studies because of leaching of radiolabel in plasma. On the contrary, ^{131}I-labeled albumin microspheres retained virtually 100% of radiolabel over a period of weeks. On this basis the latter system was chosen for clinical studies. To perform this work the standard technique of microsphere manufacture[32] was adapted for use under sterile conditions and to produce larger batches incorporating adequate activity for imaging purposes[31] (0.8 to 8.7 MBq per patient in the following studies).

Examples of the uses of radiolabeled biodegradable albumin microspheres in defining tumor vascularity are given next.

V. MICROSPHERE FATE AFTER REGIONAL ADMINISTRATION

A. ARTERIOVENOUS SHUNTING

The configuration of tumor vasculature became particularly important with the advent of regional anticancer treatment. There are two levels at which the tumor blood supply can be evaluated:

1. The vessel from which tumors within a particular organ derive their blood supply (and by implication, the vessel that is of greatest value for access to the tumor during regional therapy)
2. The local vascular patterns in and around the tumor, and the functional implications of arteriovenous connections

The work of Breedis and Young in the late 1940s and 1950s demonstrated that liver tumors gained their blood supply almost exclusively from the hepatic artery.[33] They used an anatomically based method of vessel injection with contrast media. More recent work by Ridge et al.[34] confirmed this finding using functional methods, which demonstrated that uptake by tumor of radiolabeled nutritional compounds administered via the hepatic artery was more than twice that recorded after similar perfusion of the portal vein.

Angiography was used by Bierman et al.[35,36] to investigate vascular patterns in the vicinity of tumors in patients with liver cancer. Their finding of rapid blood flow through large blood vessels adjacent to hepatic metastases led to the hypothesis that connections, or shunts, existed between the arterial and systemic venous sides of the tumor circulation.

If significant arteriovenous shunts (AVS) were to occur in patients with intrahepatic tumors, arterially administered substances would bypass the microvasculature of the tumor-bearing organ and enter the systemic circulation directly. Not only would this phenomenon cause a reduction in the regional advantage of intra-arterial drug administration, but it could also increase systemic or, in the case of microsphere bound therapy, pulmonary toxicity.

The phenomenon of AVS has been investigated using arterially administered radiolabeled microparticles in patients with intrahepatic tumor. Particles with a diameter of approximately 40 μm should embolize at an arteriolar level within the tumor-bearing target organ when injected arterially. However, in the presence of arteriovenous connections a proportion of the injectate would travel to the lungs with the venous return and impact throughout the pulmonary vascular tree. The use of radiolabeled particles allows their entrapment to be monitored within the target organ and lung fields. The proportion of radioactive particles shunting to the lungs, relative to that retained in the target organ, provides an indication of shunt magnitude.

Particle labeling with gamma emitting isotopes allows activity in the upper abdomen and thorax to be monitored by gamma camera. Technetium is the most convenient isotope for use in patients because it has a short half-life and is widely available.[37,38]

In many studies of arteriovenous shunting, biodegradable macroaggregates of albumin were used, in which the particle size ranged from 10 to 90 μm. With this technique ^{99m}Tc-macroaggregated albumin was infused via a hepatic arterial catheter, followed by a flush of saline. Posterior gamma camera images of the liver and thorax were acquired, and the percentage ratio of lung activity to the summation of liver and lung activity from these two images was defined as the percent shunt index:

$$\text{Percent shunt index} = \frac{\text{Activity in lungs}}{\text{Activity in liver} + \text{Activity in lungs}} \tag{1}$$

Shunt levels greater than 30% were reported after injection of a tracer dose of particles in patients with hepatic metastases in one series.[38,39] However, criticism was leveled at their technique. Failure to subtract background levels of radiation and blood pool activity from the thoracic scan could have caused gross overestimation of AVS. When comparing the relatively low activity level within the thorax with the high level of activity within the liver after regional administration of radioactive microspheres, it is important to subtract background levels of radiation from both thoracic and abdominal scans so that the relative thoracic activity is not greatly overestimated.

After an arterial injection of radiolabeled microspheres for shunt assessment, the radioactivity should only be detected within the target organ and the lung fields. If activity is found within the blood pool (heart and great vessels), then the integrity of the radiopharmaceutical is brought into question. Such a finding would suggest either that some of the isotope had dissociated from the particle or that the smallest particles had failed to be trapped by lung capillaries. Both factors would lead to overestimation of arteriovenous shunting. The presence of activity within abdominal organs other than the target organ would suggest either that the target organ artery had patent branches or that flow phenomena were responsible for retrograde flow of injectate.

A different technique was used by Starkhammar et al.[40] to evaluate AVS in the clinical setting. They devised a system for measuring AVS and regional advantage during the treatment of intrahepatic tumor by the intra-arterial chemotherapeutic agent mitomycin C, mixed with embolizing biodegradable starch microspheres (Spherex,® Pharmacia, Sweden). The rationale for this type of treatment was that hepatic arterial blood flow would be temporarily arrested by the microspheres, thereby trapping the coadministered cytotoxic within the target organ. Pilot studies had shown that the tolerated dose of particles varied widely, both between patients and for the same patient, during subsequent therapeutic sessions. Variation in microsphere dosage was thought to depend upon several factors, including the size of the liver, vascularity of the tumors, and the magnitude of AVS. This dynamic system enabled estimation of the dosage of microspheres required for the arrest of hepatic arterial flow.[40] This was necessary because of the observation that when the optimal dose of particles was exceeded, the backflow of injectate into the gastroduodenal tissues led to side effects.

The methods of Starkhammar et al.[40] consisted of continuously monitoring the escape from the liver of a soluble arterially administered radiolabeled marker substance, ^{99m}Tc-methylene diphosphonate (^{99m}Tc-MDP), mixed with microspheres and cytotoxic drug. ^{99m}Tc-MDP was chosen because of its similarity to many low molecular weight cytotoxic drugs, being nonionic, diffusible, and not actively taken up by the liver. The monitoring system comprised a 50×50 mm sodium iodide detector with a straight bore collimator, which was positioned over the clavicular area of the subject. The system was assembled to enable the continuous recording of activity in the lung apex onto a dedicated computer. Corrections were made for radioactive decay and the time lag between injection and the appearance of activity at the apex of the lung.

Before administering therapy, a reference dose of 20 to 40 MBq ^{99m}Tc-MDP was given alone for calibration purposes, with the net increase in counts per second representing 100% passage of the marker substance. During a treatment session, three repeated injections of admixed ^{99m}Tc-MDP, starch microspheres (300 mg), and cytotoxic drug were given, with the increase in recorded counts per second after each injection (corrected for the dose of activity given) being expressed as a percentage of the reference value and termed the passing fraction.

The change in AVS with starch microsphere administration was studied by recording the passage of ^{99m}Tc-macroaggregated albumin through the liver into the apex of the lung. Two estimates were made, one before the first and one after the last of the injections of mixed microspheres and cytotoxic agent. Intra-arterial boluses of particles, (90% between 20 to 70 μm, average 45 μm) were administered. A major limitation of this technique was that arbitrary units were used to express the relative change in AVS after microsphere administration.

Nevertheless, Starkhammar et al.[40] found that although passing fraction was significantly reduced by repeatedly coadministering microspheres (representing increased retention of ''cytotoxic drug'' by the target organ), the effect was associated with an increase in AVS levels in 15 of 19 patients.[41] Other groups have confirmed the finding of increasing AVS in association with administration of microspheres using a similar technique,[42-44] although others have not found this to be the case.[45]

To some extent, Starkhammar et al.[40] were able to relate their arbitrary shunt units to the baseline percent shunt index described by Kaplan et al.[37] In a small number of patients, the clavicular detector was used to relate the shunting to lung after a hepatic arterial injection of radiolabeled macroaggregated albumin, to that of an intravenous injection of the same radiopharmaceutical (representing a 100% shunt). Their "estimated percent shunt index" (the ratio of lung activity after intra-arterial to that following intravenous injection) in their study of 10 patients ranged from 1.0 to 12.8% at baseline (median = 4.1%, mean = 5.4%).[41]

In contrast to the aforementioned studies, in which macroaggregated albumin was used, recent data of absolute values of AVS (at baseline and during the administration of therapeutic quantities of microspheres) have been acquired using radiolabeled microspheres. These data suggest that shunting may be much less of a problem than was previously thought with regard to reducing the regional advantage of arterial therapy.

In their first study of baseline shunting, Goldberg et al.[46] used ^{99m}Tc-albumin microspheres (TDK-5, Sorin Biomedica) instead of macroaggregated albumin to perform hepatic arterial perfusion scintigraphy (HAPS). The radiolabeled microspheres were of a size comparable with both therapeutic degradable starch and albumin microspheres (mean diameter 40 ± 5 μm and between 20 to 40 μm, respectively). In addition, the effect of the vasoactive agent angiotensin II on baseline AVS was evaluated. This drug had been shown to alter the hemodynamics of intrahepatic tumors by Sasaki et al.,[47] and it was proposed as a potential mechanism for targeting regional therapy to tumors within the liver. Sasaki et al.[47] demonstrated that an arterial infusion of angiotensin II in patients with liver cancer resulted in a transient reduction in arterial perfusion of liver parenchyma but greatly increased perfusion of the tumors. It was hypothesized that this mechanism might be of clinical value in improving the selectivity and, hence, the potency of regional therapy. It was therefore important to establish that angiotensin II did not also increase AVS.

The methods used for quantitative assessment of AVS were based on those of Kaplan et al.[37] and Zeissman et al.[38] The activity in the thorax (less that of the blood pool) was expressed as a percentage of the sum of activities in thorax and liver after infusion of radiolabeled microspheres into the hepatic artery (Equation 1). However, for this method to achieve accuracy, three conditions were considered necessary:

1. Low background activity
2. Efficient binding of radiolabel to the particle, so that the presence of activity within the lung fields would accurately represent the presence of trapped particles and not circulating unbound activity
3. Efficient delivery of large numbers of radiolabeled particles to the target organ with minimal extrahepatic perfusion

It was found, however, that a number of errors could be inadvertently introduced leading to a gross overestimate of AVS. The small proportion of unbound activity in the radiopharmaceutical (approximately 5%) achieved great significance when the number of radioactive microspheres in the liver was low. This circumstance occurred because there was an unexpectedly high affinity of protein microspheres (and the bound activity) for the plastic injection equipment. This in turn resulted in a significant reduction in the proportion of microsphere-bound activity reaching the target organ and a corresponding increase in the proportion of unbound activity in the injectate. This factor prevented condition 2 from being fulfilled and resulted in high levels of circulating "free" radioactivity being detected in the lung fields (hence a relatively high numerator for the shunt equation), with low particle-bound activity in the liver (hence a relatively low denominator in the shunt equation). The presence of a high level of extrahepatic flow in some studies had similar consequences.

The distribution of microsphere-bound activity to spleen or upper gastrointestinal tract resulted in the small proportion of unbound radioactivity in the lung fields reaching even greater significance in the shunt equation due to a concomitant reduction in microsphere-bound activity within the liver. If measured, however, the proportion of microsphere-bound activity reaching the liver (which is dependent upon the proportion of the dispensed radiopharmaceutical injected and extrahepatic flow) could be adjusted for mathematically, leading to a corrected AVS value. "Measured" values of AVS using this technique were as high as 18%. However, once these factors had been accounted for mathematically, the corrected baseline AVS was negligible.[46] The effect of angiotensin II on AVS was to cause a minimal increase (Figure 3, Table 2).

In an attempt to improve the accuracy of measurement of AVS and to investigate the effect of therapeutic quantities of microspheres on shunting, a second study was performed. Baseline shunting was measured as in the previous study, only under more ideal conditions of administration. In addition, the shunted fraction of a "therapeutic quantity" of microspheres was assessed on a separate occasion in the same patients using albumin microspheres labeled with [131]I. In the initial scan a tracer dose of surface-labeled ^{99m}Tc-albumin microspheres was used. Careful attention was paid to preparation and handling, and glass, rather than plastic, injection equipment was used during the study to reduce the relative amount of circulating free pertechnetate. Values of baseline AVS were again found to be consistently low, with only an exceptional value as high as 6% and 5 of 7 values less than 1.5% (Table 3). To assess the possibility that free pertechnetate had been unusually high in the dose of the study yielding a result of 6%, a region over the sternum was defined that would be expected to contain a quantity of blood pool activity. Repeating the shunt calculation in this study after subtracting the blood pool activity gave a shunt percentage of 3.2%.[48]

On a separate occasion, a much larger quantity of particles was administered via the hepatic artery catheter to the same group of patients. The microsphere dosage was comparable with that used in the therapeutic setting. The number of particles used had been found to be near the limit of tolerance in separate studies for coad-

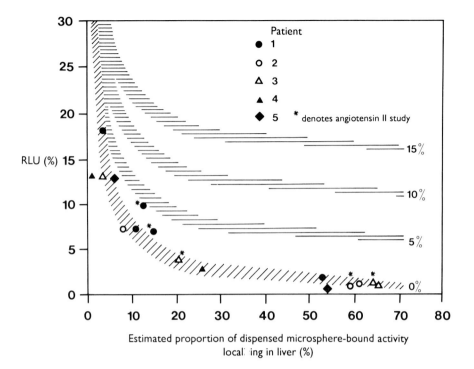

FIGURE 3. Hepatic arterial perfusion scintigraphy using ^{99m}Tc-labeled albumin microspheres to estimate arteriovenous shunting. The proportion of the dispensed dose of radiopharmaceutical reaching the liver as microsphere-bound activity is plotted on the x-axis. The ratio of activity in the thorax to the sum of thoracic and hepatic activity (RLU) is recorded on the y-axis. Mathematically derived theoretical error regions for 0 (oblique shading), 5, 10, and 15% (horizontal shading) arteriovenous shunting are shown. Data points are shown for 16 studies in five patients. Angiotensin II studies are indicated. (From Goldberg et al., *Nucl. Med. Commun.*, 8, 1033, 1987. With permission.)

ministered chemotherapy and biodegradable microspheres (4 to 8 × 10⁷ [= 200 to 400 mg]).[49] The radiopharmaceutical was custom-designed especially for the study of AVS. The requirements were for sterile radioactive microspheres (diameter 20 to 40 μm), which were biocompatible, could be imaged by gamma camera, made in batches containing between 4 and 8 × 10⁷ particles, and from which the activity would not leach.

[131]I-labeled albumin microspheres were made for this study by a technique based on glutaraldehyde stabilization of a water-in-oil emulsion.[50] The radiopharmaceutical had a high technical specification, being stable in air, phosphate-buffered saline, and plasma. The isotope ^{131}I was covalently bound to the protein and distributed evenly throughout the matrix of the microspheres, resulting in minimal leaching of free radioactivity.

In this study, baseline shunt of ^{99m}Tc-labeled microspheres (5 × 10⁵) was 2.2 ± 1.8% (mean ± SD, n = 7); the percentage shunt after injection of a therapeutic quantity (4 to 8 × 10⁷) of microspheres was 3.0 ± 0.8% (Table 3). Although the

TABLE 2
The Measured and Corrected[a] Shunt Levels, Activity, and Extrahepatic Flow in Studies of Three Patients, with or without Angiotensin II

Patient no.	Without angiotensin II			With angiotensin II		
	Activity injected (MBq)	Measured shunt (%)	Corrected shunt (%)	Activity injected (MBq)	Measured shunt (%)	Corrected shunt (%)
1	58	1.8	0	74	10.0[b]	4
	31	7.4	0	57	6.9[c]	1
2	66	1.3	0	64	0.9	0
3	70	1.2	0	69	1.4	0

[a] "Corrected" shunt values indicate the true magnitude of arteriovenous shunting, once the proportion of particle-bound activity and extrahepatic flow has been taken into account. The mathematical basis for the correction is described elsewhere.[46]

[b] More than 80% extrahepatic flow occurred during this study.

[c] Repeat study on patient 1: extrahepatic flow was 69% on the second occasion.

From Goldberg, J. A., Bradnam, M. S., Kerr, D. J., Haughton, D. M., McKillop, J. H., Bessent, R. G., Willmott, N., and McArdle, C. S., *Nucl. Med. Commun.*, 8, 1033, 1987. With permission.

TABLE 3
Arteriovenous Shunt in Seven Patients with Advanced Liver Metastases: Estimation after a Tracer Dose (Baseline) or Therapeutic Dose of Radiolabeled Microspheres

Patient no.	Baseline shunt (%) (5×10^5 microspheres)	Therapeutic dose shunted (%) (4 to 8×10^7 microspheres)
1	1.2	2.4
2	6.0	3.8
3	1.4	3.6
4	1.3	2.6
5	1.1	2.8
6	3.1	4.1
7	1.2	1.8

From Goldberg, J. A., Thomson, J. A. K., McCurrach, G., Anderson, J. H., Willmott, N., Bessent, R. G., McKillop, J. H., and McArdle, C. S., *Br. J. Cancer*, 63, 466, 1991. With permission.

number of patients was small, these studies demonstrate the low risk of clinically significant AVS at baseline and that the vasoactive drug angiotensin II or therapeutic doses of microspheres would be unlikely to increase AVS during regional therapy.[48]

Arteriovenous shunting is a phenomenon with the potential to significantly reduce the regional advantage of hepatic arterial therapeutic techniques and increase systemic or pulmonary toxicity. Although there is little support for the presence of large functional AVS at baseline in most patients with intrahepatic tumor, there is evidence from some centers that AVS may become a significant problem when microspheres are given in therapeutic quantities. Although this has not been a universal finding, it is recommended that AVS be monitored, using suitable radio-labeled microspheres, in patients who are to receive therapeutic quantities of microspheres regionally.

B. MICROSPHERE BIODISTRIBUTION AND DEGRADATION EVALUATED BY WHOLE BODY IMAGING AND BIOPSY

The biodistribution and handling of therapeutic microspheres is of great importance when considering regional therapy using drug-loaded particles. Early in the development of arterial drug administration, it became apparent that the ability to target cytotoxic substances preferentially to neoplasms within the tumor-bearing organ might enhance efficacy. Furthermore, by encapsulating the anticancer agent into particles of an appropriate size, regionally administered cytotoxics might become trapped within the tumor tissue, to be released in high concentration in the vicinity of cancer cells. This strategy, it was hoped, would greatly improve tumor exposure to therapeutic agents without causing unacceptably high systemic side effects.[51] Clearly, techniques for improving tumor targeting merited further investigation, and more data were required detailing the subsequent *in vivo* breakdown of embolized drug-loaded particles.

Radioisotopes have been widely used to evaluate the arterial perfusion of tumors and the biodistribution of microparticles administered via the arterial route. Much of the recent work examining the arterial perfusion and delivery of microspheres to tumors has taken place as part of studies attempting to manipulate blood flow and microsphere distribution to therapeutic advantage by the use of vasoactive drugs.

The first clear evidence that human tumor blood vessels responded differently from normal vessels when exposed to certain pharmacological agents was provided by Abrams in 1964,[52] who observed that intra-arterial epinephrine caused cessation of blood flow through normal tissue but that dense opacification of tumor vasculature occurred during selective renal angiography in a patient with hypernephroma. Abrams[52] suggested that such a phenomenon might have therapeutic implications for the selective chemotherapeutic perfusion of the tumor. Subsequent work with animal models demonstrated that other substances, such as bradykinin, noradrenaline, and angiotensin II, could similarly alter arterial perfusion of experimental tumors[53,54] and that the mechanism of action was largely due to a lack of autoregulation associated with tumor neovasculature.[55] The apparent increase in tumor perfusion under the influence of vasoactive drugs was shown by Hafstrom et al.[56] to be due to vasoconstriction in the surrounding normal blood vessels, causing diversion of arterial blood flow from normal tissue to tumor.

In an elegant study by a group working in Osaka, Japan, the magnitude and nature of the change in tumor blood flow by an arterial infusion of angiotensin II was studied in a group of patients with liver cancer.[47] The technique used to make these observations involved the infusion of a very short half-life radioisotope (^{81m}Kr, half-life 13 s) into the hepatic artery at a constant rate, until a state of dynamic equilibrium was reached between the rate of isotope decay and infusion. This resulted in stable activity within liver and intrahepatic tumor as detected by gamma camera, the tissues having been previously identified by tin colloid imaging. The preangiotensin II activity ratio (tumor/normal ratio) demonstrated tumor hypervascularity in 9 of 14 readings from 9 patients (mean ratio ± SD, 1.47 ± 0.88). The relative increase in tumor perfusion was shown to be by a factor of between 1.5- and 5-fold under the influence of angiotensin II. The majority of patients in this study were suffering from hepatocellular carcinoma.

Studies by our group in Glasgow, Scotland have evaluated the potential of vasoactive drugs for tumor targeting in patients with liver metastases using radioactive microspheres. In the first of two studies, a double-isotope technique was used in patients undergoing placement of a hepatic artery catheter for regional chemotherapy. Albumin microspheres, labeled either with ^{131}I or ^{99m}Tc, were used (mean diameter of individual preparations was between 20 and 40 μm). The ^{99m}Tc-microspheres were obtained commercially (Sorin Biomedica), whereas ^{131}I microspheres were manufactured "in house" by a technique of glutaraldehyde stabilization of an oil-in-water emulsion of albumin and subsequently labeled with ^{131}I by the Chloramine T method.[26,27]

At the time of laparotomy, after placement of the hepatic artery catheter, a tracer dose of ^{131}I microspheres was infused via the hepatic artery. An arterial infusion of angiotensin II (17 μg over 100 s) was then administered, followed immediately by a tracer dose of ^{99m}Tc-microspheres. This rate of infusion of angiotensin II and timing of microsphere administration was thought most likely to result in maximal tumor targeting, as suggested by the data of Sasaki et al.[47] Biopsies of tumor and adjacent normal liver were obtained (mean weight 0.8 g; range 0.3 to 1.8 g) and the activity attributable both to ^{131}I and ^{99m}Tc estimated by gamma scintillation counting.

Prior to administration of angiotensin II, the number of particles per gram of tumor was found to be less than that in normal liver for each patient. Following angiotensin II administration, the uptake of microspheres by tumor was greater than that of normal liver in 4 of 9 individuals. The median improvement in tumor/normal ratio was by a factor of 2.8 (range 0.8 to 11.7, $p < 0.05$). The uptake of microspheres more than doubled in 5 patients, was more modestly improved in 2, unchanged in 1, and slightly reduced in 1 (Table 4).

In further studies by our group, hepatic arterial perfusion scintigraphy (HAPS) was used to evaluate tumor targeting by angiotensin II.[57,58] Three scintigrams (IGE Medical Systems, Slough, U.K.) were acquired with tomography for each of 11 patients with advanced colorectal liver metastases and indwelling hepatic arterial perfusion catheters. The studies were performed 3 or more days apart, and the series was completed within 2 weeks. The first acquisition was performed after an intravenous injection of ^{99m}Tc-colloid to identify tumor regions and estimate disease burden. Another acquisition was performed after a hepatic arterial injection of ^{99m}Tc-

TABLE 4
Uptake of Microspheres by Tumor and Normal Liver before and after Angiotensin II

Patient no.	Weight liver biopsy (g)	Weight tumor biopsy (g)	Pre-AII[a] T[b]/N[c] ratio (activity ^{131}I/g of tissue)	Post-AII T/N ratio (activity ^{99m}Tc/g of tissue)	Improvement factor with AII (T/N post-AII)/(T/N pre-AII)
1	0.9	1.2	0.31	3.62	11.7
2	0.7	0.5	0.26	1.16	4.5
3	0.7	1.4	0.47	0.75	1.6
4	0.5	1.3	0.11	0.42	4.0
5	1.0	1.0	0.25	0.32	1.3
6	0.6	1.8	0.90	8.11	9.1
7[d]	0.5	0.6	0.60	1.68	2.8
8	0.3	0.8	0.51	0.41	0.8
9	1.0	0.9	0.11	0.10	1.0

[a]   Angiotensin II.
[b]   Intrahepatic tumor.
[c]   Normal liver parenchyma.
[d]   Unknown primary.

From Goldberg, J. A., Murray, T., Kerr, D. J., Willmott, N., Bessent, R. G., McKillop, J. H., and McArdle, C. S., *Br. J. Cancer*, 63, 308, 1991. With permission.

Sorin Biomedica). The third acquisition was performed after infusion of a similar dose of ^{99m}Tc-microspheres, this time administered immediately after an infusion of angiotensin II (17 μg over 100 s).

SPECT data were reconstructed by computer (Data General Nova) using commercial software (Link Analytical Ltd.). Corresponding transverse slices from the colloid study and one or other HAPS study were aligned and superimposed. In this way, a qualitative appreciation of the power of tumor targeting by angiotensin II could be made by noting the degree of correspondence between the "cold spots" on the colloid scan, i.e., the tumor deposits, and the "hot spots" appearing after the HAPS studies with microspheres.* (See color Plate.)

A quantitative evaluation was also possible by drawing regions of interest to define tumor and normal liver parenchyma (identified from slices of the colloid scan) on corresponding slices from both HAPS studies. Ratios of activity in tumor and normal liver were calculated for individual tumors, before and after enhancement by the vasoactive agent. Standardization was achieved by evaluating each metastasis at the slice of its largest diameter, i.e., at the "equator" of the tumor.

Two of the 11 patients included in the above study had such markedly hypervascular tumors that the effect of angiotensin II was impossible to quantitate, there being no measurable activity in the normal liver regions after angiotensin II had been administered. In the remaining nine patients, 48 tumors were individually assessed, ranging in diameter from 4.5 to 10 cm. In contrast to the biopsy-based study described earlier, all of these tumors were hypervascular relative to the surrounding liver parenchyma before exposure to angiotensin II (median ratio of activity, tumor/normal, 3.4:1; range 1.3 to 6.0). The corresponding median ratio after angiotensin II was 7.3:1 (range 1.5 to 8.8; $p < 0.05$, Wilcoxon test). The median improvement in tumor/normal liver ratio was by a median factor of 1.8 (range 0.5 to 3.4). There was no apparent relationship between tumor size or disease burden and success in tumor targeting with angiotensin II (Table 5).

In addition to the tumors described above, it was noted that three tumors had hypovascular cores and hypervascular shells, an observation that had been noted by other investigators.[59] All of these "hollow" metastases were greater than 5 cm in diameter (Figure 4). Quantitation of the angiotensin II effect in these tumors was difficult because the resolution of the acquisition system was not sufficiently accurate to define the boundary between core and shell regions within the tumor. However, the effect of angiotensin II on these tumors did appear to be positive in the hypervascular shell. Whether or not the hypovascular tumor cores were composed of viable tissue was not known, but it is likely that any live tumor cells within these regions would escape treatment by arterially administered therapy, even with the use of angiotensin II enhancement.

The intriguing question remains as to why the tumors in the biopsy-based study appeared universally "hypovascular" in their baseline microsphere distribution pattern, whereas the majority of tumors in the HAPS/SPECT study were "hyper-

---

* Color plate follows page 70.

TABLE 5
Improvement in Tumor Uptake of Microspheres in Nine Patients after Angiotensin II: Evaluation by Hepatic Arterial Perfusion Scintigraphy and Single Photon Emission Computed Tomography

Patient no.	T^a/N^b ratio pre-AII[c] (median)	T/N ratio post-AII (median)	Improvement in ratio post-AII (median)
1	1.60	3.36	2.98
2	3.96	7.62	1.92
3	6.04	8.10	1.11
4	3.73	1.54	0.52
5	3.40	8.82	3.41
6	2.57	7.61	3.03
7	1.33	2.64	1.77
8	4.65	7.32	1.74
9	2.44	2.61	0.86

Note: The median values are based on evaluation of all tumors at the tomographic slice of their maximal diameter. Tumor regions were defined as areas of low uptake on the ^{99m}Tc-colloid tomographic slice; the remainder of the organ was taken to be normal liver parenchyma. A region of interest approximately 5 pixels in diameter was defined over an area of uniformly high uptake on each colloid slice and used as a sample of normal liver to quantitate the activity ratios of tumor and normal liver.

[a]   Tumor.
[b]   Normal liver.
[c]   Angiontensin II.

From Goldberg, J. A., Thomson, J. A. K., Bradnam, M. S., Fenner, J., Bessent, R. G., McKillop, J. H., Kerr, D. J., and McArdle, C. S., *Br. J. Cancer*, 64, 114, 1991. With permission.

vascular.'' Five of the patients were common to both studies, which allows a direct comparison of relative tumor vascularity as measured by the two different techniques, albeit with the data acquired on different occasions (Table 6).[60]

Work in a rabbit tumor model may shed some light on this paradox. In their study of the relative vascularity of hepatic tumor implants, Burton et al.[61] demonstrated a dependence upon whether or not blood flow was measured during laparotomy. The tumors were greatly hypervascular when microspheres were administered to the intact animal (corresponding to conditions for acquisition of SPECT data) but were slightly hypovascular when microspheres were administered with the liver exposed (corresponding to conditions for acquisition of biopsy data). These findings were associated with a reduction in the surface temperature of both liver and tumor during laparotomy, with the decrease being significantly more pronounced in tumor tissue than in liver.

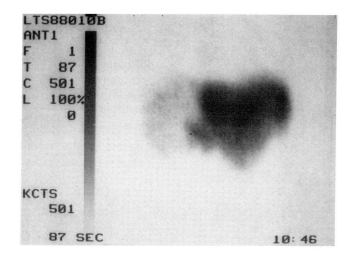

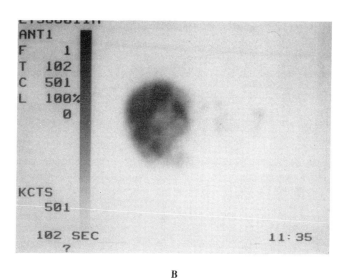

FIGURE 4. A large intrahepatic tumor mass demonstrating a hypovascular core. (A) ^{99m}Tc-colloid image of the liver, demonstrating a large tumor mass in the right lobe (cold spot). (B) Hepatic arterial perfusion scintigraphy using ^{99m}Tc-labeled albumin microspheres, demonstrating a hypervascular shell and hypovascular core in the tumor.

The validity of various techniques for investigating microsphere distribution *in vivo* has been demonstrated for the human kidney in a study by Anderson et al.[62] The relationship between organ perfusion scintigraphy (*in vivo* and *ex vivo* imaging) and biopsy techniques was correlated for accuracy of tumor/normal ratios of activity in a patient with hypernephroma. A selective angiography catheter was placed within

TABLE 6
Relative Microsphere Uptake by
Tumor and Normal Tissue
Assessed by Two Techniques

Patient no.	T/N ratio[a] by biopsy	Median T/N ratio[b] by SPECT[c]
1	0.31	1.53
2	0.26	3.96
3	0.25	2.44
4	0.90	3.73
5	0.51	1.98

[a] T/N ratio obtained using ^{131}I microspheres during laparotomy.
[b] T/N ratio obtained using ^{99m}Tc microspheres in the intact patient.
[c] Single photon emission computed tomography.

From Willmott, N., Goldberg, J. A., Anderson, J. H., Bessent, R. G., McKillop, J. H., and McArdle, C. S., *Int. J. Radiat. Biol.*, 60, 195, 1991. With permission.

the renal artery under local anesthesia using the Seldinger technique. A tracer bolus of ^{131}I-albumin microspheres was infused, followed by an infusion of angiotensin II (15 μg over 90 s), then a tracer dose of ^{99m}Tc-albumin microspheres. The patient was imaged by gamma camera in both [131]I- and ^{99m}Tc-channels. Under general anesthesia the kidney was removed, reimaged by gamma camera, then tissue samples taken for both histology and well gamma counting.

It was interesting to note that part of the tumor was necrotic, and samples were taken of both viable and nonviable tumor, as well as normal renal tissue. There was good correlation between *in vivo* and *ex vivo* organ imaging, in terms of tumor vascularity relative to normal tissue and enhancement of tumor/normal ratio of activity by angiotensin II. The tumor was marginally hypervascular compared with the surrounding renal tissue by all three methods of assessment. The well gamma counting suggested that targeting enhancement by angiotensin II in the viable tumor had actually been underestimated by imaging methods. It was observed that levels of activity were only marginally lower in the necrotic tumor than in viable tumor and that targeting was also enhanced in necrotic tumor by angiotensin II, although the enhancement ratio was less than for viable tissue (Table 7, Figure 5).

Any technique that improves the relative exposure of tumor regions to arterially administered therapeutic agents is likely to improve the regional advantage if the thresholds for drug extraction or metabolism are not exceeded. The technique has been applied to internal radiation therapy (using [90]Yttrium-labeled glass microspheres) in a clinical trial.[63] The temporary nature of the angiotensin II targeting

TABLE 7
The Effect of Angiotensin II on Distribution of Microspheres in a Hypernephroma-Bearing Kidney: A Comparison of Three Techniques for Evaluation (*In Vivo* and Post-Resection Imaging of the Intact Organ and Well Gamma Counting of Tissue Samples)

	Pre-AII[a] (^{131}I)		Post-AII (^{99m}Tc)		
	Counts	T[b]/N[c]	Counts	T/N	Enhancement
Posterior *in vivo* gamma camera images (counts/min/ROI[d])					
Normal kidney	2078		10498		
Viable tumor	2333	1.1	29302	2.8	2.5
Nonviable tumor	2038	1.0	22581	2.2	2.2
Posterior postresection gamma camera images (counts/min/ROI)					
Normal kidney	1218		5700		
Viable tumor	1759	1.4	21713	3.8	2.6
Nonviable tumor	968	0.8	8486	1.5	1.9
Tissue samples (counts/min/g)					
Normal kidney	593699		309964		
Viable tumor	863057	1.5	1790458	5.8	4.0
Nonviable tumor	515532	1.4	585941	1.9	1.4

[a] Angiotensin II.
[b] Tumor.
[c] Normal renal tissue (see Figure 6).
[d] ROI = Region of interest.

From Anderson, J. H., Willmott, N., Bessent, R. G., Angerson, W. J., Kerr, D. J., and McArdle, G. S., *Br. J. Cancer,* 64, 365, 1991. With permission.

mechanism is ideally suited to administration of particles incorporating active agents as a bolus, and other vasoactive agents are under investigation.[64]

Biodegradable microspheres have been used in two ways to improve the regional advantage of arterial chemotherapy. Microspheres, particularly starch, have been mixed with cytotoxic agents, the rationale being that they slow down blood flow through the target organ, thereby allowing more drug to be taken up by the tissues[25,65-69] (see also Chapter 7). Microspheres have also been developed as drug carriers, which can release their drug payload when targeted to tumors by the arterial route (Chapter 3). Adriamycin-loaded albumin microspheres[70,71] and mitomycin C-loaded albumin microspheres[72] have been described. The drug payload is relatively low, but there is evidence to suggest that potency is enhanced when the cytotoxic drug is in microspherical form.[73,74]

Clearly, the differential handling of biodegradable microspheres by tumor and normal tissues and the variability of breakdown rate between individuals are issues

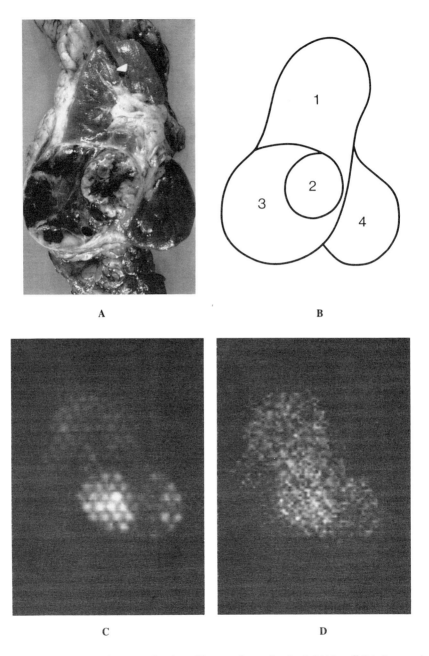

FIGURE 5.   Coronal section, posterior view of hypernephroma-bearing left kidney.[62] (A) photograph; (B) line drawing showing [(1) normal superior pole, (2) viable tumor, (3) nonviable tumor, (4) normal inferior pole]; (C) postresection, preangiotensin II gamma camera image of ^{131}I-microsphere distribution; and (D) postresection, postangiotensin II gamma camera image of ^{99m}Tc-microsphere distribution. (From Anderson et al., *Br. J. Cancer,* 64, 365, 1991. With permission.)

that are of clinical importance. Radioactive isotopes have been used to examine differential degradation rates of albumin microspheres *in vivo* in patients with liver metastases. In a study by our group[75] ^{131}I-albumin microspheres were made under sterile conditions by the same technique as described above involving glutaraldehyde stabilization of a water-in-oil emulsion of iodinated protein.[31] This produced a radiopharmaceutical in which the iodine was covalently bound to the albumin and was incorporated throughout the matrix of the microsphere. The radiolabel was therefore released uniformly during degradation of the microsphere. In these studies, the mean diameter of batches of microspheres was between 20 and 40 μm.

Stability of the particles on storage and in plasma was checked by incubating microspheres in serum at 37°C. After 10 days the particles were separated from supernatant and the radioactivity in both measured. The amount of ^{131}I released was expressed as a percentage of total activity. The radiopharmaceutical was stable in phosphate-buffered saline; more than 99.7% of the activity remained particle-bound after 2 weeks. The preparation was also remarkably stable in plasma: between 92 and 96% of the original activity remained microsphere-bound after 10 days (median of 95%, n = 6).

Another *in vitro* experiment was performed to measure the sensitivity of albumin microspheres to protease digestion. Microspheres were incubated in a 0.4% trypsin solution at 37°C and degradation and solubilization of particles recorded. The *in vitro* breakdown pattern of microspheres by protease enzyme featured a lag phase followed by swelling of the particles and then degradation, which was complete after 4 h.[50]

In vivo biodegradation was studied in eight patients with advanced metastatic liver disease. The severity of disease was assessed by ^{99m}Tc-colloid scan. All patients had previously undergone insertion of a hepatic artery catheter, which had been checked to ensure perfusion of the whole liver and exclude extrahepatic perfusion. HAPS using a tracer dose of commercial ^{99m}Tc-albumin microspheres had been performed more than 2 weeks previously and low baseline arteriovenous shunting (<5%) was observed. The patients were started on a regimen of potassium iodate 2 days prior to the administration of ^{131}I-microspheres to prevent uptake of released radioactivity by the thyroid gland. This was continued for 14 days after microsphere administration.

The patient was positioned supine on the couch of a gamma camera (IGE 400A tomographic gamma camera with high energy, parallel hole multipurpose collimator) and anterior and posterior images of the abdomen acquired. Regions of interest were drawn around the liver on the images. Scanning was performed on the day of injection and at 24-h intervals for 5 or more consecutive days. The anterior views from the studies were aligned and the same region of interest superimposed to estimate the rate of decay of activity in the liver region during the study period. The same technique was used on the posterior views. The effective half-life was derived from these results and the biological half-life obtained by using the physical half-life of ^{131}I and the following equation:

$$\frac{1}{T^{BIOL}} = \frac{1}{T^{EFFECT}} - \frac{1}{T^{PHYS}} \qquad (2)$$

TABLE 8
Biological Half-Life (days) of Hepatic Arterially Administered ^{131}I-Labeled Albumin Microspheres in Eight Patients with Advanced Liver Metastases

Patient no.	Whole liver anterior and posterior geometric mean	Tumor anterior view	Normal liver anterior view
1	3.30	6.23	3.27
2	2.33	1.93	2.00
3	1.66	1.18	1.51
4	2.07	1.56	1.55
5[a]	1.52	—	—
6	2.73	3.23	1.64
7[a]	11.70[b]	—	—
8	2.48	0.97	0.89

Note: The activity in 200 mg of freshly prepared ^{131}I-albumin microspheres (containing approximately 4×10^7 particles) was measured. The preparation was drawn into a glass syringe and infused into the hepatic artery catheter. The syringe was flushed with saline to maximize delivery of particles. The activity in both dispensing vial and administration equipment was measured following injection to determine the amount of activity injected (range 0.78 to 8.67 MBq). Anterior and posterior images were acquired by gamma camera on successive days, enabling rates of microsphere degradation to be estimated.

[a] In these patients there were insufficient counts in normal liver to enable the degradation rate in a region of normal liver to be estimated.

[b] In this patient, the half-life from a log-linear fit was used because the activity did not decrease to one half the initial value during the study period.

From Goldberg, J. A., Willmott, N., Anderson, J. H., McCurrach, G., Bessent, R. G., McKillop, J. H., and McArdle, C. S., *Nucl. Med. Commun.,* 12, 57, 1991. With permission.

Where T^{BIOL}, T^{EFFECT}, and T^{PHYS} are the biological half-life of the microspheres, the effective half-life of the liver activity, and the physical half-life of ^{131}I, respectively.

The biological half-life of microspheres in the whole liver was estimated from the geometric means of the anterior and posterior images. In patients with sufficient counts in normal liver, regions of interest were positioned around a tumor region on the anterior view, as identified from the colloid scan, and a corresponding area of normal liver (>180 pixels in size). The half-life of microspheres in these two regions was calculated. The median biological half-life of the microspheres in the tumor-bearing liver (calculated from the anterior images) was 1.8 days (range 0.95 to 11.7, Table 8).

The biological half-life of albumin microspheres varied considerably between individuals. It was interesting to note the variation in half-life in tumor regions relative to normal liver, with some tumors being more efficient at degrading particles than the corresponding normal liver.

V. CONCLUSION

This chapter has shown that, when administered regionally, particles of a suitable size will embolize in solid tumor tissue with little arteriovenous shunting: if made of biodegradable material, e.g., albumin, the embolized particles will biodegrade over a period of days. The regional advantage gained is different depending on the method of assessment. Thus, T/N ratios are higher by whole body imaging than when biopsy samples are examined, which may be explained in terms of tumor response to laparotomy in the latter case. It is our opinion that whole body imaging will better reflect the distribution of microspheres administered with therapeutic intent via an indwelling arterial catheter (Portacath® System 320 Pharmacia, Milton Keynes, U.K. or Infusaid® arterial catheter, Shirley Infusaid Inc., Norwood, U.S.A.) consisting of a silicone catheter and a subcutaneous resealable injection port. Taken together, these data show the suitability of microspheres as a tumor targeting vehicle in regional cancer therapy.

ACKNOWLEDGMENTS

Dr. Rodney Bessent of the Department of Clinical Physics and Bioengineering, Royal Infirmary, Glasgow is gratefully acknowledged for generously supplying Figures 1 and 2.

REFERENCES

1. **Parker, R. P., Smith, R. H. S., and Taylor, D. M.,** *Basic Science of Nuclear Medicine,* 2nd ed., Churchill Livingstone, Edinburgh, 1984.
2. **Heymann, M. A., Payne, B. D., Hoffman, J. I. E., and Rudolph, A. M.,** Blood flow measurements with radionuclide-labelled particles, *Prog. Cardiovasc. Dis.,* 20, 55, 1977.
3. **Hertz, S., Roberts, A., and Evans, R. D.,** Radioactive iodine as an indicator in the study of thyroid physiology, *Proc. Soc. Exp. Biol. Med.,* 38, 510, 1938.
4. **Cassen, B., Curtis, L., Reed, C., and Libby, R.,** Instrumentation for ^{131}I use in medical studies, *Nucleonics,* 9, 46, 1951.
5. **Anger, H. O.,** Scintillation camera, *Rev. Sci. Instrum.,* 29, 27, 1958.
6. **Chilton, H. M. and Witcofski, R. L.,** *Nuclear Pharmacy: An Introduction to the Clinical Application of Radiopharmaceuticals,* Lea & Febiger, Philadelphia, 1986.
7. Administration of Radioactive Substances Advisory Committee, Notes for guidance on the administration of radioactive substances to persons for purposes of diagnosis, treatment or research, Department of Health, London, 1992.
8. **Wagner, H. N.,** Clinical PET: its time has come, *J. Nucl. Med.,* 32, 561, 1991.

9. **Phelps, M. E., Mazziotta, J. C., and Schelbert, H. R.,** *Positron Emission Tomography and Autoradiography,* Raven Press, New York, 1986.
10. **Ell, P. J. and Holman, B. L., Eds.,** *Computed Emission Tomography,* Oxford, Oxford, 1982.
11. **Williams, E. D., Ed.,** *An Introduction to Emission Computed Tomography,* Report 44, Institute of Physical Sciences in Medicine, London, 1985.
12. **George, M. S., Ring, H. A., Costa, D. C., Ell, P. J., Kouris, K., and Jarritt, P. H.,** *Neuroactivation and Neuroimaging with SPET,* Springer-Verlag, Berlin, 1991.
13. **Hoffman, E. J.,** 180x compared with 360x sampling in SPECT, *J. Nucl. Med.,* 23, 745, 1982.
14. **Herman, G. T.,** *Image Reconstructions from Projections: The Fundamentals of Computerised Tomography,* Academic Press, London, 1980.
15. **Jaszczak, R. J., Greer, K. L., and Coleman, R. E.,** SPECT, in *Physics of Nuclear Medicine: Recent Advances,* Rao, D. V., Chaudra, R., and Graham, M. C., Eds., American Institute of Physics, New York, 1984, 457.
16. **Chang, L. T.,** A method for attenuation correction in radionuclide computer tomography, *IEEE Trans. Nucl. Sci.,* 25, 638, 1978.
17. **Gilland, D. R., Tsui, B. M. W., McCartney, W. H., Perry, J. R., and Berg, J.,** Determination of the optimum filter function for SPECT imaging, *J. Nucl. Med.,* 29, 643, 1988.
18. **Heller, S. L. and Goodwin, P. N.,** SPECT instrumentation: performance, lesion detection and recent innovations, *Semin. Nucl. Med.,* 17, 184, 1987.
19. **Koral, K. F., Swailem, F. M., Buchbinda, S., Clinthorne, N. H., Rogers, W. L., and Tsui, B. M. W.,** SPECT dual-energy-window Compton correction: scatter multiplier required for quantification, *J. Nucl. Med.,* 31, 90, 1991.
20. **Kouris, K., Elgazzar, A., Affana, R., and Abdel-Dayem, H. M.,** Methodology and performance assessment of zoom SPECT, *J. Nucl. Med. Technol.,* 18, 198, 1990.
21. **Mueller, S. P., Polak, J. F., Kijewski, M. F., and Holman, B. L.,** Collimator selection for SPECT brain imaging: the advantage of high resolution, *J. Nucl. Med.,* 27, 1729, 1986.
22. **Williams, E. D., Harding, L. K., and McKillop, J. H.,** Checklists for quality assurance and audit in nuclear medicine, *Nucl. Med. Commun.,* 10, 595, 1989.
23. **Graham, L. S.,** A national quality assurance program for SPECT instrumentation, in *Nuclear Medicine Annual 1989,* Freeman, L. M. and Weissmann, H. D., Eds., Raven Press, New York, 1989, 81.
24. **Dakhil, S., Ensminger, W. D., Cho, K., Neiderhuber, J., Doan, K., and Wheeler, R.,** Improved regional selectivity of hepatic arterial BCNU with degradable microspheres, *Cancer,* 50, 631, 1982.
25. **Ensminger, W. D., Gyves, J. W., Stetson, P., and Walker-Andrews, S.,** Phase I study of hepatic arterial degradable starch microspheres and mitomycin, *Cancer Res.,* 45, 4464, 1985.
26. **Lee, T. K., Sokolski, T. D., and Royer, G.,** Serum albumin beads: an injectable, biodegradable system for the sustained release of drugs, *Science,* 213, 233, 1981.
27. **Hunter, W. M. and Greenwood, F. C.,** Preparation of iodine ^{131}I-labelled human growth hormone of high specific activity, *Nature,* 194, 495, 1962.
28. **Goldberg, J. A., Murray, T., Kerr, D. J., Willmott, N., Bessent, R. G., McKillop, J. H., and McArdle, C. S.,** The use of angiotensin II as a potential method of targeting cytotoxic microspheres in patients with intrahepatic tumor, *Br. J. Cancer,* 63, 308, 1991.
29. **Paik, C. H., Hong, J. J., Ebert, M. A., Heald, S. C., Reba, R. C., and Eckelman, W. C.,** Relative reactivity of DTPA, immunoreactive antibody-DTPA conjugates and nonimmunoreactive antibody-DTPA conjugates toward indium-111, *J. Nucl. Med.,* 26, 482, 1985.
30. **Hnatowich, D. J., Layne, W. W., and Childs, R. L.,** The preparation and labelling of DTPA-coupled albumin, *Int. J. Appl. Radiat. Isot.,* 33, 327, 1982.
31. **Willmott, N., Murray, T., Carlton, R., Chen, Y., Logan, H., McCurrach, G., Bessent, R. G., Goldberg, J. A., Anderson, J. H., McKillop, J. H., and McArdle, C. S.,** Development of radiolabeled albumin microspheres: a comparison of gamma-emitting isotopes of Iodine (^{131}I) and Indium (^{111}In/[113m]In), *Nucl. Med. Biol.,* 18, 687, 1991.

32. **Willmott, N., Cummings, J., Stuart, J. F. B., and Florence, A. T.,** Adriamycin-loaded albumin microspheres: preparation, *in vivo* distribution and release in the rat, *Biopharm. Drug Dispo.,* 6, 91, 1985.
33. **Breedis, C. and Young, G.,** The blood-supply of neoplasms in the liver, *Am. J. Pathol.,* 30, 969, 1954.
34. **Ridge, J. A., Bading, J. R., Gelbard, A. S., Benua, R. S., and Daly, J. M.,** Perfusion of colorectal hepatic metastases: relative distribution of flow from the hepatic artery and portal vein, *Cancer,* 59, 1547, 1987.
35. **Bierman, H. A., Miller, E. R., Byron, R. L., Dod, K. S., Black, D., and Kelly, K. H.,** Intra-arterial catheterization of viscera in man, *Am. J. Roentgenol.,* 66, 555, 1951.
36. **Bierman, H. R., Byron, R. L., Kelley, K. H., and Grady, A.,** Studies on the blood-supply of tumors in man: III, vascular pattern of the liver by hepatic angiography *in vivo, J. Natl. Cancer Inst.,* 12, 107, 1951.
37. **Kaplan, W. D., Come, S. E., Laffin, S. M., and Takvorian, R. W.,** The clinical significance of pulmonary Tc 99m-MAA following radionucleide hepatic artery (HA) perfusion, *J. Nucl. Med.,* 24, 51, 1983.
38. **Zeissman, H. A., Thrall, J. H., Gyves, J. W., Ensminger, W. D., Niederhuber, M., Tuscan, M., and Walker, S.,** Quantitative hepatic arterial perfusion scintigraphy and starch microspheres in cancer therapy, *J. Nucl. Med.,* 24, 871, 1983.
39. **Zeissman, H. A., Gyves, J. W., Juni, J. E., Wahl, F. L., Thrall, J. H., Ensminger, W. D., Goldstein, H. A., and Dubiansky, V.,** Atlas of hepatic arterial perfusion scintigraphy, *Clin. Nucl. Med.,* 10, 675, 1985.
40. **Starkhammar, H., Hakansson, L., Morales, O., and Svedberg, J.,** Intra-arterial mitomycin C treatment of unresectable liver tumors: preliminary results on the effect of degradable starch microspheres, *Acta Oncol.,* 26, 295, 1987.
41. **Starkhammar, H., Hakansson, L., Morales, O., and Svedberg, J.,** Effect of microspheres in intra-arterial chemotherapy: a study of arterio-venous shunting and passage of a labeled marker, *Med. Oncol. Tumor Pharmacother.,* 4, 87, 1987.
42. **Nott, D. M., Yates, J., Grime, J. S., Maltby, P., O'Driscoll, P. M., Baxter, J. N., Jenkins, S. A., and Cooke, T. G.,** Induced hepatic arterial blockade by degradable starch microspheres in the rat, *Nucl. Med. Commun.,* 8, 1019, 1987.
43. **Mavor, A. I. D., Parkin, A., Riley, A., Smye, S., O'Brien, T., Robinson, P. J., and Giles, G.,** Initial clinical experience with degradable starch microspheres, *Nucl. Med. Commun.,* 8, 1011, 1987.
44. **Chang, D., Jenkins, S. A., Nott, D. M., and Cooke, T. G.,** Biodegradable emboli increase the delivery of cytotoxic drug to hepatic tumors, *Br. J. Surg.,* 76, 631, 1989.
45. **Civalleri, D., Gianandria, R., Simoni, G. M., Mallarini, G., Repetto, M., and Bonalumi, U.,** Redistribution of arterial blood-flow in metastases-bearing livers after infusion of degradable starch microspheres, *Acta Chir. Scand.,* 151, 613, 1985.
46. **Goldberg, J. A., Bradnam, M. S., Kerr, D. J., Haughton, D. M., McKillop, J. H., Bessent, R. G., Willmott, N., and McArdle, C. S.,** Arteriovenous shunting of microspheres in patients with colorectal liver metastases: errors in assessment due to free pertechnetate and the effect of angiotensin II, *Nucl. Med. Commun.,* 8, 1033, 1987.
47. **Sasaki, Y., Imaoka, S., Hasegawa, Y., Nakano, S., Ishikawa, O., Ohigashi, H., Taniguchi, K., Koyama, H., Iwanaga, T., and Terasawa, T.,** Changes in distribution of hepatic blood-flow induced by intra-arterial infusion of angiotensin II in human hepatic cancer, *Cancer,* 55, 311, 1985.
48. **Goldberg, J. A., Thomson, J. A. K., McCurrach, G., Anderson, J. H., Willmott, N., Bessent, R. G., McKillop, J. H., and McArdle, C. S.,** Arteriovenous shunting in patients with colorectal liver metastases, *Br. J. Cancer,* 63, 466, 1991.
49. **Goldberg, J. A., Kerr, D. J., Willmott, N., McKillop, J. H., and McArdle, C. S.,** Pharmacokinetics and pharmacodynamics of locoregional 5-fluorouracil (5FU) in advanced colorectal liver metastases, *Br. J. Cancer,* 57, 186, 1988.

50. **Willmott, N., Chen, Y., Goldberg, J. A., McArdle, C. S., and Florence, A. T.**, Biodegradation rate of embolised protein microspheres in lung, liver and kidney of rats, *J. Pharm. Pharmacol.*, 41, 433, 1989.

51. **Widder, K. J., Senyei, A. E., and Ranney, D. F.**, Magnetically responsive microspheres and other carriers for the biophysical targeting of antitumor agents, *Adv. Pharmacol. Chemother.*, 16, 213, 1979.

52. **Abrams, H. L.**, Altered drug response of tumor vessels in man, *Nature*, 201, 167, 1964.

53. **Ackerman, N. B. and Henchmer, P. A.**, Effects of pharmacological agents on the microcirculation of tumors implanted in the liver, *Bibl. Anat.*, 15, 301, 1977.

54. **Burton, M. A., Gray, B. N., Self, G. W., Heggie, J. C., and Townsend, P. S.**, Manipulation of experimental rat and rabbit tumor blood-flow with angiotensin II, *Cancer Res.*, 45, 5390, 1985.

55. **Suzuki, M., Hori, K., Abe, I., Saito, S., and Sato, H.**, A new approach to cancer chemotherapy: selective enhancement of tumor blood-flow with angiotensin II, *J. Natl. Cancer Inst.*, 67, 663, 1981.

56. **Hafstrom, L., Nobin, A., Persson, B., and Sundqvist, K.**, Effects of catecholamines on cardiovascular response and blood-flow distribution to normal tissue and liver tumors in rats, *Cancer Res.*, 40, 481, 1980.

57. **Goldberg, J. A., Bradnam, M. S., Kerr, D. J., McKillop, J. H., Bessent, R. G., McArdle, C. S., Willmott, N., and George, W. D.**, Single photon emission computed tomographic studies (SPECT) of hepatic arterial perfusion scintigraphy (HAPS) in patients with colorectal liver metastases: improved tumor targeting with angiotensin II, *Nucl. Med. Commun.*, 8, 1025, 1987.

58. **Goldberg, J. A., Thomson, J. A. K., Bradnam, M. S., Fenner, J., Bessent, R. G., McKillop, J. H., Kerr, D. J., and McArdle, C. S.**, Angiotensin II as a potential method of targeting cytotoxic-loaded microspheres in patients with colorectal liver metastases, *Br. J. Cancer*, 64, 114, 1991.

59. **Gyves, J. W., Zeissman, H. A., Ensminger, W. D., Thrall, J. H., Neiderhuber, J. E., Keyes, J. W., and Walker, S.**, Definition of hepatic tumor microcirculation by single photon emission computerised tomography (SPECT), *J. Nucl. Med.*, 25, 972, 1984.

60. **Willmott, N., Goldberg, J. A., Anderson, J. H., Bessent, R. G., McKillop, J. H., and McArdle, C. S.**, Abnormal vasculature of solid tumors: significance for microsphere-based targeting strategies, *Int. J. Radiat. Biol.*, 60, 195, 1991.

61. **Burton, M. A., Kelleher, D. K., Gray, B. N., and Morgan, C. K.**, Alteration of experimental liver tumor blood-flow: II, effect of laparotomy, *Cancer J.*, 3, 351, 1990.

62. **Anderson, J. H., Willmott, N., Bessent, R. G., Angerson, W. J., Kerr, D. J., and McArdle, C. S.**, Regional chemotherapy for inoperable renal carcinoma: a method of targeting therapeutic microspheres to tumor, *Br. J. Cancer*, 64, 365, 1991.

63. **Anderson, J. H., Goldberg, J. A., Bessent, R. G., Kerr, D. J., McKillop, J. H., Cooke, T. G., and McArdle, C. S.**, Glass yttrium-90 microspheres for patients with colorectal liver metastases, *Radiother. Oncol.*, 25, 137, 1992.

64. **Hemingway, D. M., Chang, D., Goldberg, J. A., Jenkins, S. A., and Cooke, T.**, Pharmacological manipulation of liver blood-flow and its implications for the treatment of hepatic metastases, *Br. J. Surg.*, 77, 702, 1990.

65. **Goldberg, J. A., Kerr, D. J., Willmott, N., McKillop, J. H., and McArdle, C. S.**, Regional chemotherapy for colorectal liver metastases: a phase II evaluation of targeted hepatic arterial 5-fluorouracil, *Br. J. Surg.*, 77, 1238, 1990.

66. **Lorelius, L. E., Benedetto, A. R., Blumhardt, R., Gaskill, H. V., Lancaster, J. L., and Stridbeck, H.**, Enhanced drug retention in VX2 tumors by the use of degradable starch microspheres, *Invest. Radiol.*, 19, 212, 1984.

67. **Flowerdew, A., Richards, H., and Taylor, I.**, Selective hepatic chemotherapy and temporary blood-flow stasis with degradable starch microspheres for liver metastases, *Br. J. Surg.*, 73, 1026, 1986.

68. **Sigurdson, E. R., Ridge, J. A., and Daly, J. M.**, Intra-arterial infusion of doxorubicin with degradable starch microspheres, *Arch. Surg.*, 121, 1277, 1986.

69. **Teder, H., Bjorkman, A. S., Lindell, B., and Ljungberg, J.,** The influence of degradable starch microspheres on uptake of 5-fluorouracil after hepatic artery injection in the rat, *J. Pharm. Pharmacol.,* 38, 939, 1986.

70. **McArdle, C. S., Lewi, H., Hansell, D., Kerr, D. J., McKillop, J. H., and Willmott, N.,** Cytotoxic-loaded albumin microspheres: a novel approach to regional chemotherapy, *Br. J. Surg.,* 75, 132, 1988.

71. **Kerr, D. J., Willmott, N., McKillop, J. H., Cummings, J., Lewi, H., and McArdle, C. S.,** Target organ disposition and plasma pharmacokinetics of doxorubicin incorporated into albumin microspheres after intra-renal arterial administration, *Cancer,* 62, 878, 1988.

72. **Fujimoto, S., Miyazaki, M., Endoh, F., Takahashi, O., Shrestha, R. D., Okui, K., Morimoto, Y., and Terao, K.,** Effects of intra-arterially infused biodegradable microspheres containing mitomycin C, *Cancer,* 55, 522, 1985.

73. **Goldberg, J. A., Willmott, N., Kerr, D. J., Sutherland, C., and McArdle, C. S.,** An *in vivo* assessment of cytotoxic-loaded microspheres, *Br. J. Cancer,* 65, 393, 1992.

74. **Morimoto, Y., Natsume, H., Sugibayashi, K., and Fujimoto, S.,** Effect of chemoembolization of albumin microspheres containing mitomycin C on AH liver metastases in rats, *Int. J. Pharm.,* 54, 27, 1989.

75. **Goldberg, J. A., Willmott, N., Anderson, J. H., McCurrach, G., Bessent, R. G., McKillop, J. H., and McArdle, C. S.,** The biodegradation of albumin microspheres used for regional chemotherapy in patients with colorectal liver metastases, *Nucl. Med. Commun.,* 12, 57, 1991.

Chapter 9

PERSPECTIVE ON MICROSPHERES IN REGIONAL CANCER THERAPY

Neville Willmott, Bruce Gray, and John Daly

There is a clear and continuing need to develop targetable devices in cancer therapy because treatment of the common, solid epithelial tumors relies heavily on inhibiting cell proliferation by potent agents (e.g., cytotoxic drugs, radiation) that have no inherent selectivity for malignant cells per se. The question then becomes: can selectivity be conferred on these agents by a suitable carrier? This constitutes the drug delivery approach to drug development, which appears an attractive alternative where the traditional medicinal chemistry approach has failed to generate compounds with adequate activity. Table 1 contrasts these approaches to achieving selectivity in drug action.

Drug delivery subsumes both targeting and controlled release; however, although work in the latter area has resulted in a variety of products at advanced stages of development (e.g., the Macromol® emulsion system for oral insulin, the Oros® system, Volmax®, for controlled release of salbutamol and the transdermal patch for nicotine addiction), this is not as yet the case for targetable devices. Antibodies in their most recent guise are undoubtedly the most advanced with regards to clinical trials and progression toward the status of pharmaceutical product.

Antibodies against putative tumor antigens have been intensively investigated as carriers for many years, without conspicuous success. Despite the manifold unsolved problems in this approach, interest in this area has continued to grow; indeed, with the advent of recombinant DNA technology, its heuristic appeal is greater than ever. The ways in which molecular biology is currently being used in this area involve (1) reduction in antibody immunogenicity by grafting onto a human antibody molecule only those mouse regions from the original monoclonal antibody that determine specificity and (2) antibody fragment engineering in which the antigen combining regions can be produced separately and combined as a molecule consisting solely of two, three, or four binding sites. Most seductive of all is the recreation in a "test tube" of the bodies way of generating high-affinity antibodies by generating diversity (e.g., mutation, shuffling of heavy and light chains) combined with subsequent cycles of selection using the recently developed phage display systems.[2]

The sophistication of this approach does not alter the fact that, despite extensive investigations on the immunology, biochemistry, biophysics, and molecular biology of malignant cells, no macromolecule has been identified that distinguishes, at the cellular level, the malignant from the normal state. Thus, there may be limited scope for effective deployment of antibody-based targeting systems, however so-

TABLE 1
Approaches to Selectivity in Cancer Chemotherapy

Medicinal chemistry	Drug delivery
Design/discover new drug molecules	Efficient delivery of existing agents
Depends on specific "locus" of drug action	Depends on localization of drug action
Chemistry-based	Physiology-based
Numerous commercial products	No commercial products

phisticated their construction or appealing the theory. Although there is little evidence for tumor specificity at the cellular level, if a solid tumor is considered an integrated functional unit, then differences between the malignant and normal state become apparent at this level of organization. The differences rely on the fact that solid tumors require an arterial blood supply to progress beyond a few millimeters in diameter and are of central importance to the therapeutic use of microspherical carriers in regional cancer therapy.

It is instructive to contrast the physiology of normal tissue vasculature (with its orderly arrangement of blood vessels responsive to a variety of mediators) with that of tumor tissue. Here, unrestrained cell growth outstrips capacity of vasculature to support it: blood vessels become aberrant, disorganized, and inefficient, leading to two important consequences. First, blood vessels of a solid tumor fail to respond to vasoactive stimuli. Attempts to exploit this using vasoactive agents to intensify the therapeutic response at the solid tumor site are reviewed in Chapter 2. A particular example, the use of the vasoconstrictor angiotensin II, which selectively reduces perfusion to normal tissue while maintaining that to tumor tissue, to target therapeutic agents incorporated within microspheres to solid tumors of liver and kidney is discussed and illustrated in Chapter 8. Second, solid tumor tissue has a reduced extraction efficiency relative to surrounding normal tissue. Thus, using positron emission tomography (see Chapter 8) to study the disposition of [^{18}F]-fluorouracil after intrahepatic arterial administration in patients with colorectal liver metastases, it was observed that tumors exhibiting greater perfusion than surrounding normal liver nevertheless had a low uptake of radiolabeled fluorouracil and appeared hypovascular.[2] Microspherical carriers, whose initial localization depends on relative tumor perfusion and not on extraction from plasma, should overcome this problem. Such systems include microspheres of a size (>10 μm) suitable for embolization (Chapters 1, 2, 5, 7, and 8) and microcarriers capable of extracorporeal guidance by magnetic fields (Chapter 4).

It is an interesting paradox that whole body imaging techniques, which reveal the deficiencies of antibody and liposome-based systems, clearly illustrate the targeting potential of microspherical systems of appropriate size in regional cancer therapy (Chapter 8). Other chapters consider how to exploit this phenomenon by discussing and comparing the properties of various microsphere matrix materials (Chapter 1) and different agents for incorporation within microspheres (Chapters 5 and 6).

Clearly, as a first approximation, it is desirable to incorporate as much active agent as possible within the microsphere matrix consistent with a degree of sustained release. Although high drug loading may lead to premature release and unacceptably high systemic concentrations of incorporated agent, preliminary data using radiolabeled doxorubicin incorporated into cation exchange resin microspheres indicate that this is not always the case (Chen, Burton, and Gray, personal communication).

Chapter 1 compares a variety of matrix materials with regard to loading of doxorubicin, and it seems that microspherical systems that are able to bind the positively charged drug via ionic association exhibit highest loading (>250 µg/mg). Although this total is impressive, it is worth pointing out that it is most meaningful when measured directly using both a high performance liquid chromatography technique to determine purity of incorporated material and radiolabeled compound to determine total drug loading. If such rigor is not possible, it is essential to assess the purity and amount of released drug for comparison with that incorporated. Techniques for characterization and quantitation of drugs frequently incorporated within microspheres are discussed and illustrated in Chapter 6.

It is of interest that a drug loading as high as 250 µg/mg may not be essential in the context of regional cancer therapy. Thus, marked pharmacological effects (e.g., tumor shrinkage, skin necrosis) were seen in a patient with locally advanced breast cancer treated with microspheres incorporating 100 µg/mg doxorubicin (Chapter 3). In this system the drug was predominantly incorporated in a form covalently bound to microsphere matrix (albumin). The implications of covalent binding for *in vivo* fate and activity of agents incorporated within microspheres are discussed in Chapter 5.

Doxorubicin has been the most frequently used agent in the context of cytotoxic drug delivery with microspheres, and relevant aspects of its chemistry and pharmacology are discussed in Chapter 6. Of particular interest is the capacity of this quinone-containing compound to participate in redox reactions under hypoxic conditions; these conditions were established in tumor tissue when the drug was administered in microspherical form.[3] It was later demonstrated that, in the case of doxorubicin, anaerobic bioreduction was a process of drug inactivation.[4] Nevertheless, there are other drugs (Chapter 5) that on reductive metabolism by the same process are indeed activated.

This class of compounds, termed hypoxia-selective cytotoxins, are obvious candidates for incorporation into microspheres because of the complementarity between their characteristics and the ischemic environment prevailing after microsphere administration. A further complementarity exists between the conditions of reduced blood flow within ischemic, embolized tissue (Chapter 5) and the application of hyperthermia, the effect of which can be amplified by reduced blood flow preventing dissipation of heat (Chapter 1).

The theoretical basis for the use of particulate systems as drug carriers in regional cancer therapy has been empirically demonstrated (Chapter 3). Thus, microspheres of requisite size can be shown to embolize at high efficiency in organ capillary beds after administration via the nutrient artery whereupon they biodegrade or, if nonbiodegradable, reside indefinitely. For microparticles incorporating cytotoxic drugs this phenomenon results in much reduced systemic exposure combined with prolonged exposure of the target organ to the incorporated agent (see Chapter 3). The question remaining to be addressed is as follows: does this translate into therapeutically useful tumor responses in terms of decreased tumor volume or, more importantly, increased survival?

Table 2 summarizes the available studies in animal models of regional cancer therapy. Only with mitoxantrone was *in vivo* activity inferior to drug in solution and with this compound problems of bioavailability would be anticipated from *in vitro* work.[6] With doxorubicin activity is apparent at low doses in appropriately designed systems delivered under optimal conditions, such as extracorporeal guidance using magnetic fields deployed over small distances. Chapter 4 illustrates the degree of targeting possible with this system, although the dose-dependent pharmacokinetics (due to saturation of extravasation mechanisms) means that optimal selectivity in drug localization is only available at low (possibly sub-therapeutic) doses. In addition, the application of this technology on a human scale requires generation of adequate magnetic fields over distances that have thus far not been achieved.

Chapter 3 reviews the clinical response data for chemoembolization and radioembolization. Tumors of kidney, breast, and head and neck have been embolized, but the data are most abundant for solid tumors of the liver (either primary hepatocellular cancer or metastasis, generally from colorectal cancer). There can be no doubt that objective responses are achieved with this approach. An example is selective internal radiation (SIR) therapy for colorectal liver metastases, which involves intrahepatic arterial administration of 32 μm diameter ion-exchange microspheres incorporating a high-energy β-emitting isotope of yttrium (^{90}Y). Of 29 treated patients, all showed a decrease in serum concentration of carcinoembryonic antigen and 82% showed a decrease in tumor volume. When SIR was alternated with cycles of regional chemotherapy, all patients demonstrated a decrease in tumor volume 3 months after treatment.[10]

The clinical data on improved local control of disease by strategies based on embolization, although largely anecdotal, can be compared with the picture emerging from the carefully controlled studies on hepatic arterial infusion of floxuridine in patients with liver metastases from colorectal cancer. These show little[11] or no[12] survival advantage for regional chemotherapy, despite significant activity against hepatic tumor. Thus, it may be that with embolization-based approaches, as with regional infusional chemotherapy, the benefits of improved local control of disease in the liver are blunted by progression of extrahepatic metastases.

This analysis should not be construed as a criticism of the regional approach to cancer therapy. Indeed, it would be wrong to criticize the approach for failing to achieve what was its purview. Moreover, it is of interest to note that current approaches to correct cellular defects at the level of DNA expression for the treatment of cystic fibrosis,[13] emphysema,[14] and Duchenne muscular dystrophy,[15] using the sophistication of molecular biological delivery vectors, such as plasmids and viruses, are predicated on a regional approach to a localized disease. In addition,

TABLE 2
Microspherical Systems for Regional Cancer Therapy: Activity Studies in the Rat

Microspherical System	Drug loading (dose)	Mode of administration	Organ harboring tumor	Result	Ref.
Doxorubicin/albumin	30 μg/mg (30 μg)	Hepatic artery	Liver	Activity superior to drug in solution	5
Doxorubicin/ion exchange	300 μg/mg (1 mg)	Descending abdominal aorta	Muscle of rear leg	Activity superior to drug in solution	6
Mitoxantrone/ion exchange	Not stated (1 mg)	Descending abdominal aorta	Muscle of rear leg	Activity inferior to drug in solution	6
Doxorubicin/ion exchange	300 μg/mg (1 mg)	Hepatic artery	Liver	Activity same as drug in solution	7
Doxorubicin/albumin	30 μg/mg (100 μg)	Intratumoral	Subcutaneous tissue	Activity same as drug in solution	Chapter 5
Mitomycin C/albumin	46 μg/mg (350 μg)	Hepatic artery	Liver	Activity superior to drug in solution	8
Doxorubicin/albumin	40 μg/mg (100 μg)	Caudal artery under extracorporeal guidance	Tail	Activity superior to drug in solution	9

in vivo transfection of tumor cells with suppressor genes, such as p53 and Rb, may also rely on a regional approach.

For diverse agents deployed regionally, microspherical systems of requisite size offer a novel and effective mode of delivery in terms of increased tumor localization and decreased systemic exposure. Because dose intensification is achieved at the cost of ignoring systemic disease in the form of occult metastases, it appears logical to use this approach in combination with systematic treatments; with regard to liver metastases from colorectal cancer, active systemic therapies are emerging.[16]

REFERENCES

1. **Chiswell, D. J. and McCaferty, J.,** Phage antibodies: will "colliclonal" antibodies replace monoclonal antibodies?, *Trends Biotechnol.,* 10, 80, 1992.
2. **Strauss, L. G. and Conti, P.,** The applications of PET in clinical oncology, *J. Nucl. Med.,* 32, 623, 1991.
3. **Willmott, N. and Cummings, J.,** Increased anti-tumor effect of adriamycin-loaded albumin microspheres is associated with anaerobic bioreduction of drug in tumor tissue, *Biochem. Pharmacol.,* 36, 521, 1987.
4. **Cummings, J., Willmott, N., Hoey, B., Marley, E. S., and Smyth, J. F.,** The consequences of doxorubicin quinone reduction *in vivo* in tumor tissue, *Biochem. Pharmacol.,* 44, 2185, 1992.
5. **Goldberg, J. A., Willmott, N., Kerr, D. J., Sutherland, C., and McArdle, C. S.,** An *in vivo* assessment of adriamycin-loaded albumin microspheres, *Br. J. Cancer,* 65, 393, 1992.
6. **Burton, M. A., Jones, C., Trotter, J. M., Gray, B. N., and Codde, J. P.,** Efficacy of ion-exchange resins for anti-tumor drug delivery, *Reg. Cancer Treat.,* 3, 36, 1990.
7. **Codde, J. P., Burton, M. A., Kelleher, D. K., Archer, S. G., and Gray, B.,** Reduced toxicity of adriamycin by incorporation into ion-exchange microspheres: a therapeutic study using a rat liver tumor model, *Anticancer Res.,* 10, 1715, 1990.
8. **Morimoto, Y., Natsume, H., Sugibyashi, K., and Fujimoto, S.,** Effect of chemoembolization of albumin microspheres containing mitomycin C on AH 272 liver metastasis in rats, *Int. J. Pharmacy,* 54, 27, 1989.
9. **Widder, K. J., Morris, R. M., Poore, G. A., Howard, D. P., and Senyei, A. E.,** Selective targeting of magnetic albumin microspheres containing low-dose doxorubicin: total remission in Yoshida sarcoma-bearing rats, *Eur. J. Cancer,* 19, 135, 1983.
10. **Gray, B. N., Anderson, J. E., Burton, M. A., Van Hazel, G., Codde, J., Morgan, C., and Kemp, P.,** Regression of liver metastases following treatment with yttrium-90 microspheres, *Aust. NZ J. Surg.,* 62, 105, 1992.
11. **Rougier, P., Laplanche, A., Huguier, M., Hay, J. M., Ollivier, J. M., Escat, J., Salmon, R., Julien, M., Audy, J.-C., Gallot, D., Gouzi, J. L., Pailler, J. L., Elisa, D., Lacaine, F., Roos, S., Rotman, N., Luboinski, M., and Lasser, P.,** Hepatic arterial infusion of floxuridine in patients with liver metastases from colorectal carcinoma: long term results of a prospective, randomized trial, *J. Clin. Oncol.,* 10, 1112, 1992.
12. **Martin, J. K., O'Connell, M. J., Wieand, H. S., Fitzgibbons, R. J., Mailliard, J. A., Rubin, J., Nagorney, D. M., Tschetter, L. K., and Krook, J. E.,** Intra-arterial floxuridine v systemic fluorouracil for hepatic metastases from colorectal cancer: a randomized trial, *Arch. Surg.,* 125, 1022, 1990.

13. **Roberts, L.,** Cystic fibrosis corrected in the lab, *Science,* 249, 1503, 1990.

14. **Hoffman, M.,** New vector delivers genes to lung cells, *Science,* 252, 374, 1991.

15. **Ascadi, G., Dickson, G., Love, D. R., Jani, A., Walsh, F. S., Gurusinghe, A., Wolff, J. A., and Davies, K. E.,** Human dystrophin expression in *mdx* mice after intramuscular injection of DNA constructs, *Nature,* 352, 815, 1991.

16. **Mayer, R. J.,** Does adjuvant therapy work in colon cancer?, *N. Engl. J. Med.,* 322, 399, 1990.

INDEX

A

B